Current Progress in Dermatology Research

Current Progress in Dermatology Research

Editor: Maximus Turner

AMERICAN
MEDICAL PUBLISHERS
www.americanmedicalpublishers.com

AMERICAN
MEDICAL PUBLISHERS
www.americanmedicalpublishers.com

Cataloging-in-Publication Data

Current progress in dermatology research / edited by Maximus Turner.
p. cm.
Includes bibliographical references and index.
ISBN 979-8-88740-034-1
1. Dermatology. 2. Dermatology--Research. 3. Skin--Diseases. 4. Skin--Diseases--Diagnosis.
5. Skin--Diseases--Treatment. I. Turner, Maximus.
RL72 .C87 2023
616.5--dc23

American Medical Publishers,
41 Flatbush Avenue,
1st Floor, New York,
NY 11217, USA

ISBN 979-8-88740-034-1 (Hardback)

Contents

Preface

This book has been a concerted effort by a group of academicians, researchers and scientists, who have contributed their research works for the realization of the book. This book has materialized in the wake of emerging advancements and innovations in this field. Therefore, the need of the hour was to compile all the required researches and disseminate the knowledge to a broad spectrum of people comprising of students, researchers and specialists of the field.

Dermatology is the branch of medicine that deals with skin problems. It is a specialty that encompasses both surgical and medical aspects. It focuses on the diagnosis and treatment of problems related with nail, skin and hair. There are several sub fields of dermatology, such as pediatric dermatology, dermatopathology, Mohs surgery, cosmetic dermatology, teledermatology, immunodermatology, dermatoepidemiology, etc. Some of the common skin conditions treated within this area of medicine are fungal infections, hand dermatitis, skin cancer, acne, warts and psoriasis. These skin conditions can be treated with treatments, such as cryosurgery, radiation therapy, photodynamic therapy, tumescent liposuction, laser therapy, systemic therapies, phototherapy, and topical therapies. Dermatology research encompasses a wide range of activities including clinical trials, molecular translational medicine and basic studies in epithelial biology. This book aims to shed light on some of the unexplored aspects of dermatology and the recent researches in this field. It traces the progress of this field and highlights some of its key concepts and applications. Those with an interest in this field would find this book helpful.

At the end of the preface, I would like to thank the authors for their brilliant chapters and the publisher for guiding us all-through the making of the book till its final stage. Also, I would like to thank my family for providing the support and encouragement throughout my academic career and research projects.

Editor

1

Cutaneous Bacteria in the Gut Microbiome as Biomarkers of Systemic Malodor and People are Allergic To Me (PATM) Conditions: Insights From a Virtually Conducted Clinical Trial

Irene S Gabashvili, PhD

Aurametrix, MEBO Research, Miami, FL, United States

Corresponding Author:
Irene S Gabashvili, PhD
Aurametrix, MEBO Research
13220 SW 35th Terrace
Miami, FL, 33175
United States

Email: irene@aurametrix.com

Abstract

Background: The skin is a dynamic ecosystem of microbes and the source of many chemical compounds that affect human health. Skin-microbiome interactions can cause persistent, psychosocially devastating body smell despite good hygiene. Since odor production is often transient, malodors may not be perceptible during medical examinations. Therefore, having odor complaints can be diagnosed as body dysmorphic disorder and referred for psychological evaluations. Development of simple at-home tests and virtual care programs could improve the diagnosis and management of socially debilitating malodor conditions.

Objective: The aim of this study was to assess potential effectiveness of at-home gut microbiome testing in the diagnosis and management of idiopathic body and breath odor and in people are allergic to me (PATM) syndrome.

Methods: We contacted participants of prior metabolic body odor (MEBO) and PATM studies and online support groups by email or social media. Individuals who consented to participate were mailed test kits for at-home collection of gut microbiome samples. Participants completed an online survey (specially developed for this study) addressing their symptoms and other quality-of-life indicators at baseline and after sampling. Participants collected stool samples after flare-ups or symptom improvements and mailed them to the laboratory to be processed and analyzed. We evaluated between-group differences in symptom severity, as well as symptom improvement observations for the same individuals. For differential abundance testing of microbial taxa, we performed nonparametric statistical analyses using Mann-Whitney *U* tests for unpaired samples and Wilcoxon signed rank test for paired samples.

Results: A total of 112 individuals from 21 countries consented to participate. About half the participants had been tested for the metabolic disorder trimethylaminuria, and about half of those tested were diagnosed with the disorder. The levels of bacteria previously associated with cutaneous body odor were significantly elevated in gut samples. For the combination of species from *Anaerococcus*, *Corynebacterium*, *Campylobacter*, and *Propionibacterium* genera, the differences were P=.002 for active (73 participants, 182 samples) versus regression or remission groups (30 participants, 51 samples); P=.01 for those experiencing symptoms most or all of the time (46 participants, 88 samples) versus those who had symptoms sometimes, rarely, or never (25 participants, 74 samples); and P<.001 for improvement of symptoms in the same individuals (22 participants, 43 sets of matched samples). Changes in microbial diversity were significant for between- but not within-participant comparisons.

Conclusions: Changes in the gut microbiome composition affect MEBO and PATM severity. In particular, an increase in intestinal bacteria producing odor when in skin flexures was associated with increased intensity of self-reported symptoms. The changes were consistent in the within-group and between-group analyses. Our findings support the feasibility of remote and decentralized clinical studies of malodor conditions. Supplementary sample collection procedures may help to meet established research quality standards.

KEYWORDS

microbiome; idiopathic body odor; systemic malodor; PATM; TMAU; MEBO; bromhidrosis; halitosis; body dysmorphic disorder; virtual care; decentralized clinical trials; diagnosis; management; patient-reported outcome; PRO; at-home test

Introduction

Background

The term people are allergic to me (PATM) was coined by a person who believed they were the cause of allergy-like symptoms in surrounding people (see this 2006 post reposted in the PATM support group [1] that received over 8800 responses; Multimedia Appendix 1 shows a screenshot of the webpage). The condition was defined as itchy nose, throat, and eyes in people exposed to the person with PATM, manifesting as sniffing, sneezing, coughing, nose-covering, and throat-clearing behavior. PATM was picked as the name for several online support groups with hundreds of members sharing similar stories (eg, this private Facebook group with over 2100 members [2]). Our molecular diagnostic study conducted in 2009-2012 [3] concluded that PATM may be a subtype of metabolic body odor (MEBO) syndrome. MEBO is another term coined by an affected person to describe idiopathic malodor due to conditions such as trimethylaminuria (TMAU) and other as-yet uncharacterized metabolic disorders. A recent study [4] identified volatile chemicals, eye and nose irritants, toluene, and xylene emitted from the skin of a person with PATM at higher concentrations. Bacterial species recently linked to underarm malodor with sour characteristics in children and teens, *Staphylococcus epidermidis* [5], was found to be overabundant in the nasal cavity of a person with PATM [4]. With the exception of these studies, however, PATM and some cases of self-reported idiopathic malodor are viewed as a dermatological nondisease [6].

The human body can shed a variety of substances that are invisible to the naked eye and are capable of creating discomfort to people in the shedder's vicinity, depending on their olfactory and immune responses. These substances include odorant molecules stemming from an altered metabolism [7], such as high levels of ketones in diabetic ketoacidosis or buildup of urea in kidney failure. Human body odor is also produced by the microbial degradation of metabolic waste excreted from the body [8,9]. Infections caused by all types of pathogenic organisms—viruses, prokaryotes, and eukaryotes—can produce volatile compounds because of infection-fighting physiological processes in the human body, as well as shifts in the intestinal microflora [9-12]. The odor can linger long after the infection is gone. Microscopic flecks of skin and hair can also become airborne and irritate the respiratory system [13]. Skin flaking can be influenced by the composition of the skin microbiome [14]. Microorganisms are informative indicators of genetic diseases linked to malodor, as well as nongenetic malabsorption and metabolic inefficiencies [15,16].

Objective

In recent years, cutaneous microbial networks responsible for localized malodors (eg, foot [17], axilla [5,18], neck and head [5]) have been mapped by using next-generation sequencing approaches. These studies used professional assessors to rate odor intensity, and were limited geographically and by numbers of study participants (30 or fewer). This patient-centric study was, to our knowledge, the largest fully virtual microbiome investigation of idiopathic body odor that was open to all of those affected who were interested in participating. Our objective was to assess the potential effectiveness of at-home gut microbiome testing in the diagnosis and management of idiopathic body and breath odor and in PATM syndrome.

Methods

Design

The experimental design of this study and the format of the paper follow the Consolidated Standards of Reporting Trials statement for reporting randomized controlled trials and the Consolidated Standards of Reporting Trials of Electronic and Mobile Health Applications and Online Telehealth (CONSORT-EHEALTH) checklist [19]. See Multimedia Appendix 2 for CONSORT-EHEALTH checklist (V 1.6.1). The trial was registered at ClinicalTrials.gov (no. NCT03582826).

Recruitment

We recruited participants from previous studies (eg, [3,20]), via social media and clinicaltrials.gov (#NCT03582826). Study participants provided electronic informed consent after they were given a complete description of the study, as described in the protocol [21], approved by MEBO Research (Miami, FL, USA) Institutional Review Board on May 11, 2018. Study information and questionnaires were provided in English and Spanish. This research was conducted according to the guidelines established by the Declaration of Helsinki and the International Ethical Guidelines for Biomedical Research Involving Human Subjects. Participants did not receive any incentives.

Data Collection

Individuals who consented to participate were mailed 3 gut microbiome sampling kits to the address they provided when enrolling. Sampling kits contained 2 sterile polyester swabs, sterile water to prewet the swabs, 2 tubes containing zirconia beads and a lysis and stabilization buffer [22], and sampling instructions (see Multimedia Appendix 1).

Participants completed an online survey (specially developed for this study) addressing their symptoms and other quality-of-life (QoL) indicators at baseline and after sampling. The QoL questionnaire was an open voluntary survey that did not collect personally identifiable information. The survey asked for unique identifiers so the study coordinator could link the data to a prior medical history protected from unauthorized access. The survey also asked for the sample kit ID associated with answers to the survey. Kits were distributed in such a way that researchers from sequence processing facilities did not have access to medical histories and identities of participants. The study coordinator had access to the identifiable information and linked medical histories with test results and answers to the QoL questionnaire.

We assessed MEBO and PATM symptoms in several ways: whether the person thought their condition was in an active state versus regression or remission (asked at the time of enrollment and when collecting a sample), by frequency of symptoms (answering the question "Have you [or your trust buddy] detected any MEBO/PATM symptoms in the past 24 hours or past few days?" on 5-point Likert scale), symptom detection distance (10-point scale), and symptom duration. We added questions assessing the severity of symptoms via related behavior, psychological symptoms (anxiety, stress, depression), social (negative) interactions, physical health, and medical comorbidities to measure internal consistency. We developed the QoL survey in January 2018 and made a few minor iterations incorporating community feedback. We administered the System Usability Scale to a few selected volunteers and found the questionnaire to be acceptable for fielding. Qualitative feedback from participants was continuously obtained through emails and private support groups. A professional health psychologist offered participants personalized behavioral intervention solutions for a wide variety of their mental health needs.

The study's primary outcome was relative abundance of bacterial classes as measured by operational taxonomic units (OTUs). We categorized these data as active versus regression and remission disease states. Secondary outcomes focused on changes in fecal gut microbiota with symptom improvement.

We used the Strengthening the Reporting of Observational Studies in Epidemiology guidelines and Checklist for Reporting Results of Internet E-Surveys [23] to ensure proper reporting of results (see Multimedia Appendix 3).

Microbiome Sequencing and Annotation

Participants collected gut microbiome samples after flare-ups or symptom improvements using the kit instructions and mailed the samples in the provided return envelope. Microbial particles were disintegrated, nucleic acid purified, amplified, sequenced in multiplex, demultiplexed, quantified, and assigned to taxonomic membership using previously described methods [24]. In the first step, cells were mechanically disrupted by grinding with glass beads. In the second step, DNA was purified from lysed samples using a liquid-handling robot by a guanidine thiocyanate silica column-based purification method. DNA was amplified with barcoded primers (515F: GTGCCAGCMGCCGCGGTAA; and 806R: GGACTACHVGGGTWTCTAAT) targeting the V4 region of the bacterial 16S ribosomal RNA (rRNA) gene. Indexed polymerase chain reaction) products were pooled by taking the same volume from each reaction, column purified, and size selected through microfluidic DNA fractionation. Consolidated libraries were quantified by quantitative polymerase chain reaction using the Kapa iCycler kit on a MyiQ (Bio-Rad Laboratories, Inc) and sequenced on the NextSeq 500 platform (Illumina, Inc), rendering 2□150 base pair paired-end sequences. After sequencing, demultiplexing of reads according to sample-specific barcodes was performed using Illumina's BCL2FASTQ algorithm. Reads were filtered using an average Q score greater than 30. After removal of primers and any leading bases, forward and reverse 16S rRNA gene reads were appended together and clustered using version 2.1.5 of the Swarm algorithm, with a distance of 1 nucleotide and the "fastidious" and "usearch-abundance" flags. Depending on the percentage identity, the most abundant forward-reverse read pair per Swarm cluster was assigned taxonomic annotation to the same species, family, order, class, or phylum as in the SILVA V.132 rRNA database [25]. Best hits for the forward and reverse reads with greater than 97% identity to the same sequence in SILVA were annotated to the same species of the hit in SILVA.

Statistical Analysis

Sequencing data were linked to QoL survey responses using unique identifiers.

We addressed the large variability of the total counts per sample through normalization of raw counts before the analysis, starting from dividing the raw abundances by the total number of counts per sample (number of reads mapped to the taxon divided by the total number of reads mapped to any 16S sequence in the SILVA database). We evaluated several normalization approaches including log ratio. Finally, we applied a centered log-ratio (CLR) transformation to account for the compositional nature of the data. Abundance-weighted phylogenetic diversity was calculated according to McCoy and Matsen [26], by weighting phylogenetic entropy contributed by each lineage by its relative abundance distribution along the rooted phylogenetic tree built for the microbial community. We also estimated other alpha diversity measures, including classical phylogenetic diversity and its partial abundance-weighted extensions.

We identified significant associations between microbial taxa and malodor through a combination of statistical tests, mainly unpaired and paired Mann-Whitney-Wilcoxon tests, herein referred to as Mann-Whitney *U* if used to compare 2 independent groups and Wilcoxon if used for paired dependent samples. OTUs with consistently significant *P* values were adjusted using the Benjamini-Hochberg procedure to avoid type I errors (false positives) and decrease the false discovery rate. All statistical analyses and visualizations were performed using Python v3.7 with the NumPy (v1.16.4), pandas (v0.25.1), scipy (v1.3.1), scikit-learn (v0.22.2), and matplotlib (v3.1.1) toolkits.

Results

Participants

Individuals who provided consent received their kits between June and December 2018, answered the QoL questionnaire [21], and sent stool samples for processing between June 2018 and July 2019.

Figure 1 shows the participant flow diagram of the study. A total of 112 individuals consented to participate and were mailed 3 gut microbiome sampling kits to the address they provided when enrolling. Volunteers represented 21 countries: the United States, United Kingdom, Argentina, Brazil, Burkina Faso, Canada, Colombia, France, Hong Kong, Italy, Kenya, Mexico, Morocco, the Netherlands, Nigeria, Pakistan, Peru, Philippines, South Africa, Spain, and Sweden. Of these, 4 participants were not able to receive the kits because of unexpected customs fees or change in address. A total of 38 did not follow up, but 1 of them submitted results of prior microbiome tests, joining 13 others who did not participate in the study but volunteered the data (from the United States, United Kingdom, and Portugal). Of these, 6 did not identify themselves with MEBO or PATM. As a result, we collected 233 samples from 84 participants, including 13 who did not enroll to participate in the study but volunteered the data and 112 who consented to participate, minus the 4 participants who did not receive the kits, 2 who opted out, and 35 who neither followed up on survey responses nor sent their samples.

Figure 1. Participant flow through the metabolic body odor/people are allergic to me (MEBO/PATM) Microbiome trial. QoL: quality of life.

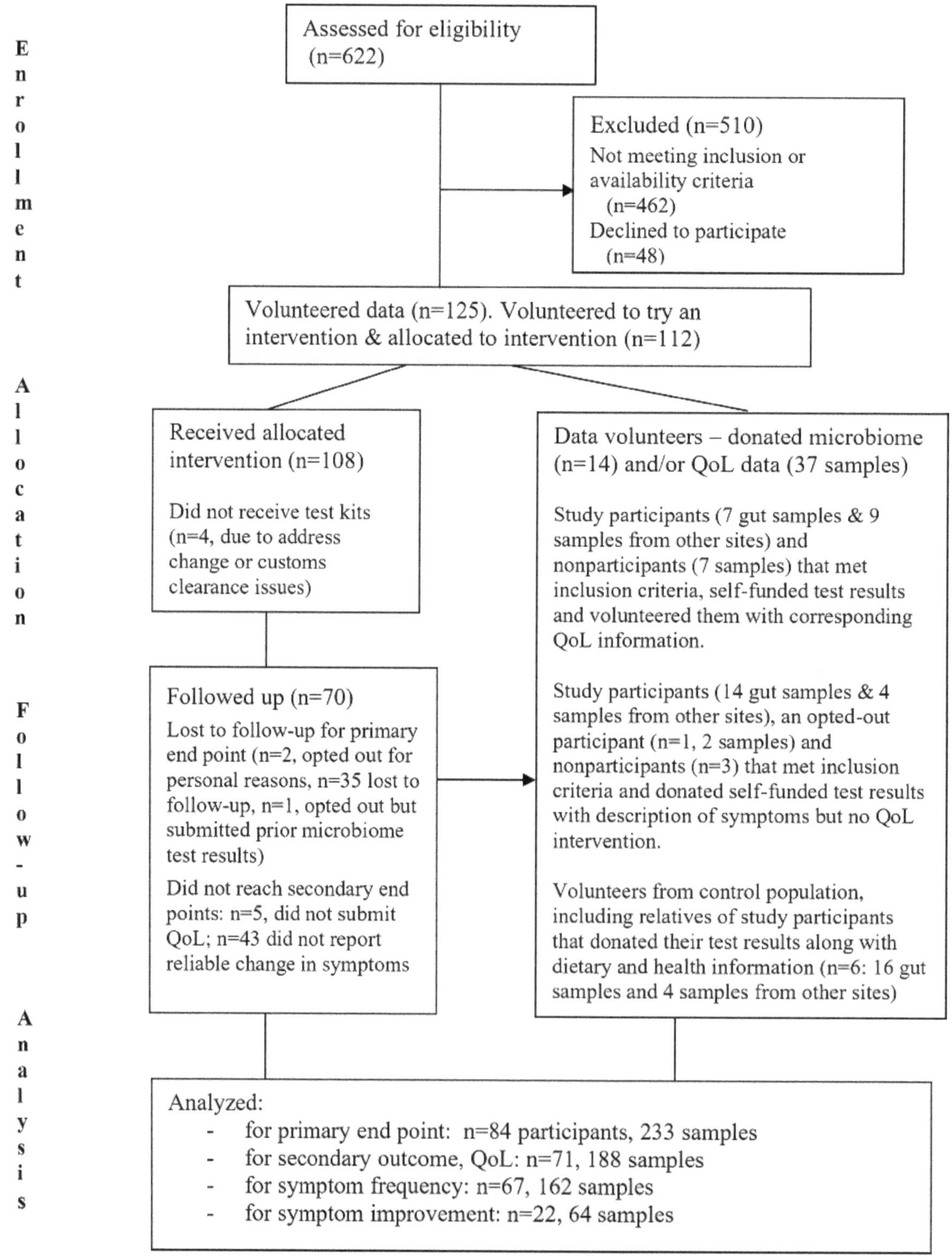

We analyzed the resulting data by first grouping them into disease states: active versus remission, regression, or healthy controls (never experienced MEBO or PATM). Of the noncontrol participants, 71 submitted answers to the QoL questionnaire [21] for 188 samples. A total of 49 participants could not comment on their symptoms because of their inability to smell, unavailability of a "trust buddy" to objectively evaluate their condition, or no change in their symptoms. The remaining 22 participants reported both flare-ups and improvements in their symptoms that we could use in a paired comparison analysis.

Baseline Characteristics

Of 336 test kits distributed to 112 consenting individuals, 189 samples were mailed for analysis by 73 participants (73/112, 65.2%; 189/336 distributed kits, 56.3%). Unfortunately, 4 of these samples (3 participants) were not processable, and 8 participants who submitted valid samples did not answer the QoL questionnaire.

Intervention dropout rates were similar to previously reported rates, and more of those who discontinued the study were women [27]. All nonrespondents received several personalized email reminders, but this did not significantly improve survey response and sample submission rates. On the other hand, 15 compliant participants from the intervention group submitted 21 additional samples using kits they purchased on their own. One participant opted out of the intervention but submitted 2 samples using previously purchased kits. In addition, 6 non-MEBO and 8 MEBO volunteers who did not participate in the intervention contributed 27 gut samples to this study. As a result, we collected 233 samples from 84 participants (Figure 1). Table 1 shows the characteristics of these individuals.

Table 1. Baseline demographic and clinical characteristics of study participants who submitted valid samples (N=84, unless otherwise stated).

Characteristics	Values
Age (years), mean (SD)	
All	40 (12)
Female	42 (11)
Male	37 (12)
Sex, n (%)	
Male	34 (40)
Female	50 (60)
Trimethylaminuria, n (%) (n=41)	
Positive	21 (51)
Negative	20 (49)
Self-diagnosis of PATM, n (%) (n=77)	34 (44)

Of the 84 study volunteers, 41 (49%; 41/78, 53% of MEBO/PATM cohort) tested for the odor-producing disorder TMAU, with 13 positives for primary TMAU and 8 for secondary TMAU, a nongenetic form arising from dysbiosis in the gut bacteria [15]. Of 78 MEBO/PATM participants, only 10 were confident about the primary source of their malodor: in 9 (12%) cases it was nose or mouth, or both, and in 1 (1%) it was the genital area. Of these individuals, 6 thought they also had body odor in other areas. A total of 43 (55%) participants described malodor or PATM toxins emanating from their entire body, not just selected areas. Many participants commented that odor has to build up to be noticed (eg, after spending more than 15 minutes in a closed room with bad air circulation). The remaining 25 (32%) study participants named body sites they thought could be contributing to their malodor: underarm, feet, genitals, scalp, and face (mostly the oily T-zone), in all possible combinations thereof. Several participants were officially diagnosed with hyperhidrosis and bromhidrosis, while in 2 cases bromhidrosis was ruled out by dermatologists. In 2 other cases, patients were treated with botulinum toxin A (Botox) injected into the underarm but they continued to experience body odor after this procedure. In all these instances, patients thought that underarm odor was not their only odor.

Evaluation of Outcomes

We performed Mann-Whitney *U* tests to identify OTUs that showed significantly different frequencies between distinct groups in our study. Remarkably, microbes known to cause malodor when present on skin were consistently significantly overabundant in active versus regression or remission states of the condition and on acute flare-up versus nonflare-up days. In particular, these included *Corynebacterium* species thought to be the primary causal agents of axillary odor dependent on secretions of the apocrine gland [18,28,29], *Anaerococcus* species also found to correlate with cutaneous odor formation [29], commensal skin bacteria *Cutibacterium* and *Propionibacterium* contributing to foot odor [30], and *Campylobacter* contributing to axillary, in addition to oral, odor in some individuals [18,31]. Figure 2 shows boxplots for microbial diversity, Corynebacteriales, and a combination of selected species from the abovementioned bacterial genera (selected cutaneous species), namely *Anaerococcus* species S9 PR-5, *Anaerococcus hydrogenalis*, *Anaerococcus lactolyticus*, *Anaerococcus octavius*, *Anaerococcus prevotii*, *Anaerococcus provencensis*, *Campylobacter hominis*, *Corynebacterium atypicum*, *Corynebacterium durum*, *Corynebacterium freiburgense*, and *Propionibacterium freudenreichii* species.

Figure 2. Changes in centered log-ratio–transformed abundances of selected bacterial species, Corynebacteriales, and microbial diversity with changes in long-term disease state (regression/remission vs active state), short-term flare-ups (24-hour symptoms observed never/rarely or sometimes vs all/most of the time), and improvement of symptoms for the same individuals. The central line in each box is the median, the upper and lower boundaries of the box mark the first and third quartiles, the thin lines show the lowest and largest data points excluding any outliers, and the diamonds show the outliers.

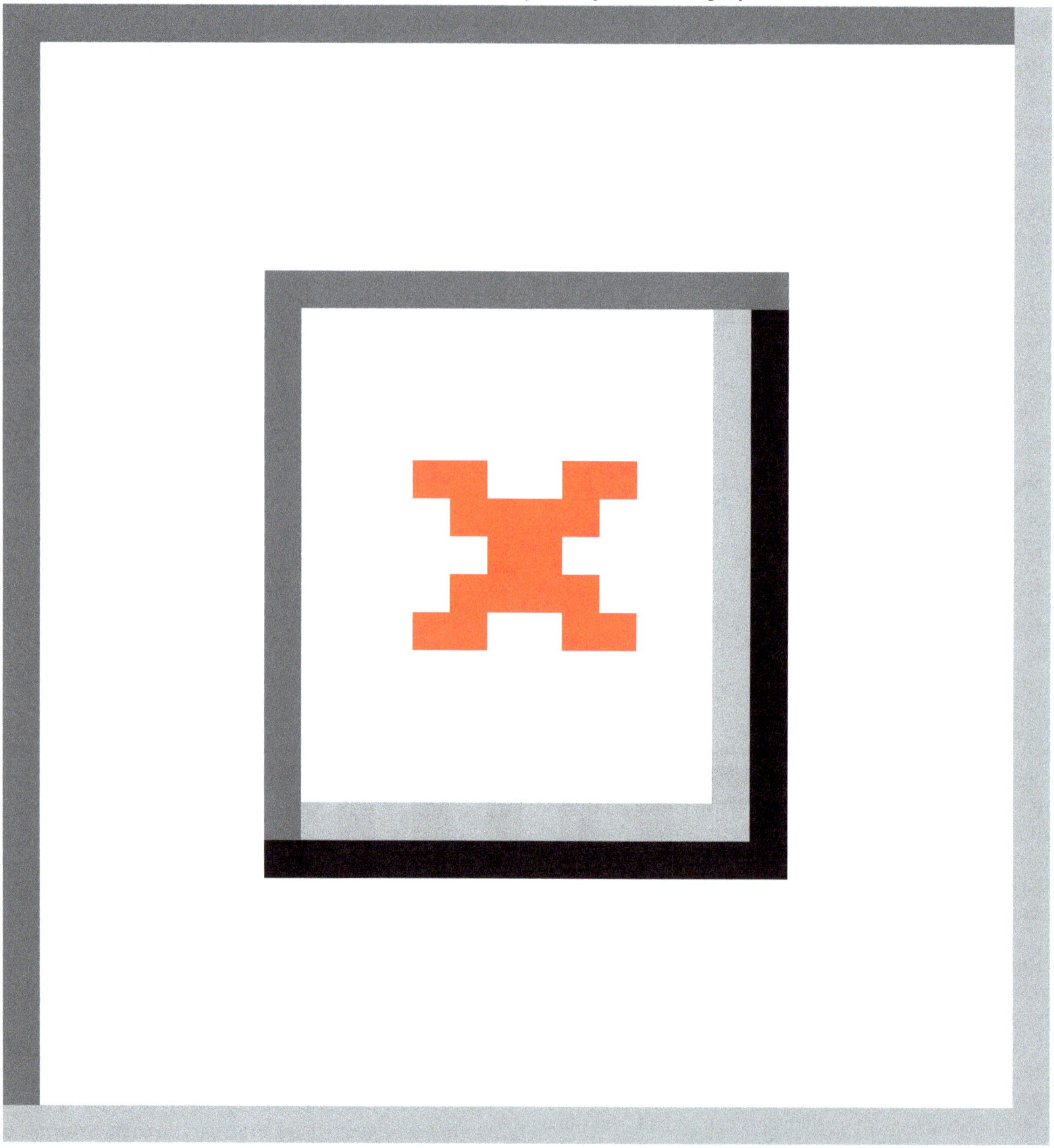

In short-term flare-ups, symptoms were grouped into 3 categories to reduce the noise of subjective self-reporting (all or most of the time vs never, rarely, or sometimes vs those who could not objectively evaluate if they experienced episodes of malodor in the past few days). It is possible to see differences among all answers on a 5-point scale ("all the time," "most of the time," "sometimes," "rarely," and "never") as Multimedia Appendix 1 shows.

Table 2 shows the results of paired and unpaired tests for different groups of participants. The difference in the selected cutaneous species defined above is statistically significant independently of analytical approaches used for data preprocessing and normalization and after the false discovery rate correction (adjusted $P<.001$). For pairwise comparison of samples before versus after improvement for the same individuals, the 95% CI is 26-163 for normalized raw counts, 0.14-1.6 for logarithm to base 10 of relative abundance in participants' stool, and 1.4-56.2 for CLR-transformed counts. For the Corynebacteriales order, the adjusted $P<.02$. Microbial diversity did not significantly change with improvement of symptoms. We note that these 22 participants submitted 73 samples, donating additional kits they purchased on their own. A total of 64 samples out of 73 were accompanied by QoL questionnaires. As a result, 6 participants submitted only 2 samples corresponding to "better" and "worse" states (6 pairs); 12 participants submitted 3 samples and 4 submitted 4 samples that could be paired in 37 different ways, since some individuals were able to recognize their symptoms at a fine-grained level. Hence, we report data for the 43 pairs of samples, although we computed Wilcoxon signed rank tests for several different pairings. *P* values were significant in all scenarios, including the smallest 22-pair set representing the largest improvement observed for each individual (P=.001for normalized counts and P=.004 for CLR-transformed counts of cutaneous bacteria). We investigated long-term disease activity by comparing participants with different overall MEBO/PATM status, self-reported in the QoL survey. We evaluated short-term effects by comparing 24-hour recalls. The selected cutaneous species index is higher for participants in the active state versus remission or regression and in those who were experiencing symptoms all or most of the time versus never or rarely or sometimes. Adjusted *P* values are higher in these cases, which could be because nonmatched individuals self-assessing their symptoms are more problematic to compare, but the difference is still significant or marginally significant (P<.01 for long term and P=.06 for short term activity). The 95% CI for CLR-transformed counts is 0.6-3.45 for long-term effects and 0-2.7 for short-term effects. For 24-hour recall, between-group comparisons of changes in Corynebacteriales and microbial diversity are significant even after false discovery rate adjustment. Table 2 also lists results for potential confounding factors, such as females versus males, younger versus older individuals, and those who mentioned underarm odor as one of their problem odors versus those who ruled the axilla out of their odor sources. Differences between these groups were not significant after false discovery rate adjustment and only marginally significant otherwise. We note that individuals who self-diagnosed PATM had significantly higher levels of cutaneous species than those who self-reported malodor only (95% CI 0.5-3.36 for CLR cutaneous species). Yet we see the same patterns for disease severity within each of the groups as within the entire population (Figure 3).

Table 2. *P* values for Mann-Whitney *U* tests for unpaired samples and Wilcoxon signed rank test for paired samples.

Test, groups, and preprocessing	Selected species	Corynebacteriales	Microbial diversity
Before and after improvement (Wilcoxon test for 43 pairs of matched samples of 22 participants)			
Normalized counts	<.001	<.001	.6
CLR[a]-transformed	<.001	.02	
Active vs regression/remission/no disease status (Mann-Whitney *U* test for 182 samples of 73 participants vs 51 samples of 30 participants)[b]			
Normalized counts	.004	.05	.3
CLR-transformed	.002	.008	
Experienced MEBO[c]/PATM[d] episodes all/most of the time vs never/rarely/sometimes (Mann-Whitney *U* test for 88 samples of 46 participants vs 74 samples of 25 participants)[b]			
Normalized counts	.01	.005	.02
CLR-transformed	.04	.002	
Females vs males: 138 vs 95 samples, 84 participants			
Normalized counts	.3	.2	.3
CLR-transformed	.09	.2	
Individuals with underarm odor vs those who ruled it out: 36 samples/13 participants vs 54 samples/15 participants			
Normalized counts	.02	.07	.08
CLR-transformed	.07	.04	
Participants with MEBO (121 samples/44 participants) vs those with self-diagnosed PATM (96 samples/34 participants)			
Normalized counts	.09	.1	.2
CLR-transformed	.008	.2	
Those who tested negative for trimethylaminuria (58 samples/20 participants) vs positive (56 samples/21 participants)			
Normalized counts	.2	.4	.3
CLR-transformed	.4	.5	
Age <40 years (115 samples/39 participants) vs ≥40 years (118 samples/45 participants)			
Normalized counts	.05	.4	.1
CLR-transformed	.05	.4	

[a]CLR: centered log-ratio.

[b]The sum of participants in active disease versus remission (73+30>84) and "most of the time" versus "sometimes" groups (46+25>67) is greater than the total number of participants because some individuals changed their answers to surveys associated with follow-up samples.

[c]MEBO: metabolic body odor.

[d]PATM: people are allergic to me.

Figure 3. Change in abundance of selected cutaneous species (log scale) with long- and short-term improvement of symptoms in metabolic body odor (MEBO) vs people are allergic to me (PATM) groups of study volunteers. Red boxes represent active state of disease or symptoms observed all or most of the time. Blue boxes show remission or regression and symptoms reported as never, rarely, or sometimes.

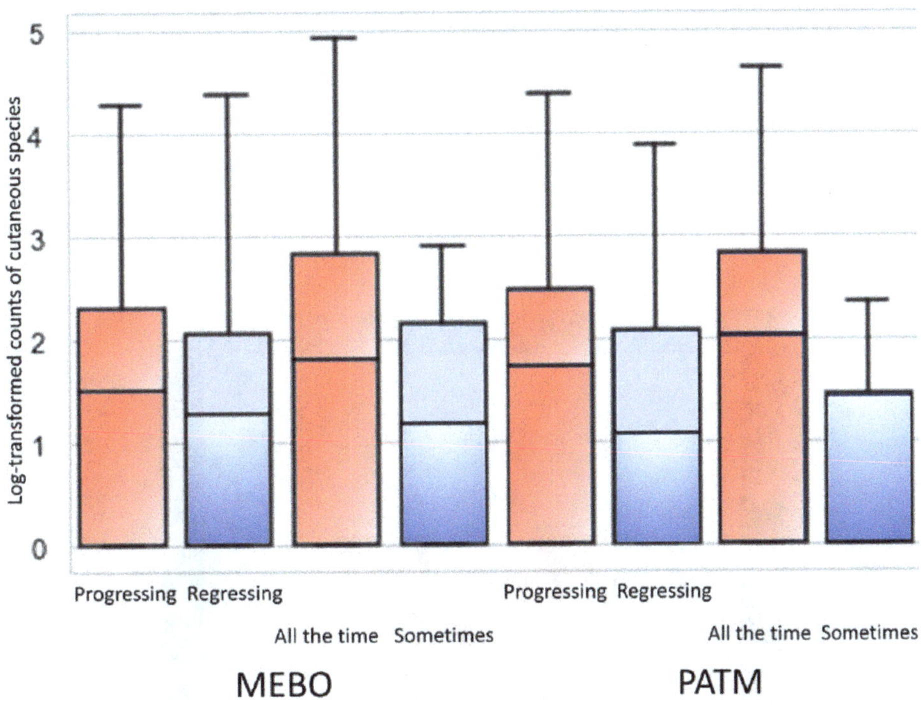

Figure 4 shows similar trends in all other groups, except cases when underarm odor was ruled out as a potential problem. Changes in abundances of cutaneous bacteria are not significant in remission only in the latter case.

Figure 5 shows how the selected cutaneous species index changed with symptom improvements in the 22 participants (12 female and 10 male) who reported flare-ups and improvements. Figure 6 shows changes in genera for 1 of the volunteers, F7, who reported fine-grained symptoms for multiple observations (refer to Multimedia Appendix 1 for more details).

Figure 4. Change in selected species of bacteria (centered log-ratio [CLR]–transformed cutaneous species) with long-term improvement of symptoms analyzed separately for different subgroups of study participants: males and females, those including or excluding underarm odor in self-reported symptoms, and participants grouped into 2 age brackets: 20-39 and 40-66 years. Red boxes represent active state of disease. Blue boxes show remission or regression.

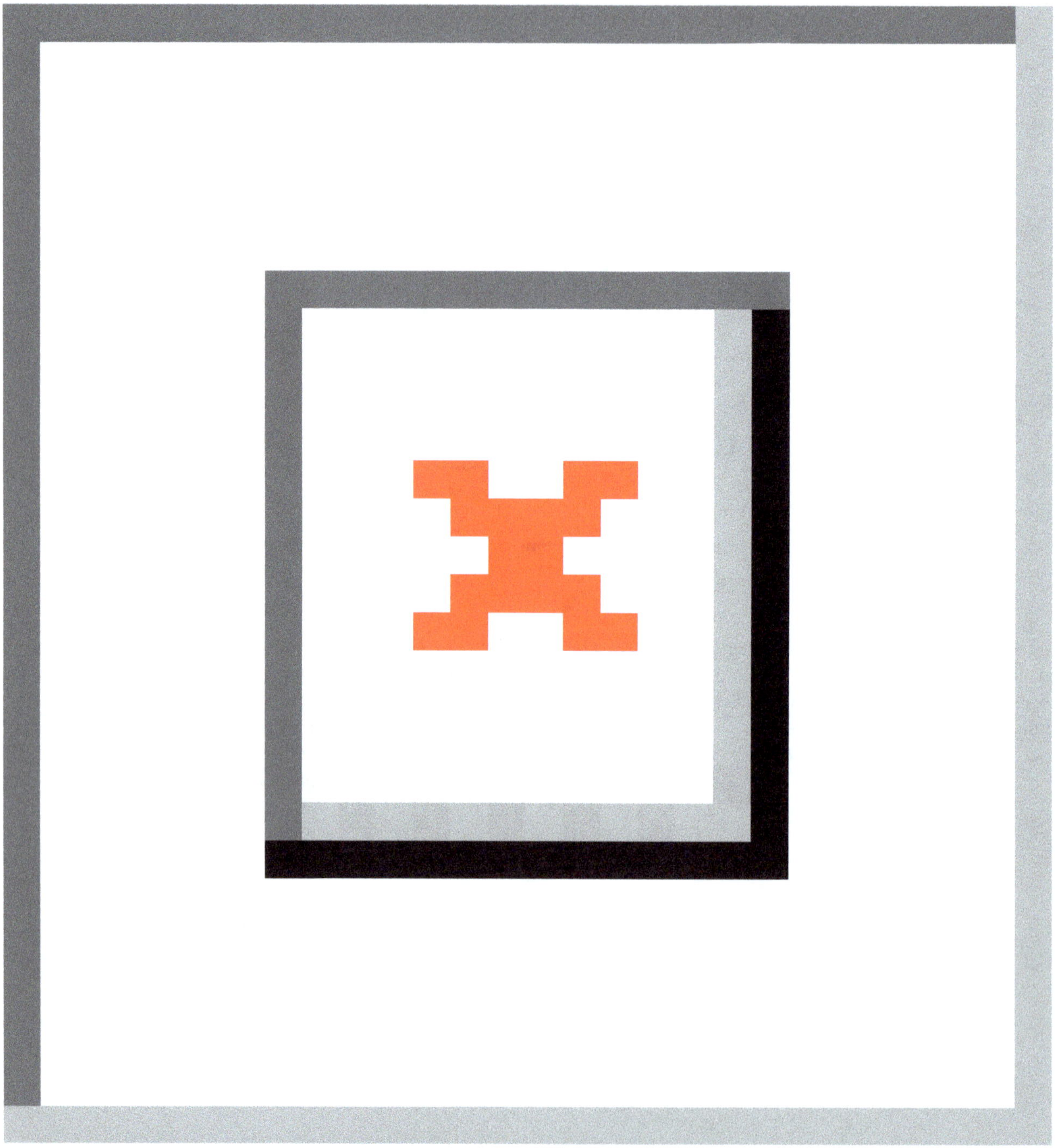

Figure 5. Changes in microbial diversity vs abundances of selected bacterial species (CSS) for 12 female (F) and 10 male (M) participants who self-reported both flare-ups (beginning of the arrow) and improvements (end of the arrow).

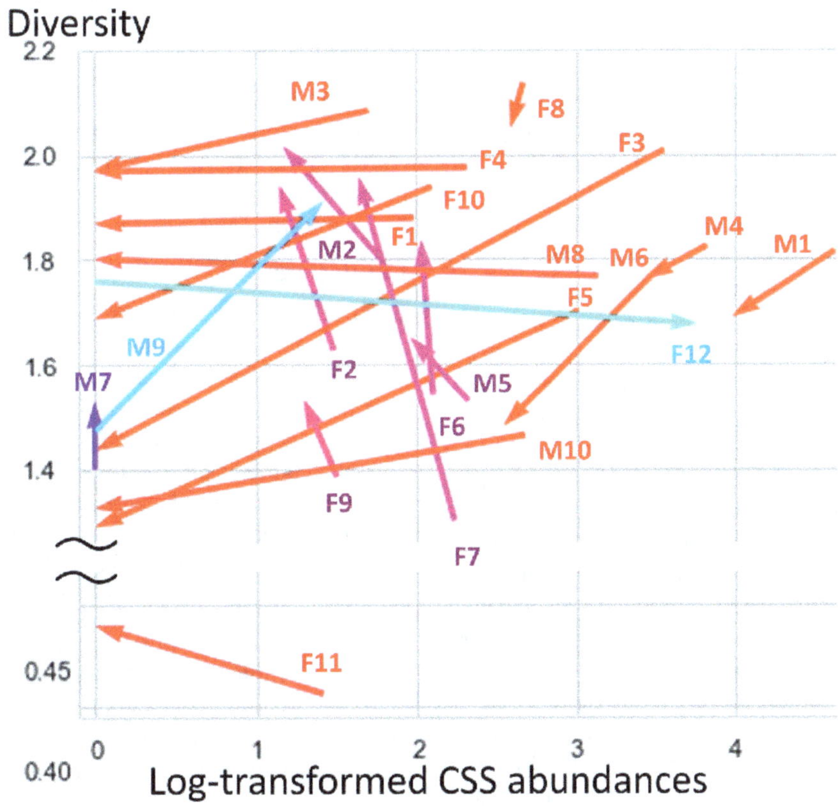

Figure 6. Changes in abundances of common dermal bacteria in the gut microbiome of participant F7. Each genus represents the total number of reads mapped to species identified in the gut sample. MEBO: metabolic body odor; OTU: operational taxonomic unit; PATM: people are allergic to me.

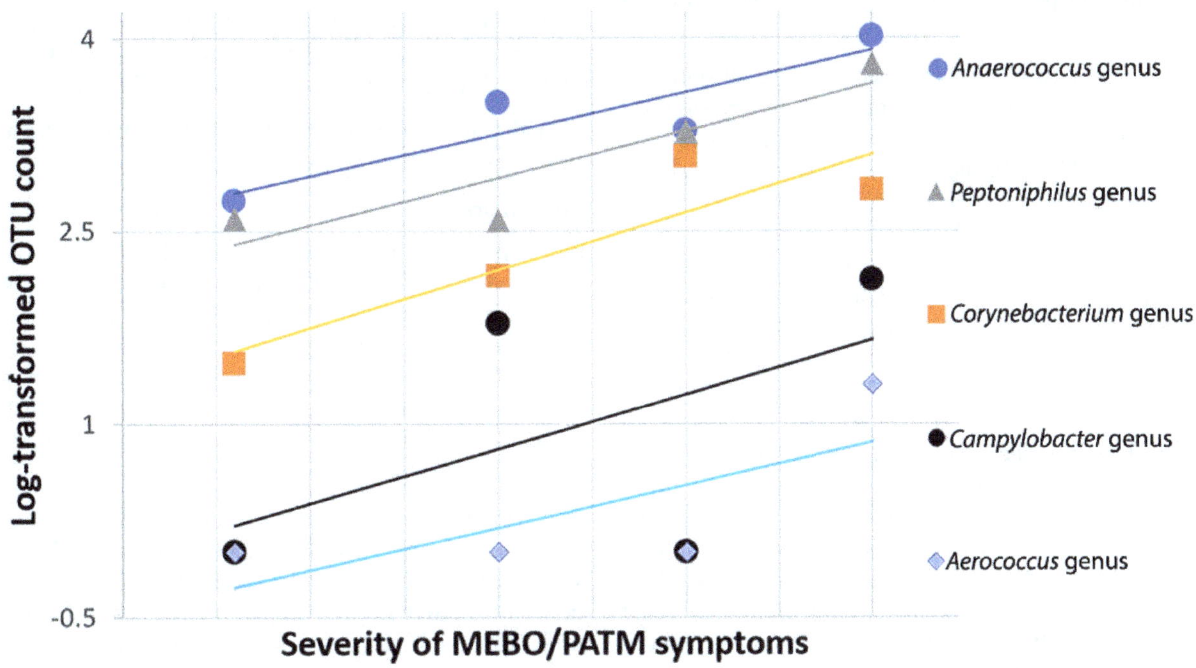

Discussion

Principal Findings and Prior Work

Previous studies have demonstrated differences in the skin and oral microbiomes of individuals experiencing body odor or halitosis [5,8,17,18,28-31]. The gut microbiota is linked to skin disorders such as psoriasis, rosacea, and atopic dermatitis [32-34] and is a target for the treatment of MEBO [35]. Yet prior studies of malodor had limited sample sizes and were lacking insights into the gut microbial community [36], focusing on skin (including vulvar) and oral microbial compositions. In this study, we observed significant differences in cutaneous gut microbes (able to colonize skin and cause skin malodor) between various groups of MEBO and PATM conditions. Levels of these bacteria were always significantly lower with improvement of symptoms, whether long- or short-term or when observed for the same individuals. There was a moderately positive relationship between answers to the QoL survey about the progression of the MEBO or PATM condition and the intensity of recent symptoms. However, since all individuals answered the question about the state of their condition (84 participants), whereas only 80% (67 participants) reported daily observations and many were not sure about some aspects of their condition, we analyzed multiple illness severity grouping systems. Remarkably, cutaneous malodor bacteria were reproducibly associated with increasing intensity of MEBO and PATM. Based on survey responses, we noticed differences in coping mechanisms between males and females and associations between answers such as "My appearance was affected because of MEBO/PATM" and "I had problems concentrating." In our future research, we plan to investigate the QoL outcomes and data sets from our past diagnostic studies at a more granular level.

Results of case-by-case studies aligned with overall statistics. As Figure 5 shows, the only exceptions to the conclusion that the fewer cutaneous bacteria in the gut, the fewer skin emanations were M7, M9, and F12. All of them observed very minor if not negligible (and easy to misinterpret) improvement of their condition (flare-ups happening from "all the time" to "most of the time"). M7 was seen by a professional dermatologist, who concluded that a diagnosis of bromhidrosis didn't seem warranted. F12 had undergone a Botox procedure to treat her hyperhidrosis about 15 years previously. M9 did not report any skin odors and noted only halitosis. It is interesting to note that, whereas those with higher abundances of cutaneous bacteria in the gut benefited from reducing their microbial diversity and bacterial counts in general, those with lower abundances benefited from increasing their microbial diversity. As in a recent study investigating differences in diversity with respect to human personality and other parameters of daily living [37], we, too, found sociability associated with higher diversity, and anxiety, depression, and stress with reduced diversity. We also analyzed differences in fiber, calcium, fat, vegetable, and heterocyclic amine intake, as well as of fermented foods and probiotic supplements. However, the impact of these factors was more profound on microbial diversity than on counts of cutaneous species in the gut microbiome. In some of these cases, such as probiotic supplements, abundances of cutaneous species were significantly lower in both flare-ups and remissions, but the impact of these bacteria remained the same: higher levels with more severe symptoms, similar to the data shown in Figures 3 and 4.

As observed earlier, abundances of common skin bacteria seemed to correlate with each other. Figure 6 shows similar effects on self-reported severity of symptoms observed for genera responsible for axillary and foot odor: *Corynebacterium*, *Anaerococcus*, *Peptoniphilus*, *Campylobacter*, and *Aerococcus*.

Limitations

The challenges of relying solely on perception of odors by nonprofessionals were previously discussed [5]. In this study [5], "malodor" and "no malodor" groups of children defined by their parents were not statistically significantly different when evaluated by professional odor assessors (Wilcoxon test $P>.1$). The self-reported nature of this study is a limitation, but medical examination may also be prone to errors and the consistency of our findings for different groups and with data from other studies demonstrates that fully remote studies of malodor are feasible.

Measuring the microbiome is not like measuring a single isolated variable pertaining to physiology. Since the data are complex and compositional, daily fluctuations get amplified, requiring multiple longitudinal sampling for patients. Multiomic measurements can improve statistical inferences, avoid false positives, and increase the overall efficiency of clinical trials.

Another limitation of this study was that we did not have data on the time period from sample collection to sequencing for all kits processed. The storage condition of gut samples introduced some biases in microbial diversity and the relative abundance of functional bacteria, even when using the best commercial stabilizers for preserving fecal samples at room temperatures [38]. However, most storage conditions and storage time had minor and acceptable impacts on nucleic acid yields or quality.

An additional limitation of this study was that we did not use incentives for participation.

Conclusions

The hypothesis of this study was that in spite of genetic heterogeneity, MEBO and PATM conditions display common patterns in the gut microbiome [21]. The collective intestinal microbiome in the study population stratified by disease severity exhibited a relative increase in bacterial species from genera associated with dermal odor. The finding was consistent in active versus remission states, and short-term flare-ups versus relative improvements.

Skin conditions often lead to difficulties in emotional, psychological, and social functioning. Our study showed that web-based research has the potential to not only offer much-needed psychosocial support [39], but also help to develop virtual care solutions for conditions resembling dermatological nondisease [40].

Our work paves the way for the development of cost-effective diagnostics of MEBO and PATM conditions based on an at-home stool test. Current methods (such as trimethylamine N-oxide urine or small intestinal bacterial overgrowth breath diagnostics) rely on tolerance tests that take many hours of preparation, testing, and recovery. External microbiome sampling may require multiple swabs, such as from the oral cavity, forearm, axilla, scalp, and feet. Simple at-home microbiome stool sampling could simplify testing.

Another implication of this work is that individuals with a high abundance of cutaneous malodor bacteria in the gut might benefit from reducing levels of these bacteria. We note that one of the common causes of both halitosis and axillar odor is a zinc deficiency. Zinc oxide is known to decrease populations of bacteria discussed in this work when applied externally [41], attenuating self-perceived malodor. Zinc also contributes to the reduction of halitosis [42]. However, not all people with MEBO and PATM are zinc deficient, and it is important to retain certain levels of cutaneous odor-producing bacteria in the body, as they prevent some skin, ear, and respiratory infections [43].

Future work will focus on incorporating more background knowledge and test results for higher precision data mining. Additional studies are needed to uncover the root causes of socially debilitating malodor and PATM conditions and, most importantly, to connect patient experiences to the development of personalized therapies.

Acknowledgments

I thank Maria de la Torre, the study coordinator, who worked hard to recruit and educate study volunteers from all over the world, and Crissan Rosalia for offering professional psychological support. We are very grateful to all participants who went the extra mile to ensure the success of this study. We thank uBiome for processing the samples and Melissa Agnello for all the help she gave us to complete this challenging project.

uBiome funded sample processing; MEBO Research funded postage to international participants; and several study volunteers self-funded their microbiome tests. The principal investigator, study coordinator, and support personnel worked pro bono.

References

1. MedHelp. People are allergic to me (PATM).: Vitals Consumer Services LLC; 2007 Apr 30. URL: https://www.medhelp.org/posts/People-Allergic-to-Me-PATM/People-Are-Allergic-To-Me-PATM/show/4415 [accessed 2020-10-26]
2. Facebook. MEBO PATM/TMAU. URL: https://www.facebook.com/groups/715913928557803 [accessed 2020-10-26]
3. Gabashvili I. Community-led research discovers links between elusive symptoms and clinical tests. bioRxiv 2017 Jan 01. [doi: 10.1101/139014]
4. Kawakami Y, Sekine Y, Kimura K, Todaka M, Hisayuki ODA. An exploratory study on "people allergic to me" syndrome based on measurement of trace gases released from skin surface and nasal microbial species in nasal cavity of a patient. Indoor Environ 2018;21(1):19-30 [FREE Full text] [doi: 10.7879/siej.21.19]
5. Lam TH, Verzotto D, Brahma P, Ng AHQ, Hu P, Schnell D, et al. Understanding the microbial basis of body odor in pre-pubescent children and teenagers. Microbiome 2018 Nov 29;6(1):213 [FREE Full text] [doi: 10.1186/s40168-018-0588-z] [Medline: 30497517]
6. Bian Y, Ma B, Wang Z, Yang F. People allergic to me and body dysmorphic disorder. Asian J Psychiatr 2019 Aug;44:61-62. [doi: 10.1016/j.ajp.2019.07.031] [Medline: 31325759]
7. Broza YY, Zuri L, Haick H. Combined volatolomics for monitoring of human body chemistry. Sci Rep 2014 Apr 09;4:4611 [FREE Full text] [doi: 10.1038/srep04611] [Medline: 24714440]
8. Shelley WB. Axillary odor. AMA Arch Dermatol Syphilol 1953 Oct 01;68(4):430. [doi: 10.1001/archderm.1953.01540100070012]
9. Elmassry MM, Piechulla B. Volatilomes of bacterial infections in humans. Front Neurosci 2020;14:257 [FREE Full text] [doi: 10.3389/fnins.2020.00257] [Medline: 32269511]
10. Ahmed WM, Lawal O, Nijsen TM, Goodacre R, Fowler SJ. Exhaled volatile organic compounds of infection: a systematic review. ACS Infect Dis 2017 Oct 13;3(10):695-710. [doi: 10.1021/acsinfecdis.7b00088] [Medline: 28870074]
11. Porter SR, Scully C. Oral malodour (halitosis). BMJ 2006 Sep 23;333(7569):632-635 [FREE Full text] [doi: 10.1136/bmj.38954.631968.AE] [Medline: 16990322]
12. Beatty JK, Akierman SV, Motta J, Muise S, Workentine ML, Harrison JJ, et al. Giardia duodenalis induces pathogenic dysbiosis of human intestinal microbiota biofilms. Int J Parasitol 2017 May;47(6):311-326 [FREE Full text] [doi: 10.1016/j.ijpara.2016.11.010] [Medline: 28237889]
13. Hampton SF, Cooke RA. The sensitivity of man to human dander, with particular reference to eczema (allergic dermatitis). J Allergy 1941 Nov;13(1):63-76. [doi: 10.1016/s0021-8707(41)90008-4]
14. Gaitanis G, Magiatis P, Hantschke M, Bassukas ID, Velegraki A. The Malassezia genus in skin and systemic diseases. Clin Microbiol Rev 2012 Jan;25(1):106-141. [doi: 10.1128/CMR.00021-11] [Medline: 22232373]
15. Fennema D, Phillips IR, Shephard EA. Trimethylamine and Trimethylamine N-Oxide, a Flavin-Containing Monooxygenase 3 (FMO3)-Mediated Host-Microbiome Metabolic Axis Implicated in Health and Disease. Drug Metab Dispos 2016 Nov

02;44(11):1839-1850 [FREE Full text] [doi: 10.1124/dmd.116.070615] [Medline: 27190056]

16. Pinheiro de Oliveira F, Mendes RH, Dobbler PT, Mai V, Pylro VS, Waugh SG, et al. Phenylketonuria and gut microbiota: a controlled study based on next-generation sequencing. PLoS One 2016;11(6):e0157513 [FREE Full text] [doi: 10.1371/journal.pone.0157513] [Medline: 27336782]
17. Wulandari NF, Suharna N, Yulinery T, Nurhidayat N. Preliminary study on bacterial diversity causing human foot odor. 2019 Presented at: International Symposium of Innovative Bio-Production Indonesia on Biotechnology and Bioengineering; October 23-24, 2019; Tangerang, Indonesia p. 23-24.
18. Troccaz M, Gaïa N, Beccucci S, Schrenzel J, Cayeux I, Starkenmann C, et al. Mapping axillary microbiota responsible for body odours using a culture-independent approach. Microbiome 2015;3(1):3. [doi: 10.1186/s40168-014-0064-3] [Medline: 25653852]
19. Eysenbach G, Consort-EHEALTH Group. CONSORT-EHEALTH: improving and standardizing evaluation reports of web-based and mobile health interventions. J Med Internet Res 2011;13(4):e126 [FREE Full text] [doi: 10.2196/jmir.1923] [Medline: 22209829]
20. Gabashvili IS. Identifying subtypes of a stigmatized medical condition. medRxiv 2019 Aug 29. [doi: 10.1101/19005223]
21. Gabashvili IS. Dynamics of the gut microbiota in MEBO and PATM conditions: protocol of a fully remote clinical study. medRxiv 2020 Aug 24. [doi: 10.1101/2020.08.21.20179242]
22. Vera-Wolf P, Cárdenas J, Morton A, Norambuena T, Torres R, Leon L, et al. Measures of reproducibility in sampling and laboratory processing methods in high-throughput microbiome analysis. bioRxiv 2018 May 15. [doi: 10.1101/322677]
23. Eysenbach G. Improving the quality of web surveys: the Checklist for Reporting Results of Internet E-Surveys (CHERRIES). J Med Internet Res 2004 Sep 29;6(3):e34 [FREE Full text] [doi: 10.2196/jmir.6.3.e34] [Medline: 15471760]
24. Agnello M, Carroll LN, Imam N, Pino R, Palmer C, Varas I, et al. Gut microbiome composition and risk factors in a large cross-sectional IBS cohort. BMJ Open Gastroenterol 2020;7(1):e000345. [doi: 10.1136/bmjgast-2019-000345] [Medline: 32518661]
25. Quast C, Pruesse E, Yilmaz P, Gerken J, Schweer T, Yarza P, et al. The SILVA ribosomal RNA gene database project: improved data processing and web-based tools. Nucleic Acids Res 2013 Jan;41(Database issue):D590-D596 [FREE Full text] [doi: 10.1093/nar/gks1219] [Medline: 23193283]
26. McCoy CO, Matsen FA. Abundance-weighted phylogenetic diversity measures distinguish microbial community states and are robust to sampling depth. PeerJ 2013;1:e157 [FREE Full text] [doi: 10.7717/peerj.157] [Medline: 24058885]
27. Kannisto KA, Korhonen J, Adams CE, Koivunen MH, Vahlberg T, Välimäki MA. Factors associated with dropout during recruitment and follow-up periods of a mHealth-based randomized controlled trial for Mobile.Net to encourage treatment adherence for people with serious mental health problems. J Med Internet Res 2017 Feb 21;19(2):e46 [FREE Full text] [doi: 10.2196/jmir.6417] [Medline: 28223262]
28. Shehadeh N, Kligman AM. The bacteria responsible for axillary odor. J Invest Dermatol 1963;41:39-43. [doi: 10.1038/jid.1963.60] [Medline: 14043010]
29. Natsch A, Emter R. The specific biochemistry of human axilla odour formation viewed in an evolutionary context. Philos Trans R Soc Lond B Biol Sci 2020 Jun 08;375(1800):20190269 [FREE Full text] [doi: 10.1098/rstb.2019.0269] [Medline: 32306870]
30. Ara K, Hama M, Akiba S, Koike K, Okisaka K, Hagura T, et al. Foot odor due to microbial metabolism and its control. Can J Microbiol 2006 Apr;52(4):357-364. [doi: 10.1139/w05-130] [Medline: 16699586]
31. Callewaert C, Hutapea P, Van de Wiele T, Boon N. Deodorants and antiperspirants affect the axillary bacterial community. Arch Dermatol Res 2014 Oct;306(8):701-710. [doi: 10.1007/s00403-014-1487-1] [Medline: 25077920]
32. Mann EA, Bae E, Kostyuchek D, Chung HJ, McGee JS. The gut microbiome: human health and inflammatory skin diseases. Ann Dermatol 2020;32(4):265. [doi: 10.5021/ad.2020.32.4.265]
33. Hidalgo-Cantabrana C, Gómez J, Delgado S, Requena-López S, Queiro-Silva R, Margolles A, et al. Gut microbiota dysbiosis in a cohort of patients with psoriasis. Br J Dermatol 2019 Dec;181(6):1287-1295. [doi: 10.1111/bjd.17931] [Medline: 30920647]
34. Dei-Cas I, Giliberto F, Luce L, Dopazo H, Penas-Steinhardt A. Metagenomic analysis of gut microbiota in non-treated plaque psoriasis patients stratified by disease severity: development of a new Psoriasis-Microbiome Index. Sci Rep 2020 Jul 29;10(1):12754 [FREE Full text] [doi: 10.1038/s41598-020-69537-3] [Medline: 32728075]
35. Schmidt AC, Leroux JC. Treatments of trimethylaminuria: where we are and where we might be heading. Drug Discov Today 2020 Sep;25(9):1710-1717 [FREE Full text] [doi: 10.1016/j.drudis.2020.06.026] [Medline: 32615074]
36. Rath S, Heidrich B, Pieper DH, Vital M. Uncovering the trimethylamine-producing bacteria of the human gut microbiota. Microbiome 2017 Dec 15;5(1):54 [FREE Full text] [doi: 10.1186/s40168-017-0271-9] [Medline: 28506279]
37. Johnson KV. Gut microbiome composition and diversity are related to human personality traits. Hum Microbiome J 2020 Mar;15:100069. [doi: 10.1016/j.humic.2019.100069]
38. Ma J, Sheng L, Hong Y, Xi C, Gu Y, Zheng N, et al. Variations of gut microbiome profile under different storage conditions and preservation periods: a multi-dimensional evaluation. Front Microbiol 2020;11:972 [FREE Full text] [doi: 10.3389/fmicb.2020.00972] [Medline: 32536906]
39. Heapy C, Montgomery K, Ersser S, Gass M, Goad N, Thompson AR. A psychosocial support website from the British

Association of Dermatologists for people living with a skin condition: mixed methods evaluation. JMIR Dermatol 2020 Jun 15;3(1):e17052. [doi: 10.2196/17052]
40. Cotterill JA. Dermatological non-disease: a common and potentially fatal disturbance of cutaneous body image. Br J Dermatol 1981 Jun;104(6):611-619. [doi: 10.1111/j.1365-2133.1981.tb00746.x] [Medline: 7248174]
41. Ågren M, Ghathian K, Frederiksen A, Bjerrum M, Calum H, Danielsen P, et al. Zinc oxide inhibits axillary colonization by members of the genus Corynebacterium and attenuates self-perceived malodour: a randomized, double-blind, placebo-controlled trial. Acta Derm Venereol 2020;100(10):a. [Medline: 32399578]
42. Lynch RJM. Zinc in the mouth, its interactions with dental enamel and possible effects on caries; a review of the literature. Int Dent J 2011 Aug;61 Suppl 3:46-54. [doi: 10.1111/j.1875-595X.2011.00049.x] [Medline: 21762155]
43. Dimitri-Pinheiro S, Soares R, Barata P. The microbiome of the nose-friend or foe? Allergy Rhinol (Providence) 2020;11:2152656720911605. [doi: 10.1177/2152656720911605] [Medline: 32206384]

Abbreviations

CLR: centered log-ratio
CONSORT-EHEALTH: Consolidated Standards of Reporting Trials of Electronic and Mobile Health Applications and Online Telehealth
MEBO: metabolic body odor
OTU: operational taxonomic unit
PATM: people are allergic to me
QoL: quality of life
rRNA: ribosomal RNA
TMAU: trimethylaminuria

2

Supporting Self-Management Among Young People with Acne Vulgaris Through a Web-Based Behavioral Intervention: Development and Feasibility Randomized Controlled Trial

Athena Ip[1,2], MSc, PhD; Ingrid Muller[1], MSc, PhD; Adam W A Geraghty[1], MSc, PhD; Kate Rumsby[1], BA, MSc; Beth Stuart[1], MSc, PhD; Paul Little[1], MD, PhD, FRCGP, FMedSci; Miriam Santer[1], MBBCHIR, MRCGP, PhD

[1]Primary Care, Population Sciences and Medical Education, University of Southampton, Southampton, United Kingdom
[2]School of Health Sciences, University of Surrey, Guildford, United Kingdom

Corresponding Author:
Athena Ip, MSc, PhD
Primary Care, Population Sciences and Medical Education
University of Southampton
Aldermoor Health Centre
Aldermoor Close
Southampton, SO16 5ST
United Kingdom

Email: a.ip@soton.ac.uk

Abstract

Background: Acne is a common skin condition that is most prevalent in young people. It can have a substantial impact on the quality of life, which can be minimized with the appropriate use of topical treatments. Nonadherence to topical treatments for acne is common and often leads to treatment failure.

Objective: The aim of this study is to develop a web-based behavioral intervention to support the self-management of acne and to assess the feasibility of recruitment, retention, and engagement of users with the intervention.

Methods: The intervention was developed iteratively using the LifeGuide software and following the person-based approach for intervention development. The target behavior was *appropriate use of topical treatments*. Barriers and facilitators identified from the qualitative research and evidence from the wider literature were used to identify techniques to improve and promote their use. Young people with acne aged 14-25 years who had received treatment for acne in the past 6 months were invited to participate through mail-out from primary care practices in the South of England in a parallel, unblinded randomized trial. Participants were automatically randomized using a computer-generated algorithm to usual care or to usual care plus access to the web-based intervention. Usage data was collected, and a series of questionnaires, including the primary outcome measure for skin-specific quality of life (Skindex-16), were collected at baseline and at the 4- and 6-week follow-ups.

Results: A total of 1193 participants were invited, and 53 young people with acne were randomized to usual care (27/53, 51%) or usual care plus intervention (26/53, 49%). The response rate for the primary outcome measure (Skindex-16) was 87% at 4 weeks, 6 weeks, and at both time points. The estimate of mean scores between groups (with 95% CI) using linear regression showed a trend in the direction of benefit for the web-based intervention group in the primary outcome measure (Skindex-16) and secondary measures (Patient Health Questionnaire-4 and the Problematic Experiences of Therapy Scale). Intervention usage data showed high uptake of the core module in the usual care plus web-based intervention group, with 88% (23/26) of participants completing the module. Uptake of the optional modules was low, with less than half visiting each (myth-busting quiz: 27%; living with spots or acne: 42%; oral antibiotics: 19%; what are spots or acne: 27%; other treatments: 27%; talking to your general practitioner: 12%).

Conclusions: This study demonstrated the feasibility of delivering a trial of a web-based intervention to support self-management in young people with acne. Additional work is needed before a full definitive trial, including enhancing engagement with the intervention, recruitment, and follow-up rates.

KEYWORDS

feasibility study; acne vulgaris; intervention study; self-management; primary care; acne; dermatology

Introduction

Acne is a common condition that is most prevalent among adolescents, affecting >85% of adolescents at some point [1-3]. It can have a substantial physical and psychological impact; however, its main effects are on quality of life (QoL) [4]. First-line treatments for acne are topical treatments that work well at improving acne [5] and have been shown to improve QoL when used appropriately [6,7]. However, studies have highlighted how adherence to topical treatments is poor [8], and discontinuing treatment is associated with a rapid increase in microcomedones, resulting in more acne lesions and subsequent treatment failure [9].

A limited number of interventions have been developed to improve adherence to acne treatments [10-15], many of which have significant shortcomings. A systematic review of the effect of mobile and electronic health technology on adherence [16] (SMS text message reminders [12], telephone call reminders [13], an internet-based education tool [11], and an internet-based survey [14]) found that a weekly internet-based survey was more effective than telephone-based reminders. However, the sample size was small and not powered to determine significance [14]. Other studies included in the review also had small sample sizes ranging between 40 and 61 participants and no power calculations, which may have limited their ability to detect statistically significant differences. To our knowledge, none of these interventions have been informed by theory or developed using robust methods. Interventions developed using theory have proven to be more effective than those without a theoretical base [17].

There is also little information on recruiting through primary care in acne trials. One randomized controlled trial (RCT) investigating the use of supplementary patient educational materials on adherence recruited patients from primary care clinics in the United Kingdom; however, there was no calculation for sample size [10]. As there is very little information regarding uptake and retention rates for this group, further feasibility trials are needed to establish this.

Feasibility trials are an essential part of complex intervention development [18]. However, few interventions for acne have been subjected to feasibility or pilot testing [11,13,19] and, as a result, these trials may have a number of issues around acceptability, delivery, recruitment, and retention and are often small in sample size [20].

In this study, we describe the development of a web-based behavioral intervention to support self-management of acne. We also present the results of a feasibility randomized trial delivering this intervention to young people with acne recruited through primary care.

Methods

Development of Web-Based Intervention

The Template for Intervention Description and Replication (TIDieR) guideline [21] was used to facilitate the appropriate reporting of intervention development.

Person-Based Approach

The intervention was developed using the Person-Based Approach (PBA) for planning, developing, and evaluating the feasibility of the intervention [22]. The aim of this method is to ground the intervention in the views and experiences of the people who will use it to ensure that it is persuasive, accessible, and engaging for the target population [22]. The PBA involves in-depth qualitative research to identify key objectives and barriers and facilitators to target behaviors [22]. We carried out a systematic review and synthesis of qualitative research to explore the qualitative literature on acne among patients, carers, and health care professionals [23]. The review protocol was registered on PROSPERO (International Prospective Register of Systematic Reviews; registration number CRD42016050525). A secondary analysis of qualitative interviews with people with acne was also carried out to understand young people's views and experiences with acne and its treatments [24].

Creating Guiding Principles

Alongside intervention planning, guiding principles were drafted and iteratively developed throughout, identifying distinctive intervention features to address these. This method involved highlighting key objectives from qualitative research (1). to support young people in gaining autonomy and competence around acne management, (2) to support and promote autonomy in making treatment choices, and (3) to provide support and acknowledge the psychological impact of acne (see Table 1 for guiding principles developed for this intervention).

Table 1. Guiding principles.

Key intervention objectives	Patient characteristics	Evidence for key behavioral issues	Guiding principles	
			Design objectives	Key (distinctive) intervention features
• To improve the lives of young people with acne • To promote self-management of acne • To promote the appropriate use of topical treatments	Young people who have mild to moderate acne vulgaris	• Little knowledge about acne and its treatments (QR)[a] • Young people can be confused with the myths and misconceptions around acne and are unaware or unwilling to acknowledge that acne requires ongoing treatment. • Low motivation to engage with long-term treatment (QR) • Certain beliefs about the causation of acne may affect people's perceived necessity of treatment. • Difficulty judging efficacy of topical treatments (QR) • Belief that topical treatments do little and are only keeping their acne at bay may result in early abandonment of treatment. • Difficulty overcoming barriers (QR) • Young people can be uncertain about how to manage side effects of treatment, financial constraints, lengthy routines, and uncertainties around how to use medication. • Confusion between cosmetic and medical treatments for acne (QR) • Young people perceive they have tried all the topical treatments available	To support young people in gaining autonomy and competence around acne management	• Offer users choice wherever possible • Minimize disruption to lifestyle • Dispel myths and misconceptions about the causes of acne • Autonomy-supportive language • Ensure they have a complete understanding of acne and the rationale behind their treatment • To build their self-efficacy for the target behaviors (eg, 4-week challenge to support patients to formulate a personal goal or action plan, advice on how to minimize side effects including skin irritation, and a video with step-by-step instructions on how and when to apply topical treatments) • Educational information or rationale supported by scientific evidence (topical treatments are equally as effective as antibiotics) • Stories and testimonials to model successful management using topical therapies • Addressing common concerns • Provide a list of topical treatments and explain how they work
		• Need for control over treatment choice and disease (SR)[b] • Young people want control over their treatment choice as well as their condition and this has been shown to improve adherence and psychological impact	To support and promote autonomy for making treatment choices	• Provide advice on how people can effectively communicate with their GP[c] • Invite, acknowledge, and value views or preferences (eg, CAM[d] therapies) • Provide a list of topical treatments and explain how they work • Offering user choice wherever possible • Autonomy-supportive language throughout

Key intervention objectives	Patient characteristics	Evidence for key behavioral issues	Guiding principles	
			Design objectives	Key (distinctive) intervention features
		• Difficulty dealing with psychological issues (SR and QR) • Young people can be unsure about how to cope with the psychological impact of acne, including depressive symptoms, stress, anxiety, and embarrassment • Difficulty presenting psychological issues to HCP[e] (SR) • Young people may be unwilling to present psychological problems to their HCP	To provide support and acknowledge the psychological impact of acne	• Acknowledge the psychological impact of acne (eg, (1) emphasize that everyone with a skin disease can be at risk of psychological symptoms and (2) provide patient stories about how they dealt with the impact of acne) • Provide advice on how people can effectively communicate with their GP • Provide advice on different coping strategies

[a]QR: qualitative research (barriers identified from the secondary analysis of qualitative interview data [24]).

[b]SR: systematic review (barriers emerged from systematic review and synthesis of qualitative papers on acne) [23].

[c]GP: general practitioner.

[d]CAM: complementary and alternative medicine.

[e]HCP: health care practitioner.

Target Behavior

The hypothesized outcome of the intervention was to improve QoL for young people with acne through the target behavior *appropriate use of topical treatments*. This target behavior was chosen as it has been shown that effective use of topical treatments can improve acne [5] and benefit QoL [6,7]. For addressing this target behavior, barriers and facilitators identified from the qualitative research were described along with the proposed intervention element.

Evidence from the literature and qualitative research (including the systematic review and synthesis of qualitative data [23] and the secondary analysis of interview data with young people [24]) highlighted several barriers to the appropriate use of topical treatments that needed to be addressed in the intervention. These included concerns about side effects, confusion about the different types of topical treatments, beliefs around the ineffectiveness of topical treatments, belief that acne is a short-term condition that will resolve on its own, confusion about how to use treatment, the time-consuming nature of topical treatments, and the belief that oral treatments were more effective than topical treatments.

Behavioral Analysis

Alongside the PBA, a behavioral analysis was carried out to map the intervention components to the behavior change taxonomy, which is a list of consensually agreed techniques for specifying interventions [25]. The behavioral analysis showed that the intervention targeted nine behavior change techniques from the 93 behavior change taxonomies [25]. A central behavior change technique was *instructions on how to perform the behavior* in terms of advice about choosing the right topical treatment and instructions and demonstrations on how to use topical treatments appropriately. The intervention components were also mapped onto the COM-B model, part of the behavior change wheel [26], to map the target constructs and functions for the intervention [26]. This included six target constructs (physical capability, psychological capability, physical opportunity, social opportunity, automatic motivation, and reflective motivation) and five intervention functions (persuasion, education, training, enablement, and modeling).

Qualitative research showed the Extended Common Sense Model of Illness [27] to be a useful model for understanding how people with acne conceptualize illness and treatment and was therefore used in the behavioral analysis to check that all important components of the model were covered in the intervention (Table 2).

Table 2. Behavioral analysis of Spotless intervention.

Barrier or facilitator for target behavior[a] and intervention component	Spotless module	Target construct (BCW)[b]	Intervention function (BCW)	Behavior change technique (using 93 BCTTv1)[c]	Target construct (ECSM)[d]
Concerns about side effects from topical treatments (eg, dry skin and bleaching; QR[e] and SR[f]). Fabbrocini et al [28]: having no side effects was reported as one of the most important attributes of topical treatments (EBL[g])					
Provide persuasive and credible information about the side effects of topicals and their safety via scientific evidence and personal stories	Core treatments	Psychological capability, reflective motivation, and social opportunity	Education, persuasion, and modeling	• 5.1. Information about health consequences • 6.2. Social comparison • 6.3. Information about others' approval • 9.1. Credible source	Beliefs about necessity and concerns over its use
Provide advice on how to choose the right topical	Core treatments	Psychological capability	Training and education	4.1. Instructions on how to perform the behavior	Beliefs about necessity and concerns over its use
Confusion about the different types of topical treatments resulting in difficulty with making own treatment choices (QR and SR)					
Provide advice on how to choose the right topical	Core treatments	Psychological capability	Training and education	4.1. Instructions on how to perform the behavior	Curability or controllability
Provide information about different topicals (eg, most common or least common topicals and how they work)	Core treatments	Psychological capability	Education	5.1. Information about health consequences	Curability or controllability
Belief that topical treatments do little to help as they are only *keeping their acne at bay* (QR)					
• Provide persuasive and credible information about the effectiveness of topicals via scientific evidence and personal stories • Provide rationale for how topicals control acne • Explain via personal stories or video that it can take time for topical treatments to work	Core treatments	Psychological capability, reflective motivation, and social opportunity	Education, persuasion, and modeling	• 5.1. Information about health consequences • 6.2. Social comparison • 6.3. Information about others' approval • 9.1. Credible source	Beliefs about necessity
Provide a chart for them to monitor how their skin is after applying topical treatments each day as part of the 4-week challenge	Core treatments	Reflective motivation	Education and persuasion	• 5.1. Information about health consequences • 2.3. Self-monitoring of outcomes of behavior	Beliefs about necessity
Belief that acne is a short-term condition caused by puberty and therefore it will go away on its own (QR); McNiven [29]: belief that acne is a cosmetic problem rather than a medical condition (EBL)					

Barrier or facilitator for target behavior[a] and intervention component	Spotless module	Target construct (BCW)[b]	Intervention function (BCW)	Behavior change technique (using 93 BCTTv1)[c]	Target construct (ECSM)[d]
• Provide information on the causes of acne and dispel misconceptions using a myth-busting quiz • Provide persuasive and credible information about how acne can be effectively managed using treatment, including scientific evidence and personal stories • Provide information about what acne is, the importance of treating it early, and information about referrals • Provide advice on when to see an HCP[h] about acne • Provide advice on speaking with an HCP about acne	Myth-busting quiz; What are spots or acne; Talking to your GP[i]	Psychological capability, reflective motivation, social opportunity, and physical opportunity	Education, modeling, persuasion, and training	• 4.1. Instructions on how to perform the behavior • 5.1. Information about health consequences • 6.2. Social comparison • 6.3. Information about others' approval • 9.1. Credible source	Cause, timeline, and identity
Lack of skills regarding how to apply topicals and for how long (QR); Myhill et al [10]: supplementary patient education materials and video about application of topical treatment led to improved adherence (EBL); Sandoval et al [19]: education via physical demonstration led to 15% overall higher adherence rates (EBL)					
• Provide written instructions and an instructional video on how to use topical treatments correctly	Core treatments	Physical capability, social opportunity, and reflective motivation	Training, modeling, and persuasion	• 4.1. Instructions on how to perform the behavior • 6.1. Demonstration of the behavior • 6.2. Social comparison • 6.3. Information about others' approval • 9.1. Credible source	Concerns over its use
4-week challenge: provide a chart to help people record their skin condition when they have used their topical treatment each day	Core treatments	Reflective motivation	Education and persuasion	• 5.1. Information about health consequences • 2.3. Self-monitoring of outcomes of behavior	Concerns over its use
Belief that topicals are time-consuming to apply (QR); Rueda [15]: simplifying regimen and considering patient preference increases adherence (EBL)					
• Provide information on how to incorporate topicals in everyday life • Reassure people that applying topicals should not be time-consuming • Advise people to plan when to apply their topical • Suggest applying their topical at the same time in the same context each day	Core treatments	Psychological capability and automatic motivation	Education and enablement	• 1.4. Action planning • 4.1. Instructions on how to perform the behavior • 5.3. Information about social and environmental consequences	Concerns over its use
Belief that tablets are easier, stronger, and quicker to take effect than topicals (QR); Santer et al [30] found that some participants preferred oral treatments as they perceived these to be *stronger* than topicals (EBL)					

Barrier or facilitator for target behavior[a] and intervention component	Spotless module	Target construct (BCW)[b]	Intervention function (BCW)	Behavior change technique (using 93 BCTTv1)[c]	Target construct (ECSM)[d]
• Provide persuasive and credible information about the effectiveness of topicals and antibiotics via scientific evidence and personal stories • Provide information about the consequences of long-term oral antibiotic use	Core treatments and antibiotics	Psychological capability, social opportunity, and reflective motivation	Education, modeling, and persuasion	• 5.1. Information about health consequences • 6.2. Social comparison • 6.3. Information about others' approval • 9.1. Credible source	Concerns over its use

[a]Target behavior: appropriate use of topical treatments.

[b]BCW: behavior change wheel.

[c]BCTTv1: behavior change technique using the Behavior Change Technique Taxonomy (v1).

[d]ECSM: Extended Common-Sense Model of Illness.

[e]QR: qualitative research (barriers identified from the secondary analysis of published interview data; evidence-based literature).

[f]SR: systematic review (barriers emerged from systematic review and synthesis of qualitative papers on acne); qualitative research.

[G]EBL: barriers and facilitators emerged from a review of literature on acne (including studies testing the effectiveness of interventions to improve adherence to acne treatments).

[h]HCP: health care practitioner.

[i]GP: general practitioner.

Web-Based Intervention

The web-based intervention, Spotless, was developed using the LifeGuide software [31]. The intervention was delivered on the web via the internet and included a compulsory core module on topical treatment. This included information about the different types of topical treatments available, how they work, how to use them appropriately, common side effects, and how to manage them. Information was adapted from accurate web-based sources, including National Health Service [32], National Institute for Health and Care Excellence [33], and the British National Formulary [34]. This was initially carried out by artificial intelligence, and the team (MS, AG, PL, and IM) provided suggestions throughout. The purpose of adapting the information was to ensure that it was easily understood by young persons. An example of this was using information about types of treatments, including how they are used and the side effects, but rewriting this in lay language. Six optional modules were highlighted as important for the self-management of acne in earlier qualitative studies (Textbox 1).

Textbox 1. Overview of intervention.

Overview

- When participants first visit the website, they are taken to a *core module* on topical treatments. In the module, they have the option to take part in a 4-week challenge using their choice of topical along with the advice from the website. After completing this module, participants are taken to a main menu page with six optional modules, which they can visit as many times as they want throughout the course of the study. These include *What are spots or acne, Myth-busting quiz, Oral antibiotics, Living with spots or acne, Talking to your general practitioner, and Other treatments* (see Figure 1 for screenshots of the website).
- After the initial visit, participants are taken directly to the main menu page, where they can choose which modules to explore with the option of looking at the *core module* again.
- The intervention includes a *Meet the team* page where participants are able to see who developed the website (general practitioners, psychologists, and academic researchers); quotes adapted from qualitative research and relevant statistics are presented throughout the intervention, and a downloadable chart is available to help participants self-monitor their progress during the 4-week challenge. The intervention also includes audio, visual, and interactive features including a *myth-busting quiz* where participants can answer questions about popular myths and misconceptions around acne.

Figure 1. Screenshots of the Spotless website.

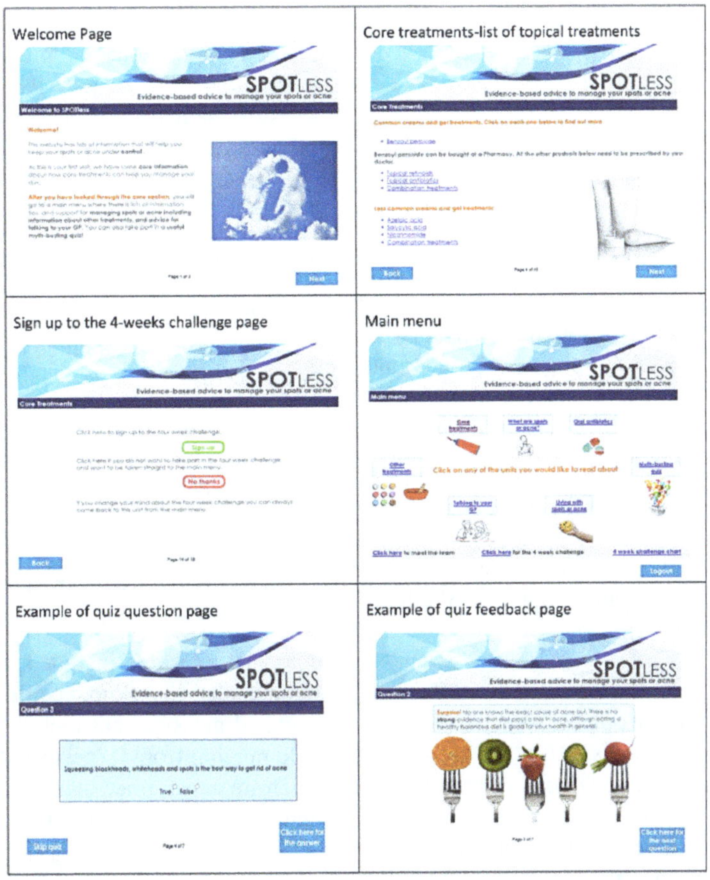

Intervention Optimization Using Think-Aloud Interviews

As part of the development stage, think-aloud interviews [35] were carried out with 19 participants with acne using the draft intervention to gather feedback and further modify the intervention. Participants were recruited through mail-out from primary care practices, opportunistic sampling using posters, and advertising via social media. The inclusion criteria for the study were young people aged 14-25 years with acne or those who had consulted about their acne or obtained a prescription for their acne in the past year. Potential participants were excluded if they were outside the age range or did not have acne. General practitioners (GPs) were also asked to screen lists to ensure that the invitation pack was not sent to patients where they felt this would be inappropriate. Face-to-face think-aloud interviews were conducted by following a semistructured interview guide to ensure that all topics were covered while also allowing participants to discuss any concerns they had about the intervention. This process involved asking participants to use the intervention while speaking out their thoughts aloud. Interviews were transcribed and analyzed using a deductive approach to code the data using the objectives of the study (engagement, persuasiveness, and usability) and identify positive and negative comments to aid intervention development.

Overall, participants found the intervention engaging, persuasive, and usable, with some suggestions for changes. Main changes made as a result of the interviews were adding pseudonyms and ages to quotes (these quotes were adapted from the qualitative interview study [24] and included to provide other peoples' experiences in managing acne); changing the context of certain quotes to make them more relatable to the intended user; providing further clarification on how people can manage sun sensitivity as a potential side effect of topical treatments; further clarification on steps for applying topical treatments (time of day and quantity) and what *sensitive areas of the face* referred to; changing the 6-week challenge to 4 weeks as some participants felt that 6 weeks would be too long to commit and based on evidence that topical treatments could take effect sooner [10]; changing the core module name from *universal core treatments* to *core treatments* so that participants would not misinterpret the website as advertising something; and changing the layout of the intervention including the banner, images, and color scheme.

Patient and Public Involvement

Two public contributors aged 24 and 26 years with experience of acne provided input throughout to enhance the usability and accessibility of the intervention. This included providing feedback to further enhance the intervention before the feasibility trial, commenting on participant facing documents, and advising on the choice of the primary outcome measure for the trial. Comments about the intervention were both positive and negative regarding the layout, content, and appropriateness of the website for the target population. One contributor commented on their preference of the primary outcome measure for the feasibility trial and opted for Skindex-16 [36] over various other skin-specific QoL measures for reasons including the appropriateness of the questions. Input on the participant facing documents led to changes in wording, making it more appropriate for a layperson and for the target population.

Feasibility Study

Trial Design

This was a randomized, unblinded feasibility trial comparing two parallel groups: usual care and usual care plus web-based intervention.

Study Population and Eligibility Criteria

The intervention was aimed at young people with acne managed through primary care in the United Kingdom. Participants were recruited through mail-outs from 20 GP practices in the South of England to people aged 14-25 years whose electronic record included a diagnosis of acne and who had received one or more prescriptions for acne in the past 6 months.

People who had previously taken part in the think-aloud study were excluded, as were people who said their acne had cleared and those taking oral isotretinoin, as it is not recommended to use topical acne treatments at the same time as isotretinoin because of the side effects of dry skin.

Procedure

Patients aged ≥16 years, who met the criteria, were sent an *adult study pack* from their GP, and patients <16 years received a *child study pack* (addressed to the parent or carer). Initially, the pack included an information sheet, a freepost envelope, and a covering letter. Those interested returned a reply slip, and a member of the study team contacted the participant, providing them with a unique participant identification number and the link to the web-based intervention. Amendments were made to the process, and these were approved by both the university and National Health Service ethics committees. Changes included an additional A5 flyer about the study to appeal to the target population and a sign-up sheet providing participants with their unique identification number and a link to the intervention. These changes were essential for assessing the feasibility of the study with a challenging population to recruit. Implied parental consent was approved for participants aged <16 years as invitation letters were sent to the parents; therefore, passing log-in details to their child implied consent. This is because young people from 14 years usually self-manage their acne and are responsible for using topical treatments themselves. The link directed all participants to further information and a web-based consent procedure. After consenting, participants were asked to complete a set of baseline questionnaires before being randomized into 1 of 2 groups. Follow-up questionnaires for the trial were conducted at 4 and 6 weeks as a recent study suggested that topical treatments could take effect within 1 to 4 weeks and that continuation after the 4 weeks would lead to further improvements [10]. Participants received an automated email followed by a reminder email a week after (5 and 7 weeks) if they had not completed these. Further text and subsequent phone follow-ups were conducted for nonresponders to complete the outcome measures, particularly the primary outcome Skindex-16.

Intervention and Comparator

The usual care group received treatment as usual from their GP, including appointments, prescriptions, and referrals to the dermatologist, if necessary. Participants in this group were given access to the intervention after they had completed the 6-week follow-up questionnaires.

Participants in the usual care plus web-based intervention group received care as usual with immediate access to the website as described to help them self-manage their acne.

Outcome Measures

We sought to assess a range of feasibility outcomes including the following:

- The rate of recruitment and the number of practices required
- Completion rates of questionnaire outcome measures
- The acceptability of measuring skin-specific QoL using Skindex-16
- The feasibility of a range of quantitative measures
- Intervention usage in terms of number of log-ins and modules accessed

Outcome measures included the following: Skindex-16 [36] was included as a skin-specific QoL measure. Skindex-16 is a validated measure that includes 16 items on a 6-point Likert scale ranging from 0 (never bothered) to 6 (always bothered), which are transformed into a 100-point scale, with higher scores indicating a lower level of QoL [36].

EQ-5D-5L [37] was included as a health-related QoL measure collected at all intervals. It comprised five domains (mobility, self-care, usual activities, pain or discomfort, and anxiety or depression) with five response levels (no problems, slight problems, moderate problems, severe problems, and extreme problems) that describe the current health state. The visual analog scale was also included alongside this [37].

The Problematic Experiences Therapy Scale (PETS) [38] was included and data collected at each interval to explore barriers to treatment adherence. This measure includes 12 items with four subscales: *problems due to symptoms*, *problems due to uncertainty about therapy*, *problems due to doubts about treatment efficacy*, and *practical problems*. Participant responses were scored on a scale ranging from 1 (disagree strongly) to 5 (agree strongly), with higher scores indicating fewer barriers to adherence [38].

Participants also completed the Credibility/Expectancy Questionnaire at baseline as a process predictor. It measures how a person thinks and feels about their therapy and its likely success [39]. These are measured using two types of rating scales, one from 1 (not at all) to 9 (very much) and another from 0% (not at all) to 100% (very much), and it provides an overall score ranging from 3-27 for each factor [40].

The Patient Health Questionnaire-4 (PHQ-4) was used to measure anxiety and depression [41] collected at all intervals. This brief screening tool has been shown to be a reliable and valid measure in young people [42] and includes 4 items measured on a 4-point Likert scale ranging from 0 (not at all) to 4 (nearly every day) [41].

Treatment monitoring questions were included in order to collect data on what topical treatments participants were using, whether they experienced side effects, how they dealt with these, how often they were using treatment, and any other treatments they were using for their acne.

Sociodemographic questions included age, gender, education, age of onset of acne, and whether living with parents or independently.

Sample Size

The target sample size was 65 participants, with 40 in the intervention group and 25 in the usual care group. This was deemed appropriate as guidance on sample sizes in feasibility trials ranged from 12 to >30 participants in each arm [43,44].

Randomization

We intended randomizing all participants into 2 groups in a 2:1 ratio using a computer-generated algorithm. However, because of an error in the randomization software, the block randomization was changed to a 1:1 ratio. The sequence was concealed as this was all done via a computer.

Data Collection and Analysis

Data were automatically collected via the LifeGuide software [31], including information about recruitment, number of log-ins, and which modules or pages participants had accessed. Descriptive statistics were used to describe the data, and outcome measures were analyzed using SPSS version 25 [45]. Linear regression, adjusting for baseline scores, age, gender, education, and age of onset of acne, was performed to provide estimates of mean scores between groups (with 95% CIs). Intention-to-treat analysis was used, including all participants who were randomized, without imputing missing data. There was no significance testing, as this was a feasibility trial and was not sufficiently powered to seek differences between groups.

Ethics Approval

The feasibility trial was approved by the National Research Ethics Service Committee east of England (ref: 18/EE/0105) and registered on the ISRCTN registry (78626638).

Results

Recruitment

Recruitment took place from September 2018 to April 2019, and the follow-up ended in June 2019. In total, 1193 invitation letters were sent from 20 primary care practices in the South of England. Of the 1193 invitations sent, we received 92 (7.71%) responses, with 63 (5.28%) agreeing to take part and 29 (2.43%) giving reasons why they could not. Of the 63 participants, 53 (84%) registered on the web and were randomized (usual care: 27/53, 51%; usual care plus web-based intervention: 26/53, 49%). Of the 53 registered participants, 46 (87%) participants completed follow-up at 4 weeks, 6 weeks, or both time points (Figure 2). Five practices carried mail-out using the amended documents, which led to a small increase in participants signing up for the study—from 4.5% to 4.8%.

Figure 2. Flow diagram of recruitment process. *Problem with LifeGuide randomization procedure incurred delay and participants did not log back in; **Felt like homework; not planning on using topicals; not interested.

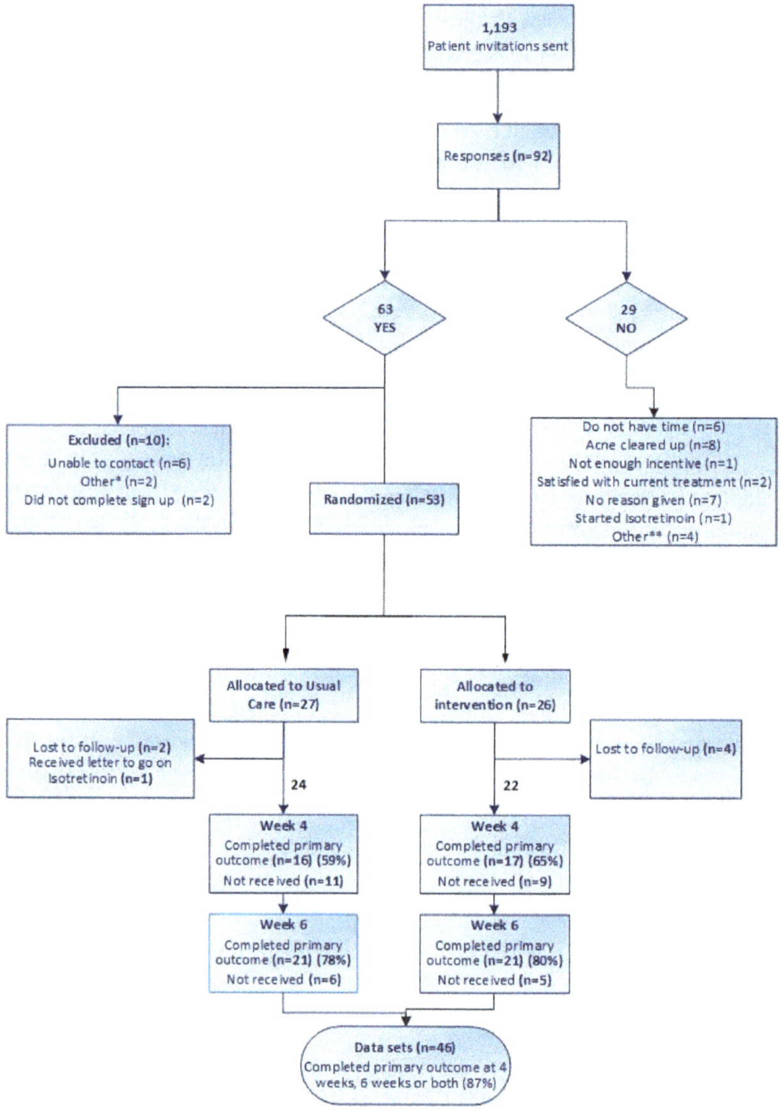

Participant Characteristics

The sample comprised 72% (38/53) female and 28% (15/53) male participants with a mean age of 19 (SD 2.6) years. The mean age at the onset of acne was reported as 14 (SD 2.1) years. Of the 53 participants, 39 (74%) reported living at home, and 44 (83%) were in full-time education (Table 3).

Table 3. Participant characteristics at baseline (N=53).

Participant characteristics	Intervention (n=26)	Usual care (n=27)	Total (n=53)
Gender, n (%)			
Female	21 (81)	17 (63)	38 (72)
Male	5 (19)	10 (37)	15 (28)
Age (years), mean (SD)	18.3 (2.6)	18.8 (3.4)	18.6 (3)
Age at onset of acne (years), mean (SD)	13.54 (2.1)	13.8 (2.5)	13.7 (2.3)
Living at home, n (%)			
Yes	21 (81)	18 (67)	39 (74)
No	5 (19)	9 (33)	14 (26)
Currently in full-time education, n (%)			
Yes	22 (85)	22 (82)	44 (83)
No	4 (15)	5 (19)	9 (17)

Questionnaire Completion

Baseline completion rates were high for all questionnaires (Table 4). Not all participants experienced side effects; therefore, the question about their management had a lower completion rate at each interval. Completion rates were higher at 6 weeks than at 4 weeks as there was a longer period to contact participants by phone to complete the questionnaires if they had not done so after receiving the reminder emails. At 4 weeks, 6% (1/17) of participants in the intervention group and 6% (1/16) of participants in the usual care group completed the primary outcome measure from the questionnaire over the phone. At 6 weeks, this was 24% (5/21) of participants in the intervention group and 14% (3/21) in the usual care group.

Table 4. Questionnaire completion rates (N=53).

Outcome measure	Baseline, n (%)	4 weeks, n (%)	6 weeks, n (%)
Overall Skindex-16	53 (100)	33 (62)	42 (79)
EQ-5D-5L	53 (100)	32 (60)	39 (74)
EQ VAS[a]	53 (100)	31 (59)	34 (64)
PHQ-4[b]	53 (100)	31 (59)	36 (68)
Credibility	53 (100)	N/A[c]	N/A
Expectancy	53 (100)	N/A	N/A
PETS[d] symptoms (n=26)	26 (100)	17 (65)	17 (65)
PETS uncertainty (n=26)	25 (96)	17 (65)	17 (65)
PETS doubts (n=26)	25 (92)	17 (65)	17 (65)
PETS practical problems (n=26)	25 (96)	17 (65)	17 (65)
What topical using	53 (100)	31 (59)	36 (68)
How often using treatment	53 (100)	31 (59)	34 (64)
Side effects	51 (96)	31 (59)	32 (60)
Management of side effects (people who reported side effects)	31 (59)	19 (36)	25 (47)
Other treatment	53 (100)	30 (57)	37 (70)

[a]EQ VAS: EuroQol Visual Analogue Scale.

[b]PHQ-4: Patient Health Questionnaire-4.

[c]N/A: not applicable.

[d]PETS: Problematic Experiences Therapy Scale.

Outcome Measures

Skindex-16

The Skindex-16 overall mean score at baseline was 55.4 (SD 21.8) across both groups. There was a substantial improvement in both groups, and the mean differences between groups, when controlling for baseline scores and covariates (gender, age, age onset, and education), suggested a trend toward benefit at both 4 and 6 weeks: at 4 weeks, the intervention group had a score 5.2 points lower (95% CI □14.58 to 4.09) than the usual care group and at 6 weeks 2.9 points lower (95% CI □13.27 to 7.47; Table 5).

Table 5. Scores at baseline and follow-up and estimate of mean differences controlling for baseline and covariates (n=53).

Score description	Baseline		4-week follow-up		4-week follow-up, controlling for baseline and other covariates, mean difference (95% CI)	6-week follow-up		6-week follow-up, controlling for baseline and other covariates, mean difference (95% CI)
	n value	Value, mean (SD)	n value	Value, mean (SD)		n value	Value, mean (SD)	
Overall Skindex-16 scores								
Usual care	27	55.4 (24)	16	54.2 (18.7)	N/A[a]	21	48 (23.8)	N/A
Web-based intervention	26	55.3 (19.8)	17	45.8 (19.9)	□5.2 (□14.58 to 4.09)	21	43.4 (22.2)	□2.9 (□13.27 to 7.47)
Skindex-16 symptom								
Usual care	N/A	41.3 (25.5)	N/A	35.5 (21.5)	N/A	N/A	37.3 (24.3)	N/A
Web-based intervention	N/A	31.9 (19.8)	N/A	30.6 (24.1)	5.4 (□8.41 to 19.22)	N/A	27 (21.5)	□0.9 (□11.76 to 10.03)
Skindex-16 emotional								
Usual care	N/A	72.7 (27.5)	N/A	74.2 (23.4)	N/A	N/A	63.6 (28.1)	N/A
Web-based intervention	N/A	76.6 (21.1)	N/A	63.7 (22.3)	□12.4 (□24.23 to □0.67)	N/A	62 (24.3)	□3.9 (□16.65 to 8.75)
Skindex-16 functioning								
Usual care	N/A	42.6 (28.3)	N/A	41.2 (22.7)	N/A	N/A	34.8 (27.8)	N/A
Web-based intervention	N/A	44.1 (27.9)	N/A	31.9 (26.8)	□6.4 (□20.52 to 7.79)	N/A	30.5 (28.9)	□3.4 (□16.75 to 9.9)
PHQ-4[b] total								
Usual care	27	4 (3.5)	16	3.9 (3.3)	N/A	18	3.7 (3.3)	N/A
Web-based intervention	26	4.6 (3.7)	15	2.3 (2.9)	□1.7 (□3.66 to 0.18)	18	3.2 (3.3)	□0.8 (□2.6 to 0.97)
PETS[c] symptoms								
Usual care	26	3.9 (1)	14	4 (1.1)	N/A	17	4.1 (0.9)	N/A
Web-based intervention	26	3.9 (0.9)	17	4.2 (1.2)	0.2 (□0.65 to 1.15)	17	4.2 (0.9)	0.2 (□0.47 to 0.82)
PETS uncertainty								
Usual care	26	4.5 (0.9)	15	4.5 (1.2)	N/A	18	4.2 (1.1)	N/A
Web-based intervention	25	4.4 (1)	17	4.7 (0.6)	0.1 (□0.51 to 0.67)	17	4.9 (0.2)	0.6 (0.19 to 1.08)
PETS doubt								
Usual care	27	3.8 (1)	19	3.7 (1.1)	N/A	18	3.7 (1.1)	N/A
Web-based intervention	24	3.4 (1.3)	17	4.2 (0.8)	0.5 (□0.23 to 1.25)	17	4.2 (1)	0.5 (□0.18 to 1.24)
PETS practical problems								
Usual care	27	3.4 (1.3)	15	3.6 (1.3)	N/A	18	3. (1.3)	N/A
Web-based intervention	25	3.8 (1)	17	4 (1.1)	0.1 (□0.44 to 0.73)	17	4.1 (1.1)	0.7 (0.02 to 1.3)

[a]N/A: not applicable.

[b]PHQ-4: Patient Health Questionnaire-4.

[c]PETS: Problematic Experiences Therapy Scale.

Individual Subscales for Skindex-16

There was no evidence of a trend toward benefit in the symptoms subscale (intervention group 5.4 points higher at 4 weeks: 95% CI □8.41 to 19.22; 0.9 points lower at 6 weeks: 95% CI □11.76 to □10.03); however, some evidence of a trend toward benefit in the emotional subscale (intervention 12.4 points lower at 4 weeks: 95% CI □24.23 to □0.67; 3.9 points lower at 6 weeks: 95% CI □16.65 to 8.75) and functioning subscale (intervention group 6.4 points lower at 4 weeks: 95% CI □20.52 to 7.79; 3.4 points lower at 6 weeks: 95% CI □16.75 to 9.9; Table 5).

Other Outcome Measures

The baseline mean score for anxiety and depression (PHQ-4) suggests that the overall scores between groups were in the mild range for anxiety and depression with a score of 4.3 (SD 3.6) and a trend toward improvement in the intervention group at 4 weeks compared with the usual care group. For all PETS subscales (symptoms, uncertainty, doubt, and practical problems), there were also suggestions of a trend toward benefit (Table 5).

Treatment Monitoring

Topical Treatment Used

More people in the usual care group reported using topicals at baseline compared with those in the intervention group. In the intervention group, the percentage of people using topicals increased from baseline to 4 weeks by 13.5% and decreased by 0.8% in the usual care group (Table 6).

Table 6. Reported topical treatment use between groups at each interval.

Topical used	Intervention		Usual care	
	n (%)	N	n (%)	N
Topical treatments				
Baseline	16 (62)	26	20 (74)	27
4 weeks	12 (75)	16	11 (73)	15
6 weeks	15 (88)	17	15 (79)	19
None				
Baseline	3 (12)	26	6 (22)	27
4 weeks	3 (19)	16	4 (27)	15
6 weeks	2 (12)	17	4 (21)	19
Other[a]				
Baseline	7 (27)	26	1 (4)	27
4 weeks	1 (6)	16	0 (0)	15
6 weeks	0 (0)	17	0 (0)	19

[a]Other topical treatments including branded products.

Topical Treatment Side Effects and Management

At 4 and 6 weeks, the usual care groups reported similar rates of side effects compared with the intervention group (Table 7). There was an increase of 13.5% from baseline to 4 weeks in the number of people reporting continuing treatment (including altering application as advised by the website) when experiencing minor side effects compared with the usual, which decreased by 2.4% at 4 weeks (Table 8). In both groups, the most common frequency of application at all intervals was *once or more than once a day or most days*. The intervention group and the usual care decreased similarly in the number of people reporting application of *once or more than once a day or most days* at 4 weeks (Table 9).

Table 7. Reported side effects from topical treatments.

Side effects	Intervention		Usual care	
	n (%)	N	n (%)	N
Topical treatments				
Baseline	15 (60)	25	16 (62)	26
4 weeks	9 (53)	17	8 (57)	14
6 weeks	10 (67)	15	12 (71)	17
None				
Baseline	10 (40)	25	10 (39)	26
4 weeks	8 (47)	17	6 (43)	14
6 weeks	5 (33)	15	5 (29)	17

Table 8. Reported management of side effects from topicals.

Management of side effects	Intervention		Usual care	
	n (%)	N	n (%)	N
Continued treatment				
Baseline	9 (64)	14	14 (82)	17
4 weeks	7 (78)	9	8 (80)	10
6 weeks	7 (64)	11	10 (71)	14
Stopped treatment				
Baseline	5 (36)	14	2 (12)	17
4 weeks	2 (22)	9	0 (0)	10
6 weeks	2 (18)	11	1 (7)	14
Other[a]				
Baseline	2 (14)	14	1 (6)	17
4 weeks	1 (11)	9	2 (20)	10
6 weeks	1 (9)	11	3 (21)	14

[a]Other management included using moisturizer, hydrating masks, or face washes.

Table 9. Reported frequency of application of topicals.

Frequency of application	Intervention		Usual care	
	n (%)	N	n (%)	N
Once or more than once a day or most days				
Baseline	19 (73)	26	19 (70)	27
4 weeks	11 (65)	17	9 (64)	14
6 weeks	13 (81)	16	12 (67)	18
Not at all or once or twice a week				
Baseline	7 (27)	26	8 (30)	27
4 weeks	6 (35)	17	5 (36)	14
6 weeks	3 (19)	16	6 (33)	18

Intervention Use

Approximately 88% (23/26) of participants in the intervention group completed the core module *core treatments*. Completion was decided based on whether participants clicked through to the end of the core module pages without logging off the web-based intervention. Approximately 69% (18/26) of participants visited the website three times or more, including baseline visits. There was a low uptake of the 4-week challenge (38%), although this was based on whether participants entered a start date; however, it is possible that some participants engaged without entering a start date. Visits to some of the optional modules were low: 42% of participants accessed the module on *living with spots or acne,* and more than a quarter viewed the *myth-busting quiz*; fewer were interested in *talking to your GP* (Table 10).

Table 10. Intervention use (N=26).

Measures of intervention use	Web-based intervention, n (%)
Core module completed	23 (88)
Total number of visits to intervention	
1	3 (12)
2	5 (19)
3	7 (27)
4	7 (27)
5	2 (8)
6	2 (8)
Signed up to 4-week challenge	10 (38)
Visits to other modules	
Living with spots or acne	11 (42)
Myth-busting quiz	7 (27)
What are spots or acne	7 (27)
Other treatments	7 (27)
Oral antibiotics	5 (19)
Talking to your GP[a]	3 (12)

[a]GP: general practitioner.

Discussion

Principal Findings

To our knowledge, this is the first web-based behavioral intervention developed for young people with acne, using the PBA along with theory and evidence [22]. The recruitment rate of 8% was lower than expected; however, retention rates for people completing the primary outcome measure at either 4 or 6 weeks were high (87%). There was a suggestive trend toward benefit in the primary (Skindex-16) and secondary outcome measures (PHQ-4 and PETS) when looking at the mean differences. More people in the intervention group reported using topical treatments, and they were also more likely to manage side effects from topical treatments by continuing treatment as opposed to stopping treatment compared with the usual care group. Completion of the core module was high (88%), although it was low for the optional modules. Although promising, these findings should be viewed with caution, as this study was not powered to determine effectiveness.

Limitations

There were several limitations and changes that should be considered based on the findings of this feasibility trial. First, the mail-out through primary care practices received a low response rate, suggesting that people who took part in the trial may be more motivated and possibly have higher literacy than those who did not respond. Therefore, the sample may not be fully representative of young people who consult primary care for their acne. A key reason for not participating was time commitment, which suggests that the level of involvement in the study may need to be made clearer. Another reason for not participating was that some participants' skin had cleared up. This could be a reflection on the search strategy or the unpredictable nature of their skin condition. The changes to the recruitment process led to a slight increase in response rate which suggests that if implemented earlier this could have potentially improved the numbers recruited. People who took part in the study also seemed to be using topical treatments already, which suggests that recruitment in a future trial should seek participants who are not already using them to benefit from the intervention. We may also need to consider other ways of reaching the target population, including other platforms such as social media, pharmacies, and schools.

Second, there was a low uptake of the optional modules, which suggests that the intervention may need to be refined further. However, the reason for including these modules as optional was that they might not be applicable to everyone at that time but were seen as important in earlier qualitative research. Uptake of the *4-week challenge* was low; however, this was only determined by people entering a date to start the challenge. In the future, this should be monitored more closely, and perhaps there should be a question in the survey to identify those who did and did not take part. It is also unclear whether people in the usual care group attended their GP practices and were prescribed treatment as usual, making it difficult to fully understand why people in the usual care increased on a number of outcome measures.

Although the target sample size was not reached, this was a feasibility study and provided useful information about the changes that need to be considered for a future trial. Owing to the randomization error, participants were randomized in a 1:1 ratio instead of 2:1 for intervention to usual care group. This resulted in less usage data for the intervention group, which could have provided further information on intervention use.

Although there was a trend toward benefit in both the primary and secondary outcome measures, a larger sample is needed to draw conclusions about the effect of the intervention.

Comparison with Prior Work

The findings from this feasibility trial reflect the results of previous trials testing the effectiveness of interventions for acne [11,13-15,19]. For example, a pilot RCT of an interactive health education tool also found that those in the intervention group had improved QoL scores compared with the control group, although these findings were not statistically significant [11]. However, this study did not specify which treatments were being used by participants in the intervention (topical or oral treatments); therefore, comparisons should be made with caution. In this study, we used PETS scores to determine adherence to topical treatments, which suggested a trend in the direction of benefit. A previous RCT investigating the effectiveness of supplementary educational materials on a combination topical treatment also found improved adherence, although using an objective measure (medication event monitoring system) [10]. There is currently no standardized or fully validated method of measurement for adherence to acne treatments [46], and further work would benefit in addressing this so that heterogeneity and adherence can be compared across trials.

The rate of follow-up in this study was high at 6 weeks (79%) in terms of those completing the primary outcome measure (Skindex-16). This is in line with a previous trial that found a follow-up rate of 84.5% when recruiting through primary care [10]. Similarly, a study investigating adherence rates using an internet-based survey for young people with acne had a follow-up rate of 75%, although it is unclear where participants were recruited from, and the sample size was small with 20 participants [14].

Conclusions

This feasibility trial demonstrates that a web-based behavioral intervention for young people with acne can be delivered with high retention, high engagement with the core module, and trends in the direction of benefit for the primary outcome measure. However, recruitment to this study was challenging, and alternative methods of seeking participants should be considered for a full-scale trial of a similar intervention, particularly when seeking a population less likely to be using effective topical treatments for acne.

Acknowledgments

We would like to thank the participants who took part in the research and the primary care practices for helping with recruitment. We would also like to thank the patient representatives who helped develop the intervention and advised on trial materials. This study was funded by the National Institute for Health Research School for Primary Care Research Studentship for Athena Ip. The views expressed are those of the authors and not necessarily those of the National Institute for Health Research or the Department of Health and Social Care.

References

1. James WD. Acne. N Engl J Med 2005 Apr 07;352(14):1463-1472. [doi: 10.1056/nejmcp033487]
2. Webster G. Acne vulgaris. Br Med J 2002;325(7362):475-479 [FREE Full text] [Medline: 12202330]
3. Cunliffe WJ, Gould DJ. Prevalence of facial acne vulgaris in late adolescence and in adults. Br Med J 1979;1(6171):1109-1110 [FREE Full text] [doi: 10.1136/bmj.1.6171.1109] [Medline: 156054]
4. Williams HC, Dellavalle RP, Garner S. Acne vulgaris. Lancet 2012;379(9813):361-372. [doi: 10.1016/s0140-6736(11)60321-8]
5. Yang Z, Zhang Y, Mosler E, Hu J, Li H, Zhang Y, et al. Topical benzoyl peroxide for acne. Cochrane Database Syst Rev 2020 Mar 16;3:CD011154 [FREE Full text] [doi: 10.1002/14651858.CD011154.pub2] [Medline: 32175593]
6. Jones-Caballero M, Pedrosa E, Peñas PF. Self-reported adherence to treatment and quality of life in mild to moderate acne. Dermatology 2008;217(4):309-314. [doi: 10.1159/000151441] [Medline: 18714158]
7. Gollnick H, Friedrich M, Peschen M, Pettker R, Pier A, Streit V, et al. Effect of adapalene 0.1%/benzoyl peroxide 2.5% topical gel on quality of life and treatment adherence during long-term application in patients with predominantly moderate acne with or without concomitant medication - additional results from the non-interventional cohort study ELANG. J Eur Acad Dermatol Venereol 2015 Jun;29 Suppl 4:23-29. [doi: 10.1111/jdv.13195] [Medline: 26059731]
8. Dréno B, Thiboutot D, Gollnick H, Finlay AY, Layton A, Leyden JJ, Global Alliance to Improve Outcomes in Acne. Large-scale worldwide observational study of adherence with acne therapy. Int J Dermatol 2010 Apr;49(4):448-456. [doi: 10.1111/j.1365-4632.2010.04416.x] [Medline: 20465705]
9. Thielitz A, Helmdach M, Röpke EM, Gollnick H. Lipid analysis of follicular casts from cyanoacrylate strips as a new method for studying therapeutic effects of antiacne agents. Br J Dermatol 2001 Jul;145(1):19-27. [doi: 10.1046/j.1365-2133.2001.04276.x] [Medline: 11453902]
10. Myhill T, Coulson W, Nixon P, Royal S, McCormack T, Kerrouche N. Use of supplementary patient education material increases treatment adherence and satisfaction among acne patients receiving adapalene 0.1%/benzoyl peroxide 2.5% gel in primary care clinics: a multicenter, randomized, controlled clinical study. Dermatol Ther (Heidelb) 2017 Dec;7(4):515-524 [FREE Full text] [doi: 10.1007/s13555-017-0203-4] [Medline: 29027127]

11. Wang AS, Wu J, Tuong W, Schupp C, Armstrong AW. Effectiveness of a novel interactive health care education tool on clinical outcomes and quality of life in acne patients: A randomized controlled pilot study. J Dermatolog Treat 2015 Oct 20;26(5):435-439. [doi: 10.3109/09546634.2015.1020915] [Medline: 25790848]
12. Boker A, Feetham HJ, Armstrong A, Purcell P, Jacobe H. Do automated text messages increase adherence to acne therapy? Results of a randomized, controlled trial. J Am Acad Dermatol 2012 Dec;67(6):1136-1142. [doi: 10.1016/j.jaad.2012.02.031] [Medline: 22521201]
13. Yentzer BA, Gosnell AL, Clark AR, Pearce DJ, Balkrishnan R, Camacho FT, et al. A randomized controlled pilot study of strategies to increase adherence in teenagers with acne vulgaris. J Am Acad Dermatol 2011 Apr;64(4):793-795. [doi: 10.1016/j.jaad.2010.05.008] [Medline: 21414505]
14. Yentzer BA, Wood AA, Sagransky MJ, O'Neill JL, Clark AR, Williams LL, et al. An Internet-based survey and improvement of acne treatment outcomes. Arch Dermatol 2011 Oct;147(10):1223-1224. [doi: 10.1001/archdermatol.2011.277] [Medline: 22006146]
15. Rueda MJ. Acne subject preference for pump over tube for dispensing fixed-dose combination adapalene 0.1%-benzoyl peroxide 2.5% gel. Dermatol Ther (Heidelb) 2014 Jun;4(1):61-70 [FREE Full text] [doi: 10.1007/s13555-014-0054-1] [Medline: 24919432]
16. Tan X, Park C, Kim G, Patel I, Chang J. Improving adherence to acne treatment: the emerging role of application software. Clin Cosmet Investigat Dermatol 2014 Feb;7:65-72. [doi: 10.2147/ccid.s46051]
17. Glanz K, Bishop DB. The role of behavioral science theory in development and implementation of public health interventions. Annu Rev Public Health 2010;31:399-418. [doi: 10.1146/annurev.publhealth.012809.103604] [Medline: 20070207]
18. Craig P, Dieppe P, Macintyre S, Michie S, Nazareth I, Petticrew M, Medical Research Council Guidance. Developing and evaluating complex interventions: the new Medical Research Council guidance. Br Med J 2008 Sep 29;337:a1655 [FREE Full text] [doi: 10.1136/bmj.a1655] [Medline: 18824488]
19. Sandoval LF, Semble A, Gustafson CJ, Huang KE, Levender MM, Feldman SR. Pilot randomized-control trial to assess the effect product sampling has on adherence using adapalene/benzoyl peroxide gel in acne patients. J Drugs Dermatol 2014;13(2):135-140. [Medline: 24509962]
20. Eldridge SM, Ashby D, Feder GS, Rudnicka AR, Ukoumunne OC. Lessons for cluster randomized trials in the twenty-first century: a systematic review of trials in primary care. Clin Trials 2004 Feb;1(1):80-90. [doi: 10.1191/1740774504cn006rr] [Medline: 16281464]
21. Hoffmann TC, Glasziou PP, Boutron I, Milne R, Perera R, Moher D, et al. Better reporting of interventions: template for intervention description and replication (TIDieR) checklist and guide. Br Med J 2014;348:g1687. [doi: 10.1136/bmj.g1687] [Medline: 24609605]
22. Yardley L, Ainsworth B, Arden-Close E, Muller I. The person-based approach to enhancing the acceptability and feasibility of interventions. Pilot Feasibility Stud 2015;1:37 [FREE Full text] [doi: 10.1186/s40814-015-0033-z] [Medline: 27965815]
23. Ip A, Muller I, Geraghty AW, Platt D, Little P, Santer M. Views and experiences of people with acne vulgaris and healthcare professionals about treatments: systematic review and thematic synthesis of qualitative research. BMJ Open 2021;11(2):e041794 [FREE Full text] [doi: 10.1136/bmjopen-2020-041794] [Medline: 33526498]
24. Ip A, Muller I, Geraghty A, McNiven A, Little P, Santer M. Young people's perceptions of acne and acne treatments: secondary analysis of qualitative interview data. Br J Dermatol 2020 Aug;183(2):349-356 [FREE Full text] [doi: 10.1111/bjd.18684] [Medline: 31701523]
25. Michie S, Richardson M, Johnston M, Abraham C, Francis J, Hardeman W, et al. The behavior change technique taxonomy (v1) of 93 hierarchically clustered techniques: building an international consensus for the reporting of behavior change interventions. Ann Behav Med 2013;46(1):81-95. [doi: 10.1007/s12160-013-9486-6] [Medline: 23512568]
26. Michie S, van Stralen MM, West R. The behaviour change wheel: a new method for characterising and designing behaviour change interventions. Implement Sci 2011;6:42 [FREE Full text] [doi: 10.1186/1748-5908-6-42] [Medline: 21513547]
27. Horne R, Weinman J. Self-regulation and self-management in Asthma: exploring the role of illness perceptions and treatment beliefs in explaining non-adherence to preventer medication. Psychol Health 2002;17(1):17-32. [doi: 10.1080/08870440290001502]
28. Fabbrocini G, Cacciapuoti S, Monfrecola G. A qualitative investigation of the impact of acne on health-related quality of life (hrql): development of a conceptual model. Dermatol Ther (Heidelb) 2018;8(1):85-99 [FREE Full text] [doi: 10.1007/s13555-018-0224-7] [Medline: 29435857]
29. McNiven A. 'Disease, illness, affliction? Don't know': ambivalence and ambiguity in the narratives of young people about having acne. Health (London) 2019 May;23(3):273-288. [doi: 10.1177/1363459318762035] [Medline: 29552892]
30. Santer M, Chandler D, Lown M, Francis N, Muller I. Views of oral antibiotics and advice seeking about acne: a qualitative study of online discussion forums. Br J Dermatol 2017 Sep;177(3):751-757. [doi: 10.1111/bjd.15398] [Medline: 28218972]
31. The LifeGuide research programme. LifeGuide Online. URL: https://www.lifeguideonline.org/ [accessed 2020-08-05]
32. Overview - acne. National Health Service. URL: https://www.nhs.uk/conditions/acne/ [accessed 2020-08-01]
33. Acne vulgaris. NICE Clinical Knowledge Summaries (CKS). URL: https://cks.nice.org.uk/acne-vulgaris#!scenarioRecommendation [accessed 2020-04-10]

34. Acne. NICE British National Formulary (BNF). URL: https://www.nice.org.uk/bnf-uk-only [accessed 2020-08-03]
35. Charters E. The Use of Think-aloud Methods in Qualitative Research An Introduction to Think-aloud Methods. Brock Edu J 2003 Jul 01;12(2):68-82. [doi: 10.26522/brocked.v12i2.38]
36. Chren M, Lasek RJ, Sahay AP, Sands LP. Measurement properties of skindex-16: A brief quality-of-life measure for patients with skin diseases. J Cutan Med Surg 2001 Mar;5(2):105-110. [doi: 10.1007/bf02737863]
37. Herdman M, Gudex C, Lloyd A, Janssen M, Kind P, Parkin D, et al. Development and preliminary testing of the new five-level version of EQ-5D (EQ-5D-5L). Qual Life Res 2011;20(10):1727-1736 [FREE Full text] [doi: 10.1007/s11136-011-9903-x] [Medline: 21479777]
38. Kirby S, Donovan-Hall M, Yardley L. Measuring barriers to adherence: validation of the Problematic Experiences of Therapy Scale. Disabil Rehabil 2014;36(22):1924-1929. [doi: 10.3109/09638288.2013.876106] [Medline: 24410171]
39. Devilly GJ, Borkovec TD. Psychometric properties of the credibility/expectancy questionnaire. J Behav Ther Exp Psychiatry 2000 Jun;31(2):73-86. [doi: 10.1016/s0005-7916(00)00012-4]
40. Smeets R, Beelen S, Goossens M, Schouten EG, Knottnerus JA, Vlaeyen JW. Treatment expectancy and credibility are associated with the outcome of both physical and cognitive-behavioral treatment in chronic low back pain. Clin J Pain 2008 May;24(4):305-315. [doi: 10.1097/AJP.0b013e318164aa75] [Medline: 18427229]
41. Kroenke K, Spitzer RL, Williams JB, Löwe B. An ultra-brief screening scale for anxiety and depression: the PHQ-4. Psychosomatics 2009;50(6):613-621. [doi: 10.1176/appi.psy.50.6.613] [Medline: 19996233]
42. Khubchandani J, Brey R, Kotecki J, Kleinfelder J, Anderson J. The psychometric properties of phq-4 depression and anxiety screening scale among college students. Arch Psychiatr Nurs 2016 Aug;30(4):457-462. [doi: 10.1016/j.apnu.2016.01.014] [Medline: 27455918]
43. Julious SA. Sample size of 12 per group rule of thumb for a pilot study. Pharmaceut Stat 2005 Oct;4(4):287-291. [doi: 10.1002/pst.185]
44. Sim J, Lewis M. The size of a pilot study for a clinical trial should be calculated in relation to considerations of precision and efficiency. J Clin Epidemiol 2012 Mar;65(3):301-308. [doi: 10.1016/j.jclinepi.2011.07.011] [Medline: 22169081]
45. IBM SPSS Statistics for Windows, Version 25.0. IBM Corp. Armonk, NY: IBM Corp; 2017. URL: https://www.ibm.com/support/pages/how-cite-ibm-spss-statistics-or-earlier-versions-spss [accessed 2020-08-03]
46. Snyder S, Crandell I, Davis SA, Feldman SR. Medical adherence to acne therapy: a systematic review. Am J Clin Dermatol 2014 Apr;15(2):87-94. [doi: 10.1007/s40257-014-0063-y] [Medline: 24481999]

Abbreviations

GP: general practitioner
PBA: Person-based approach
PETS: Problematic Experiences Therapy Scale
PHQ-4: Patient Health Questionnaire-4
PROSPERO: International Prospective Register of Systematic Reviews
QoL: quality of life
RCT: randomized controlled trial
TIDieR: Template for Intervention Description and Replication

3

The Contact Dermatitis Quality of Life Index (CDQL): Survey Development and Content Validity Assessment

Mary K Hill[1], MD; Melissa R Laughter[2], PhD; Cecile I Harmange[2], BSc; Robert P Dellavalle[1,3,4], MD, PhD, MSPH; Chandler W Rundle[5], BS; Cory A Dunnick[1,3], MD

[1]Department of Dermatology, University of Colorado Anschutz Medical Campus, Aurora, CO, United States

[2]School of Medicine, University of Colorado, Aurora, CO, United States

[3]Dermatology Service, United States Department of Veterans Affairs, Eastern Colorado Health Care System, Aurora, CO, United States

[4]Department of Epidemiology, Colorado School of Public Health, University of Colorado Anschutz Medical Campus, Aurora, CO, United States

[5]School of Medicine, Loma Linda University, Loma Linda, CA, United States

Corresponding Author:
Cecile I Harmange, BSc
School of Medicine
University of Colorado
1665 Aurora Court, MS 703
Aurora, CO, 80045
United States

Email: cecile.harmange@cuanschutz.edu

Abstract

Background: There is limited measurement and reporting of quality of life (QoL) outcomes for patients with contact dermatitis (CD).

Objective: The purpose of this study is to develop a standardized Contact Dermatitis Quality of Life index (CDQL) for adult patients.

Methods: A list of 81 topics was compiled from a review of QoL measures used previously in CD research. A total of 2 rounds of web-based Delphi surveys were sent to physicians who registered to attend the 2018 American Contact Dermatitis Society meeting, asking that they rank the relevance of topics for measuring QoL in CD using a 4-point scale. Items met consensus for inclusion if at least 78% of respondents ranked them as relevant or very relevant, and their median score was ≥3.25.

Results: Of the 210 physicians contacted, 34 physicians completed the initial survey and 17 completed the follow-up survey. A total of 22 topics met consensus for inclusion in the CDQL, addressing symptoms, emotions, functions of daily living, social and physical functions, work/school functions, and treatment.

Conclusions: This study was limited by the following factors: few open-ended questions in the initial survey, a lack of direct patient feedback, and long survey length, which likely contributed to lower survey participation. The CDQL is a comprehensive, CD-specific QoL measure developed on the basis of expert consensus via a modified Delphi process to be used by physicians and other health care professionals who care for adult patients with contact dermatitis.

KEYWORDS

contact dermatitis; allergic contact dermatitis; irritant contact dermatitis; quality of life; outcomes instruments; health outcomes

Introduction

Measures of quality of life (QoL) have become a fundamental component in evaluating the benefits of dermatologic interventions, especially for chronic, incurable diseases. Supplementary to the objective clinical indices used to assess disease severity, QoL instruments incorporate patients' impressions of their functioning and well-being, allowing for a more complete picture of their health status. Unlike generic questionnaires, disease-specific instruments are more responsive to changes over time in QoL [1,2].

The negative impact of contact dermatitis (CD) on QoL has been established in existing literature [3-13]. Worse QoL is associated with the presence of several features, including pruritus, discomfort, and trouble working with one's hands or carrying out everyday activities [14]. Chronically, the impact of dermatologic diseases on QoL can result in considerable emotional and functional impairment [15]. The extent of CD's effect on QoL is not always adequately reflected by disease severity, possibly due to the psychological stress and embarrassment caused by visual manifestations of the disease [14]. It is therefore essential to use a standardized tool for quantitatively assessing QoL in patients with CD. However, as revealed by a systematic review of outcomes instruments used for CD in randomized controlled trials (RCTs) published between 2005 and 2015 [16], only a small minority of RCTs (6%) assessed QoL, and among those studies, there was a lack of consensus on what tool to use for this purpose.

A standardized measure of QoL for adult patients with CD would be beneficial in guiding individual treatment strategies and to potentially help prevent the risks associated with chronically depressed QoL. Additionally, such a universal tool would allow for greater comparability among articles in the CD literature. The purpose of this study, therefore, was to develop the Contact Dermatitis Quality of Life index (CDQL), a QoL measure specific to CD that quantifies the impact of the disease on functioning and well-being from a patient perspective. This tool was created for use by physicians and other health care professionals caring for patients with contact dermatitis.

Methods

The process of developing the CDQL consisted of initial topic generation via a literature review, followed by a 2-step modified Delphi method to establish the content validity of the instrument.

Preliminary topics compiled for the questionnaire were based on a review of QoL outcome measures used in previous studies of CD. A systematic review [16] of CD outcome measures in RCTs published from 2005 to 2015 found that QoL was evaluated using the Dermatology Life Quality Index (DLQI) [17] and various general assessments of pruritus. According to a 2003 literature review [12], other QoL tools used for patients with CD include the Dermatology-Specific Quality of Life (DSQL) instrument [15], the Skindex-29 [18,19], and the 36-item Short Form Health Survey [20]. Additionally, the Skindex-16 [21] was previously modified for use in allergic CD, with the addition of 5 questions specific to the effect on one's occupation [22]. A subsequent QoL measure for CD incorporated modifications of both the Skindex-16 and the DLQI, as well as 6 additional items addressing feelings and functioning [14].

A total of 81 topics were generated from a review of the aforementioned QoL instruments. Similar to the Skindex-16 [21], each topic was worded to ask patients how often the event in the topic bothered them. Expert consensus was sought regarding questionnaire topics in accordance with a modified Delphi technique, with 2 rounds of surveys conducted to maximize consensus [23]. Following institutional review board approval, the initial voluntary, anonymous web-based surveys were sent to the 210 registrants of the 2018 annual meeting of the American Contact Dermatitis Society (ACDS), asking that dermatology physicians rank the relevance of each questionnaire topic using the following 4-point Likert scale: (1) not relevant, (2) somewhat relevant, (3) relevant, or (4) very relevant (Multimedia Appendix 1). Topics derived from the Skindex-16 were italicized. Survey respondents were also asked to provide their opinion regarding the time frame which the CDQL should be designed to address, keeping in mind both the potentially intermittent nature of CD [15] and the goal of maximizing patient recollection [17].

Definitions of consensus vary throughout the literature. A prior systematic review investigating consensus in Delphi studies found that consensus is most often defined by the percentage of agreement, followed by the proportion of subjects' ratings falling within a specified range [24]. Thresholds set for consensus definitions based on percentages or proportions range from 50% to 97%, with a median of 75%. Green et al [25,26] suggested that consensus is achieved when at least 70% of Delphi respondents rank the item as 3 or 4 on a 4-point Likert scale, and the median is at least 3.25. Lynn et al [27,28] suggested that with at least 6 professionals ranking the relevance of a topic for a new instrument, the content validity index (CVI) of the topic (the proportion of professionals ranking it as a 3 or 4 on a 4-point scale) should be ≥0.78 in order to reduce the possibility of agreement due to chance. A combination of these criteria was used for this study, with items meeting consensus for inclusion in the CDQL if at least 78% of respondents ranked them as relevant or very relevant (a score of 3 or 4), and the median score was at least 3.25. Also in line with precedent [29-34], items rated as relevant or very relevant by less than 50% of respondents were excluded.

In response to expert comments from the initial survey recommending less repetition and a shorter questionnaire length to improve practicality for clinical use, similar questionnaire topics were combined and/or excluded. The remaining topics with CVIs of 50% to 77% were compiled in a second survey, which listed the initial CVI for each item and asked respondents of the first survey to rank topic relevance on a 4-point scale again (Multimedia Appendix 2). A total of 7 new topics were included in the second survey based on preliminary results from a study aimed at developing a QoL index for allergic CD [35]. Additionally, based on comments from the initial survey, 4 other new topics were included under a treatment domain. Survey respondents were asked to provide a brief explanation for their ranking of relevance if the initial CVI for a topic was <60% or if they ranked an item with a CVI of >60% as somewhat relevant or not relevant. Again, individual items from the second survey were included as items in the final CDQL if the CVI among respondents was ≥0.78 and the median score was ≥3.25.

In order to further establish the CDQL's content validity, the CVI for the total scale was calculated. Different ways of quantifying this value exist, although it is recommended (especially when larger numbers of experts are involved, as in this study) that it be calculated by taking the average of the CVIs for the individual questionnaire topics [28]. A total scale CVI of ≥0.90 has been previously deemed acceptable [28,36].

Survey data were collected and managed using REDCap (Research Electronic Data Capture; Vanderbilt University) electronic data capture tools hosted at the University of Colorado Denver [37]. REDCap is a secure, web-based application designed to support data capture for research studies, providing the following: (1) an intuitive interface for validated data entry, (2) audit trails for tracking data manipulation and export procedures, (3) automated export procedures for seamless data downloads to common statistical packages, and (4) procedures for importing data from external sources. Statistical analysis was performed using Excel (Microsoft Corporation).

This study was reviewed and approved by The Colorado Multiple Institutional Review Board.

Results

Of the 210 individuals contacted, 43 (20.5%) completed the initial Delphi survey. A total of 8 surveys were completed by nonphysicians and were therefore excluded. Additionally, 13 partially completed surveys were excluded. A total of 34 physicians completed the initial survey, of whom 33 were attending dermatologists and 1 was a fellow. Of the 34 physicians who completed the survey, 27 (79%) patch tested >41 patients per year; only 1 physician did not do any patch testing. All but 2 of the physicians were members of the ACDS, American Academy of Dermatology, and/or American Academy of Allergy, Asthma, and Immunology.

A total of 12 topics from the first Delphi survey with a CVI of <50% were excluded. Of the remaining topics, 22 were deemed repetitive and also excluded. Initially, 23 topics from the first Delphi survey met consensus for inclusion in the CDQL; however, based on expert feedback, several redundant topics were either removed or combined, ultimately resulting in 19 topics meeting consensus for inclusion (Table 1). The CVIs and median relevance scores for these topics ranged from 0.79 to 1.0 and 3.5 to 4.0, respectively.

The follow-up Delphi survey consisted of 35 questionnaire topics not yet meeting consensus for inclusion or exclusion (including 11 new topics). Of the 43 individuals contacted (those who had responded to the initial survey), 23 (53%) completed the second Delphi survey. The final analysis included a total of 17 surveys fully completed by physicians who had also completed the initial survey. Following completion of the second survey, an additional 4 topics met consensus for inclusion, with CVIs ranging from 0.82 to 1.0, and a median relevance score of 4.0 for all 4 questions (Table 2).

Based on the first survey, 20 (59%) of the 34 respondents felt the questionnaire should ask about QoL over the past 6 months, 8 (24%) felt it should address the past month, 4 (12%) felt it should address the past year, and 2 (6%) felt it should address the past week. Agreement improved in the follow-up survey, with 16 (70%) of the 23 respondents suggesting that the CDQL inquire about the past 6 months.

The resulting CDQL consists of 23 items, asking patients how often they have been bothered by each item over the past 6 months (Multimedia Appendix 3). Responses are structured on a 4-point Likert scale: (1) never bothered, (2) sometimes bothered, (3) often bothered, or (4) always bothered. For ease of use, this was simplified from the Skindex-16 [21], which uses a continuous bipolar scale with 7 answer choices.

The CDQL can be broken down into 6 different domains: symptoms (1 item), emotions (9 items), functions of daily living (3 items), social and physical functions (2 items), work/school functions (4 items), and treatment-related items (4 items). The CVI for the total scale was 0.85. A total of 10 topics were at least in part derived from the Skindex-16 [21], 9 topics were derived from the Skindex-29 [18,19], 7 topics were derived from the DSQL [15], 5 topics were derived from the DLQI [17], 6 topics were derived from the CD-specific quality of life measure by Ayala et al [14], 2 topics were derived from the 36-item Short Form Health Survey [20], 2 topics were derived from the modified Skindex-16 by Kadyk et al [22], and 3 topics were based on expert recommendations from the first survey.

Table 1. Topics meeting consensus for inclusion after the initial Delphi survey.

Topics[a]	Content validity index[b]	Median (SD)[c]
Symptoms		
Itching of your skin[d,e,f,g]	1.0	4.0 (0.24)
Emotions		
Your skin condition persisting or reoccurring[d]	0.94	4.0 (0.58)
Your skin condition's appearance[d]	0.91	4.0 (0.65)
Frustration because of your skin condition[d,e,f]	0.91	4.0 (0.66)
Feeling embarrassed[d,e,f,g] or ashamed[e] because of your skin condition[h]	0.82-0.91	3.5-4.0 (0.66-0.84)
Feeling uncomfortable because of your skin condition[i]	0.91	4.0 (0.75)
Feeling annoyed or irritated because of your skin condition[d,e,i]	0.85	3.5 (0.87)
Feeling depressed because of your skin condition[d,e]	0.85	4.0 (0.82)
Lack of self-confidence because of your skin condition[f]	0.82	4.0 (0.85)
Concern about what others think about you because of your skin condition[f]	0.82	4.0 (0.86)
Functions of daily living		
Effects of your skin condition on your daily activities[d]	0.97	4.0 (0.38)
Your skin condition interfering with your sleep[e,i]	0.97	4.0 (0.53)
Social and physical functions		
Effects of your skin condition on your social or leisure activities[e,f,g,k]	0.88	4.0 (0.70)
Effects of your skin condition on your interactions with others (for example, your partner, friends, or relatives)[d,e]	0.85	4.0 (0.81)
Work/school functions		
Difficulties using your hands at work because of your skin condition[i,j]	0.91	4.0 (0.75)
Difficulties working or studying because of your skin condition[d,e,g,k]	0.85	4.0 (0.75)
Concerns that you may lose your job (either because you need to quit or are fired) due to your skin condition[i,j,l]	0.85	4.0 (0.82-0.83)
Effects of your skin condition on your finances[i]	0.79	4.0 (0.94)
Treatment		
Problems from the treatment of your skin condition (for example, taking up time or being messy)[g,m]	0.88	3.5 (0.77)

[a]Topics are intended to ask patients how often they have been bothered by them.

[b]The proportion of physicians ranking a topic's relevance as 3 or 4 on a 4-point Likert scale: (1) not relevant, (2) somewhat relevant, (3) relevant, or (4) very relevant. All values are based on a total of 34 physicians completing the survey.

[c]Values are based on relevance scoring using a 4-point scale, as noted previously.

[d]Topics derived from the Skindex-16 [21].

[e]Topics derived from the Skindex-29 [18,19].

[f]Topics derived from the Dermatology-Specific Quality of Life (DSQL) instrument [15].

[g]Topics derived from the Dermatology Life Quality Index (DLQI) [17].

[h]The following topics were combined: "embarrassment because of your skin condition" and "feeling ashamed of your skin condition." Listed values display the range of values for the combined topics.

[i]Topics derived from a contact dermatitis (CD)-specific quality of life measure from Ayala et al [14].

[j]Topics derived from the 36-item Short Form Health Survey [20].

[k]Topics derived from a modified Skindex-16 from Kadyk et al for use in allergic CD [22].

[l]The following topics were combined: "concerns that you may need to quit your job because of your skin condition" and "concerns about being fired from your job because of your skin condition." The range of standard deviations is listed; other values for the two combined topics were the same.

[m]Prior to the development of a treatment domain in the second round of surveying, this topic was initially categorized under functions of daily living.

Table 2. Topics meeting consensus for inclusion after the second Delphi survey.

Topics[a]	Content validity index[b]	Median (SD)[c]
Functions of daily living		
Limitations in shaving or wearing makeup because of your skin condition[d]	0.88	4.0 (0.86)
Treatment		
Lack of treatment success using recommended remedies for your skin condition[e]	1	4.0 (0.51)
Difficulty finding products that are safe for your skin[e]	0.94	4.0 (0.62)
The cost of products that are safe for your skin[e]	0.82	4.0 (0.93)

[a]Topics are intended to ask patients how often they have been bothered by them.

[b]The proportion of physicians ranking a topic's relevance as 3 or 4 on a 4-point Likert scale: (1) not relevant, (2) somewhat relevant, (3) relevant, or (4) very relevant. All values are based on a total of 34 physicians completing the survey.

[c]Values are based on relevance scoring using a 4-point scale, as noted previously.

[d]Topics derived from the Dermatology-Specific Quality of Life (DSQL) instrument [15].

[e]Topics added to the second survey round based on expert recommendations from the first survey.

Discussion

There are multiple tools to assess QoL in dermatology; however, few of these tools have been validated for use in CD. The 36-item Short Form Health Survey is frequently used in dermatology as a broad questionnaire to assess a wide variety of skin concerns. The DLQI, DSQL instrument for CD, Skindex-16 and its modified versions, and Skindex-29 are more commonly used tools for measuring QoL specifically in CD [38]. However, there are many aspects important for assessing QoL that are not completely incorporated into these questionnaires [39]. Some areas lacking in these questionnaires include psychosocial impact, impact on occupation, and treatment concerns. For these reasons, we developed a new QoL tool specific to CD that can adequately assess all important aspects of QoL in one complete questionnaire. This tool aims to increase detection of QoL changes related to CD in order to better assess disease-related QoL, disease progression, and response to therapies.

Previously validated tools such as the Skindex-16 and the Skindex-29 were used to aid the creation of our new tool. Topics such as those exploring stinging or burning of the skin, irritation of the skin, and worry caused by the skin condition are all validated questions present in the Skindex-16 and also included in the CDQL; these overlapping topics are indicated in Table 1. In terms of more recently published QoL measures, the disease-specific questionnaire for allergic contact dermatitis proposed by Botto et al [35] explores a variety of topics that are also included in the CDQL, such as "concern for infecting others because of your skin condition" and "I am bothered by cracking of my skin." While the CDQL includes similar types of questions under the categories of function, emotions, and symptoms, it also further addresses topics of "functions of daily living" and "work and school function," allowing for a more complete understanding of the impact this skin condition has on patients' daily lives. For example, we include impacts on types of clothes worn, the ability to participate in certain sports, and the duration of time needed to find treatment or care for their condition. Additionally, our tool examines contact dermatitis more broadly, rather than focusing on the specific subset of allergic contact dermatitis, allowing for a more universal application of the tool.

The Delphi technique, a series of successive questionnaires aimed at determining opinion consensus among a group of experts [40], was used to formulate the CDQL. The strength of this technique comes from its ability to efficiently achieve consensus on topics of uncertainty [41]. Furthermore, the controlled feedback following each round of the questionnaire can broaden thinking and stimulate new ideas among experts [42]. However, the weakness of the Delphi technique typically stems from a lack of agreement on how consensus is defined [43]. Varying interpretations and methodology to define consensus and validity can diminish the credibility of this technique.

The precedent is to deem the content validity of an instrument excellent if the following criteria are met: (1) The CVIs for individual topics are ≥0.78 when at least 6 experts are assessing the relevance of the topics, and (2) the CVI of the total scale (when calculated in the same manner as for this study) is ≥0.90 [27,28,36]. The final individual topics included in this tool had CVIs ranging from 0.79 to 1.0. However, the CVI of the total scale was 0.85, falling slightly below the previously determined 0.90 standard to be considered excellent. Of note, some studies recommend a minimum total scale CVI of 0.80 [44]. While this may be a more realistic benchmark for the total CVI, some researchers have argued that a total scale CVI of 0.90 would better protect against exceedingly low individual CVIs (eg, <0.4) [36]. As the CDQL had final individual topic CVIs ranging from 0.79 to 1.0, a total scale CVI ≥0.80 may be a suitable indication of content validity.

One limitation of this study was the long length of the surveys, which likely played a role in the lower survey completion rate. Additionally, while a typical Delphi method would have consisted of an initial survey with a series of open-ended questions intended to generate a list of QoL issues [45], this was replaced by a literature search in this study. Nevertheless, experts were still given the opportunity in the first survey to note additional topics that they felt were relevant. Additionally, while this study did not directly incorporate patient feedback during development of the scale, the second round of surveying incorporated unique topics from another recent study [35] aimed at developing a QoL index for allergic CD based on patient interviews. This index is intended for use in conjunction with another more comprehensive QoL scale, whereas the CDQL is designed to be sufficient by itself for assessing QoL in CD. Furthermore, 1 respondent to the initial survey felt that the questionnaire was limited by its lack of items incorporating intensity and localization of CD. However, these factors are specific to disease severity and the CDQL is meant to be used in combination with, not in lieu of, a validated disease severity tool. As previously noted, the degree of impact of CD on QoL may not always correlate with disease severity [14].

Future studies are planned to further establish the CDQL's validity, reliability, and responsiveness to changes in QoL. It is hoped that the resulting validated outcomes instrument will be suitable for use in both clinical practice and research to quantitatively determine the effect of health care interventions on QoL among patients with CD.

Funding Sources

None.

Authors' Contributions

MKH performed data collection, data analysis, and manuscript writing. MRL performed data analysis and manuscript writing. RPD performed manuscript editing and direction for the study. CWR performed manuscript writing and editing. CIH performed manuscript editing. CAD conceived of the study and performed manuscript editing and direction for the study.

References

1. Murawski MM, Miederhoff PA. On the generalizability of statistical expressions of health related quality of life instrument responsiveness: a data synthesis. Qual Life Res 1998 Jan;7(1):11-22. [doi: 10.1023/a:1008828720272] [Medline: 9481147]
2. Augustin M, Langenbruch AK, Gutknecht M, Radtke MA, Blome C. Quality of life measures for dermatology: definition, evaluation, and interpretation. Curr Dermatol Rep 2012 Aug 9;1(3):148-159 [FREE Full text] [doi: 10.1007/s13671-012-0020-z] [Medline: 30311153]
3. Anderson RT, Rajagopalan R. Effects of allergic dermatosis on health-related quality of life. Curr Allergy Asthma Rep 2001 Jul;1(4):309-315. [doi: 10.1007/s11882-001-0041-3] [Medline: 11892052]
4. Hachem JP, De Paepe K, Sterckx G, Kaufman L, Rogiers V, Roseeuw D. Evaluation of biophysical and clinical parameters of skin barrier function among hospital workers. Contact Dermatitis 2002 Apr;46(4):220-223. [doi: 10.1034/j.1600-0536.2002.460406.x] [Medline: 12081700]
5. Holness DL. Results of a quality of life questionnaire in a patch test clinic population. Contact Dermatitis 2001 Mar;44(2):80-84. [doi: 10.1034/j.1600-0536.2001.440204.x] [Medline: 11205408]
6. Hutchings CV, Shum KW, Gawkrodger DJ. Occupational contact dermatitis has an appreciable impact on quality of life. Contact Dermatitis 2001 Jul;45(1):17-20. [doi: 10.1034/j.1600-0536.2001.045001017.x] [Medline: 11422262]
7. Meding B, Swanbeck G. Consequences of having hand eczema. Contact Dermatitis 1990 Jul;23(1):6-14. [doi: 10.1111/j.1600-0536.1990.tb00076.x] [Medline: 2144814]
8. Nethercott JR, Holness DL. Disease outcome in workers with occupational skin disease. J Am Acad Dermatol 1994 Apr;30(4):569-574. [doi: 10.1016/s0190-9622(94)70064-8] [Medline: 8157783]
9. Rajagopalan R, Anderson RT. The profile of a patient with contact dermatitis and a suspicion of contact allergy (history, physical characteristics, and dermatology-specific quality of life). Am J Contact Dermat 1997 Mar;8(1):26-31. [Medline: 9066845]
10. Rajagopalan R, Anderson RT, Sarma S, Kallal J, Retchin C, Jones J, et al. An economic evaluation of patch testing in the diagnosis and management of allergic contact dermatitis. Am J Contact Dermat 1998 Sep;9(3):149-154. [Medline: 9744907]
11. Rajagopalan R, Anderson RT, Sarma S, Retchin C, Jones J. The use of decision-analytical modelling in economic evaluation of patch testing in allergic contact dermatitis. Pharmacoeconomics 1998 Jul;14(1):79-95. [doi: 10.2165/00019053-199814010-00008] [Medline: 10182197]
12. Skoet R, Zachariae R, Agner T. Contact dermatitis and quality of life: a structured review of the literature. Br J Dermatol 2003 Sep;149(3):452-456. [doi: 10.1046/j.1365-2133.2003.05601.x] [Medline: 14510974]
13. Thomson KF, Wilkinson SM, Sommer S, Pollock B. Eczema: quality of life by body site and the effect of patch testing. Br J Dermatol 2002 Apr;146(4):627-630. [doi: 10.1046/j.1365-2133.2002.04692.x] [Medline: 11966694]
14. Ayala F, Nino M, Fabbrocini G, Panariello L, Balato N, Foti C, et al. Quality of life and contact dermatitis: a disease-specific questionnaire. Dermatitis 2010 Apr 23;21(2):84-90 [FREE Full text] [doi: 10.2310/6620.2010.09057] [Medline: 20233546]

15. Anderson RT, Rajagopalan R. Development and validation of a quality of life instrument for cutaneous diseases. J Am Acad Dermatol 1997 Jul;37(1):41-50. [doi: 10.1016/s0190-9622(97)70210-x] [Medline: 9216522]
16. Braunberger T, Lynn D, Reimer C, Doctor M, Hill MK, Mounessa J, et al. Disease severity and quality of life measurements in contact dermatitis: a systematic review 2005-2015. Dermatitis 2016;27(6):362-371. [doi: 10.1097/DER.0000000000000235] [Medline: 27775978]
17. Finlay AY, Khan GK. Dermatology Life Quality Index (DLQI)--a simple practical measure for routine clinical use. Clin Exp Dermatol 1994 May;19(3):210-216. [Medline: 8033378]
18. Chren MM, Lasek RJ, Quinn LM, Mostow EN, Zyzanski SJ. Skindex, a quality-of-life measure for patients with skin disease: reliability, validity, and responsiveness. J Invest Dermatol 1996 Nov;107(5):707-713 [FREE Full text] [doi: 10.1111/1523-1747.ep12365600] [Medline: 8875954]
19. Chren MM, Lasek RJ, Quinn LM, Covinsky KE. Convergent and discriminant validity of a generic and a disease-specific instrument to measure quality of life in patients with skin disease. J Invest Dermatol 1997 Jan;108(1):103-107 [FREE Full text] [doi: 10.1111/1523-1747.ep12285650] [Medline: 8980297]
20. Ware JE, Sherbourne CD. The MOS 36-item short-form health survey (SF-36). I. Conceptual framework and item selection. Med Care 1992 Jun;30(6):473-483. [Medline: 1593914]
21. Chren MM, Lasek RJ, Sahay AP, Sands LP. Measurement properties of Skindex-16: a brief quality-of-life measure for patients with skin diseases. J Cutan Med Surg 2001;5(2):105-110. [doi: 10.1007/BF02737863] [Medline: 11443481]
22. Kadyk DL, McCarter K, Achen F, Belsito DV. Quality of life in patients with allergic contact dermatitis. J Am Acad Dermatol 2003 Dec;49(6):1037-1048. [doi: 10.1016/s0190-9622(03)02112-1] [Medline: 14639382]
23. Yousouf MI. The Delphi technique. Essays in Education 2007;20(8):80-89. [doi: 10.1108/17538370910930545]
24. Diamond IR, Grant RC, Feldman BM, Pencharz PB, Ling SC, Moore AM, et al. Defining consensus: a systematic review recommends methodologic criteria for reporting of Delphi studies. J Clin Epidemiol 2014 Apr;67(4):401-409. [doi: 10.1016/j.jclinepi.2013.12.002] [Medline: 24581294]
25. Green P. The Content of a College-Level Outdoor Leadership Course. 1982 Presented at: the Conference of the Northwest District Association for the American Alliance for Health, Physical Education, Recreation, and Dance; 1982; Spokane, Washington p. 140678032.
26. Hsu C, Sandford B. The Delphi technique: making sense of consensus. Practical assessment, research & evaluation 2007;12:1-8. [doi: 10.4018/978-1-4666-0074-4.ch011]
27. Lynn MR. Determination and quantification of content validity. Nurs Res 1986;35(6):382-385. [Medline: 3640358]
28. Polit DF, Beck CT. The content validity index: are you sure you know what's being reported? Critique and recommendations. Res Nurs Health 2006 Oct;29(5):489-497. [doi: 10.1002/nur.20147] [Medline: 16977646]
29. Bulathsinhala L, Eleangovan N, Heaney LG, Menzies-Gow A, Gibson PG, Peters M, et al. Development of the International Severe Asthma Registry (ISAR): a modified Delphi study. J Allergy Clin Immunol Pract 2019 Feb;7(2):578-588.e2. [doi: 10.1016/j.jaip.2018.08.016] [Medline: 30179741]
30. Ghorbani N, Ahmadi M, Sadoughi F, Abadi A, Ghanei M. Developing Research Information System in Health Sector: a Delphi Study. Aust J Basic & Appl Sci 2012;6(8):124-132 [FREE Full text] [Medline: 23641388]
31. Ayesa-Arriola R, Terán JMP, Moríñigo JDL, Rivero MC, Setién-Suero E, Al-Halabi S, et al. The dynamic relationship between insight and suicidal behavior in first episode psychosis patients over 3-year follow-up. Eur Neuropsychopharmacol 2018 Oct;28(10):1161-1172. [doi: 10.1016/j.euroneuro.2018.05.005] [Medline: 30097249]
32. Uegaki K, de Bruijne MC, Anema JR, van der Beek AJ, van Tulder MW, van Mechelen W. Consensus-based findings and recommendations for estimating the costs of health-related productivity loss from a company's perspective. Scand J Work Environ Health 2007 Apr;33(2):122-130 [FREE Full text] [doi: 10.5271/sjweh.1115] [Medline: 17460800]
33. Farzandipour M, Ahmadi M, Sadoughi F, Karimi Irajk I. Adopting confidentiality principles for electronic health records in iran: a delphi study. J Med Syst 2011 Jun;35(3):333-343. [doi: 10.1007/s10916-009-9370-x] [Medline: 20703556]
34. Ahmadi M, Mohammadi A, Chraghbaigi R, Fathi T, Shojaee Baghini M. Developing a minimum data set of the information management system for orthopedic injuries in iran. Iran Red Crescent Med J 2014 Jul;16(7):e17020 [FREE Full text] [doi: 10.5812/ircmj.17020] [Medline: 25237576]
35. Botto N, Raffi J, Trivedi M, Ramirez F, Allen IE, Chren M. Validating a quality-of-life instrument for allergic contact dermatitis. Dermatitis 2019;30(5):300-305. [doi: 10.1097/DER.0000000000000515] [Medline: 31524758]
36. Waltz CF, Strickland OL, Lenz ER. Measurement in Nursing and Health Research, 3rd Edition. New York, NY: Springer Publishing Company; 2005.
37. Harris PA, Taylor R, Thielke R, Payne J, Gonzalez N, Conde JG. Research electronic data capture (REDCap)--a metadata-driven methodology and workflow process for providing translational research informatics support. J Biomed Inform 2009 Apr;42(2):377-381 [FREE Full text] [doi: 10.1016/j.jbi.2008.08.010] [Medline: 18929686]
38. Swietlik J, Reeder M. Current quality-of-life tools available for use in contact dermatitis. Dermatitis 2016;27(4):176-185. [doi: 10.1097/DER.0000000000000192] [Medline: 27427819]
39. Lau MYZ, Burgess JA, Nixon R, Dharmage SC, Matheson MC. A review of the impact of occupational contact dermatitis on quality of life. J Allergy (Cairo) 2011;2011:964509 [FREE Full text] [doi: 10.1155/2011/964509] [Medline: 21603173]

40. Linstone HA, Turoff M. The Delphi Method: Techniques and Applications. Boston, MA: Addison Wesley Publishing Company; 1975.
41. Murphy MK, Black NA, Lamping DL, McKee CM, Sanderson CF, Askham J, et al. Consensus development methods, and their use in clinical guideline development. Health Technol Assess 1998;2(3):i-88 [FREE Full text] [Medline: 9561895]
42. Pill J. The Delphi method: substance, context, a critique and an annotated bibliography. Socio-Econ Plan Sci 1971 Feb;5(1):57-71. [doi: 10.1016/0038-0121(71)90041-3]
43. Powell C. The Delphi technique: myths and realities. J Adv Nurs 2003 Feb;41(4):376-382. [Medline: 12581103]
44. Davis LL. Instrument review: getting the most from a panel of experts. Appl Nurs Res 1992 Nov;5(4):194-197 [FREE Full text] [doi: 10.1016/S0897-1897(05)80008-4]
45. Thangaratinam S, Redman CW. The Delphi technique. Obstet Gynaecol 2011 Jan 24:120-125.

Abbreviations

ACDS: American Contact Dermatitis Society
CD: contact dermatitis
CDQL: Contact Dermatitis Quality of Life index
CVI: content validity index
DLQI: Dermatology Life Quality Index
DSQL: Dermatology-Specific Quality of Life instrument
NIH/NCRR CSTI: National Institutes of Health/National Center for Research Resources Colorado Clinical and Translational Science Institute
QoL: quality of life
RCT: randomized controlled trial
REDCap: Research Electronic Data Capture

4

Factors Contributing to Diagnostic Discordance Between Store-and-Forward Teledermatology Consultations and In Person Visits

Michelle S Lee[1], BA; Robert Stavert[2], MD, MBA

[1]Harvard Medical School, Boston, MA, United States

[2]Department of Dermatology, Cambridge Health Alliance, Somerville, MA, United States

Corresponding Author:
Michelle S Lee, BA
Harvard Medical School
25 Shattuck Street
Boston, MA, 02115
United States

Email: michelle_lee3@hms.harvard.edu

Abstract

Background: Use of asynchronous store-and-forward (SAF) teledermatology can improve access to timely and cost-effective dermatologic care and has increased during the COVID-19 pandemic. Previous research has found high diagnostic concordance rates between SAF teledermatology and face-to-face clinical diagnosis, but to our knowledge, none have used specific cases to illustrate factors contributing to diagnostic discordance.

Objective: To identify and illustrate characteristics that may have contributed to diagnostic discordance between store-and-forward teledermatology and in-person clinical diagnosis in a series of patients.

Methods: We identified 7 cases of diagnostic discordance between teledermatology and in-person visits where the favored diagnosis of the in-person dermatologist was not included in the differential diagnosis formulated by the teledermatologist. Cases were identified from a previously published retrospective chart review of 340 SAF teledermatology consultations, which was previously performed at an academic community health care system in the greater Boston area, Massachusetts, from January 1, 2014, through December 31, 2017. Of 99 patients who completed an in-person dermatology appointment after their teledermatology consultation, 7 had diagnostic disagreement between the teledermatologist and in-person dermatologist where the diagnosis in the in-person consultation was not included in the differential diagnosis in the original teledermatology consult. These 7 cases were examined by 2 author reviewers to identify factors that may have contributed to diagnostic discordance.

Results: Factors contributing to diagnostic discordance between SAF teledermatology consultations and in-person visits included poor image quality, inadequate history or diagnostic workup, inability to evaluate textural characteristics, diagnostic uncertainty due to atypical presentations, and evolution in appearance of skin conditions over time.

Conclusions: We identified multiple factors that contributed to diagnostic discordance. Recognition and mitigation of these factors, when possible, may help to improve diagnostic accuracy and reduce the likelihood of misdiagnosis. Continuing education of referring providers and implementation of standardized guidelines for referrals may also be helpful in reducing the risk of misdiagnosis due to inherent limitations of teledermatology services.

KEYWORDS

teledermatology; eHealth; dermatology; telemedicine; diagnosis

Introduction

Store-and-forward (SAF) teledermatology systems utilize asynchronous evaluation of clinical images and information to provide diagnostic and management guidance directly to patients or other health care providers. In contrast to real-time telemedicine such as video encounters, SAF encounters involve collecting clinical information from a referring provider to be sent electronically to another site or provider, often a specialist, for review at a later time. SAF teledermatology platforms can increase access to dermatologic care, provide financial savings for patients and health systems, and provide a comparable quality of care to in-person evaluation for numerous dermatologic conditions [1-8]. Utilization of both synchronous video and asynchronous SAF telemedicine has increased significantly during the 2020 COVID-19 pandemic [9,10]. SAF teledermatology may play a particularly vital role in the provision of safe and efficient dermatologic care as it requires less resources and coordination to implement compared to live interactive teledermatology [11].

Evaluation of diagnostic concordance for patients who receive both a teledermatology and in-person consultation is one method of assessing the diagnostic quality of SAF teledermatology consultations. Complete diagnostic concordance occurs when the first diagnosis matches between the in-person dermatologist and teledermatologist [12-17]. Previous research has found 79%-94% concordance rates between teledermatology and face-to-face clinical diagnosis, with some variation based on factors including skin condition and whether or not dermatoscopy is utilized [12-17]. High rates of diagnostic concordance help to ensure that the diagnoses patients receive from SAF teledermatology platforms are comparable to those that patients would receive during an in-person encounter.

Although previously published work has examined rates and patterns of discordance [12-17], to our knowledge, none have previously used cases to identify and illustrate specific characteristics that may contribute to diagnostic discordance. We analyzed a series of 7 cases of diagnostic discordance, identifying contributing factors in hopes of identifying opportunities to improve teledermatology systems and mitigate potential risks that can occur from misdiagnosis.

Methods

Previously, a retrospective chart review of 340 SAF teledermatology consultations performed at our institution from January 1, 2014, through December 31, 2017, was conducted [18]. All SAF teledermatology cases were ordered alphabetically by patient's last name, and the first 340 cases were reviewed. Among these 340 teledermatology cases, there were 99 patients who also completed an in-person dermatology visit, and further chart review was performed to determine the level of management concordance between teledermatologist and in-person dermatologist, defined by five categories: (1) fully concordant, (2) partially concordant, (3) discordant, (4) unable to assess because treatment was not specified by the referring provider, and (5) treatment not specified by teledermatology provider and an in-person appointment is requested for further evaluation. The definition of diagnostic discordance for this study was based on previous literature, which has defined diagnostic concordance as complete agreement (where the first diagnosis matched between in-person dermatologist and teledermatologist), partial agreement (where diagnoses overlapped between in-person dermatologist and teledermatologist), and discordant (where diagnoses did not match between teledermatologist and in-person dermatologist) [18-20]. Analysis of the 99 patients with both teledermatology and in-person visits found that diagnoses in 76 (77%) encounters were fully concordant, 16 (16%) were partially concordant, and 7 (7%) were fully discordant. We further evaluated these 7 diagnostically discordant cases to identify factors contributing to diagnostic discordance. Both authors (MSL and RS) performed retrospective chart review of the cases and discussed causes of the diagnostic discordance to come to a consensus.

Images from the teledermatology consult were submitted by the referring provider and taken using the Epic Haiku mobile app (Epic Systems Corporation). The teledermatologist was different than the in-person dermatologist in all but the second case reviewed. This project was exempt from full review by our Institutional Review Board.

Results

Overview

A summary of the cases, teledermatology and in-person differential diagnoses, in-person diagnosis, and factors contributing to diagnostic discordance is provided in Table 1.

Table 1. Summary of cases and factors contributing to diagnostic discordance.

Case	Age (yrs) and gender	Telederm[a] differential diagnosis	Treatment after telederm visit	In-person differential diagnosis	In-person diagnosis (diagnostic test)	Contributing factors to diagnostic uncertainty
1	31, male	Superficial morphea, superficial dermatophyte infection, pityriasis rotunda, psoriasis, parapsoriasis, CTCL[b], Hansen	None	Confluent and reticulated papillomatosis of Gougerot and Carteaud, morphea, tinea corporis, and discoid erythrasma	Eczematous dermatitis (punch biopsy)	Image quality compromised by patient positioning and lighting leading to shine artifact; unusual morphology, presentation; lack of historical details provided
2	60, male	Sarcoid, mycobacterial, hypersensitivity, lichenoid reaction, pseudolymphoma, arthropod bite, folliculitis	Betamethasone dipropionate 0.05% cream twice a day	Tinea corporis, sarcoid, annular lichen planus	Tinea corporis (KOH prep[c] confirmed)	Image quality compromised by limited view of anatomic area; evolution of rash from time of telederm to time of in-person visit from papular to characteristic annular with scale
3	26, male	Impetigo, tinea faciei, Majocchi, contact dermatitis, rosacea	Empiric doxycycline 100 mg orally twice a day for 2 weeks, continue clotrimazole	VZV[d] reactivation (herpes zoster)	Herpes zoster (physical exam)	Limited single-image view made it more difficult to appreciate dermatomal distribution; lack of adequate testing including superficial bacterial culture and KOH prep; evolution of rash from telederm consult to time of in-person visit
4	63, male	Actinic keratoses, excoriated papulopustular rosacea, squamous cell carcinoma	None prescribed	Telangiectasias due to sun damage	Nonspecific telangiectasias due to sun damage (clinical diagnosis)	Inability to palpate lesion to determine textural characteristics; image artifact showing overlying scale; no dermatoscopic images taken during initial consultation
5	69, male	HSV[e], erythema multiforme, contact dermatitis, or pemphigus vulgaris, and paraneoplastic pemphigus	None prescribed	Allergic contact dermatitis vs actinic cheilitis	Lichenoid dermatitis (biopsy)	HSV/VZV viral culture would have been helpful when evaluating vesicles on mucosal surfaces; diagnostically challenging case; lack of historical details provided
6	41, male	HSV, LGV[f]	None prescribed	Condyloma acuminata	Epidermal inclusion cyst (biopsy)	Nonclassic presentation resulting in diagnostic uncertainty; viral and bacterial swab cultures would be helpful for initial consult; difficulty in distinguishing between vesicles, pustules, cysts via telederm
7	65, male	Unable to determine	None prescribed	Irritated seborrheic keratosis vs melanoma	BCC[g] (shave biopsy)	Dermatoscopic images were out of focus, and nondermatoscopic images were not included

[a]Telederm: teledermatology.
[b]CTCL: cutaneous T-cell lymphoma.
[c]KOH prep: potassium hydroxide preparation.
[d]VZV: varicella zoster virus.
[e]HSV: herpes simplex virus.
[f]LGV: lymphogranuloma venereum.
[g]BCC: basal cell carcinoma.

Case 1

A 31-year-old male presented to his primary care provider with a several-year history of well-circumscribed, hyperpigmented, nonpruritic, thin, scaly plaques with skin tightening on his back, trunk, and chest, as well as associated gynecomastia. The patient had tried applying moisturizing lotion without relief. Teledermatology consultation resulted in a broad differential diagnosis including superficial morphea, superficial dermatophyte infection, pityriasis rotunda, psoriasis, parapsoriasis, cutaneous T-cell lymphoma, and Hansen disease. The submitted images showed several sharply demarcated hyperpigmented thin plaques with overlying xerotic scale on the back as well as well-circumscribed tan thin plaques with overlying scale on the collar distribution of the neck and the upper chest (Figures 1 and 2). The teledermatologist noted that the image quality was limited by patient positioning and lighting, leading to shine artifact, and noted that further history about potential exposures and travel history would have been helpful, particularly to rule out Hansen disease. Due to the broad differential and no leading diagnosis, he was referred for an in-person consultation. His in-person exam revealed well-demarcated geographic hyperpigmented atrophic and wrinkly patches on the back (Figure 3) and the anterior bilateral shoulders, left flank, and upper arms, as well as gynecomastia. The differential diagnosis included confluent and reticulated papillomatosis of Gougerot-Carteaud, morphea, tinea corporis, and discoid erythrasma. A punch biopsy was performed, which revealed findings most consistent with an eczematous dermatitis. The patient was treated with triamcinolone 0.1% cream and did not return for scheduled follow-up appointments.

Figure 1. Case 1. Submitted teledermatology image showing patient's back with hyperkeratotic plaque and xerotic scale. Image quality compromised by patient positioning and lighting leading to shine artifact.

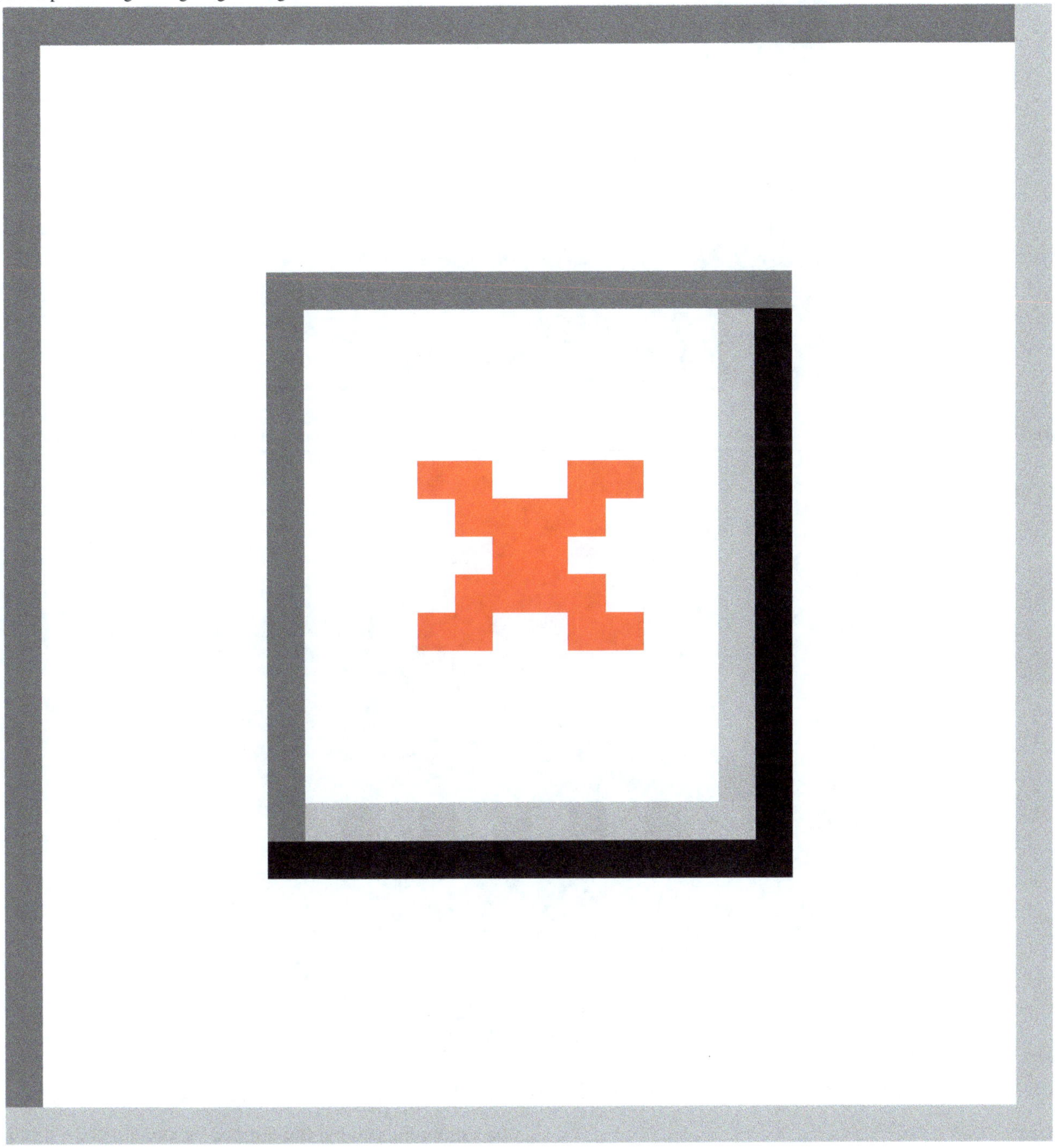

Figure 2. Case 1. Submitted teledermatology image showing patient's neck and clavicular region with hyperkeratotic plaque and xerotic scale. Image quality compromised by patient positioning and lighting leading to shine artifact.

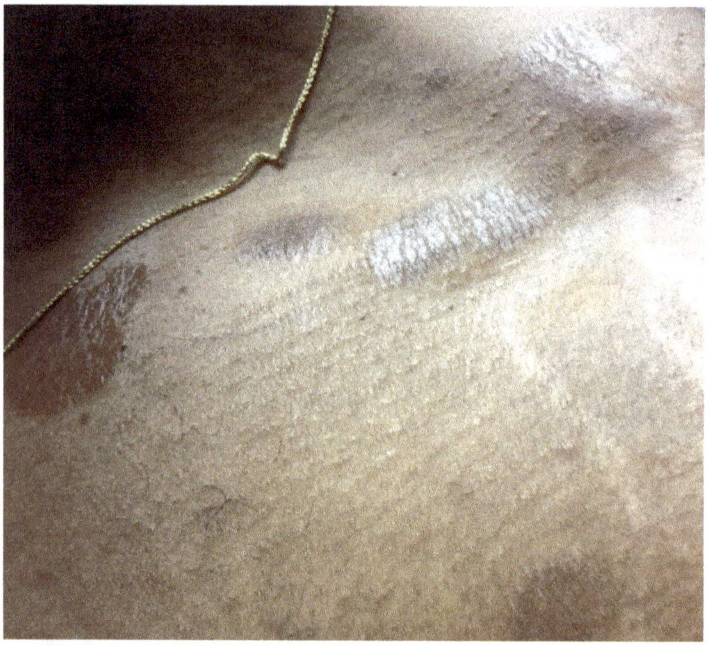

Figure 3. Case 1. Image for in-person visit showing well-demarcated, geographic, hyperpigmented, atrophic, and wrinkly patches on the back.

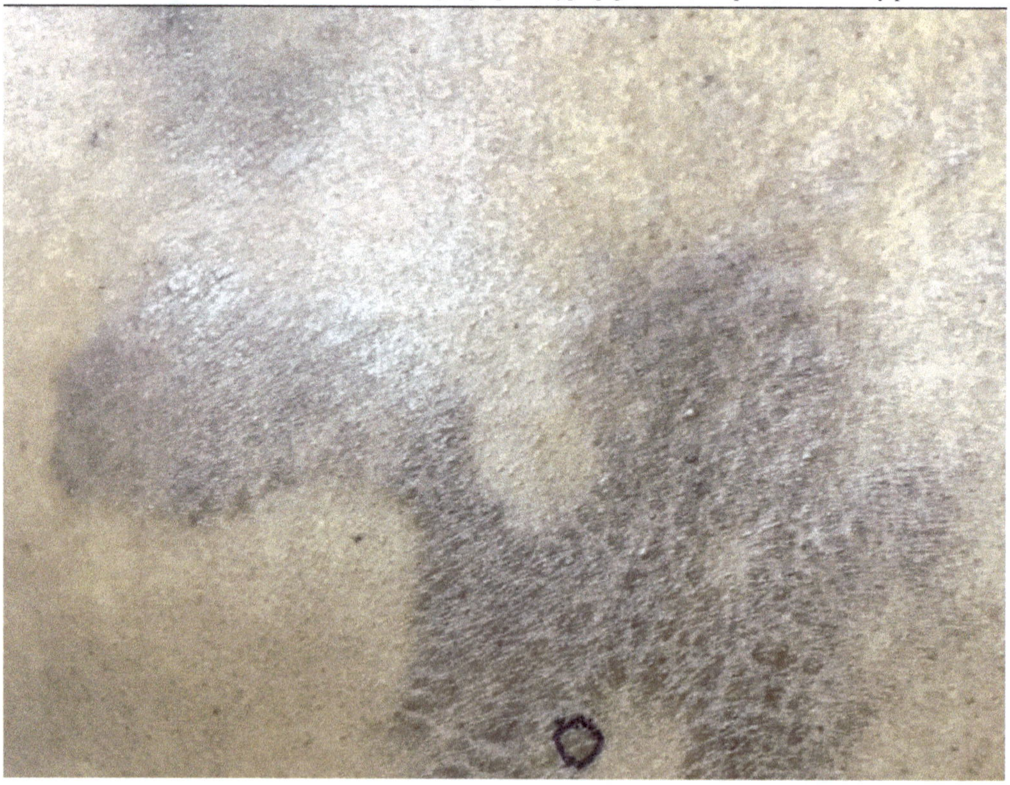

Case 2

A 60-year-old man with 3 weeks of pruritic pink papules on the left forearm next to tattooed skin was referred to teledermatology. Submitted photos showed a 1-2 cm light pink patch containing three discrete 4-6 mm pink papules, and the differential diagnosis included sarcoidosis, atypical mycobacterial infection, hypersensitivity reaction, lichenoid reaction, and pseudolymphoma, as well as arthropod assault and folliculitis. The teledermatologist noted that image quality was compromised by the limited anatomic view provided (Figure 4). The patient was prescribed betamethasone dipropionate 0.05% cream twice daily for 2 weeks. In the office 3 weeks later, he was noted to have a pink-red annular plaque with overlying scale (Figure 5) that was suspicious for tinea corporis, which was confirmed with a potassium hydroxide preparation (KOH prep) showing hyphae. The patient was treated with topical ketoconazole 1% cream, and his rash resolved without recurrence.

Figure 4. Case 2. Submitted teledermatology image showing left forearm with 1-2 cm light pink patch containing three discrete 4-6 mm pink papules. Image quality compromised by limited anatomic view.

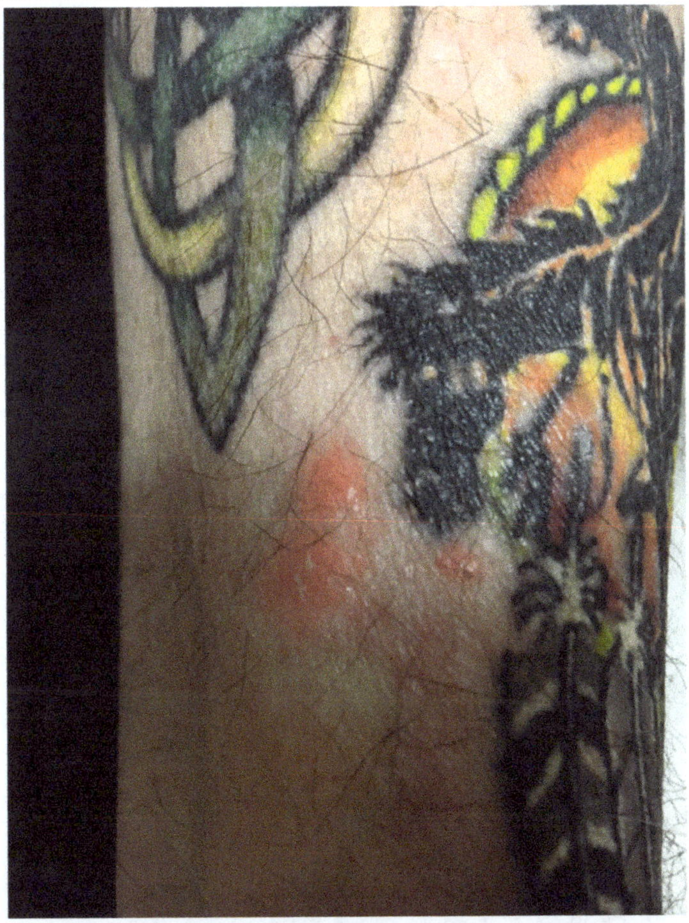

Figure 5. Case 2. In-office photo obtained from same patient, demonstrating left forearm with pink-red annular plaque with scale (tinea corporis).

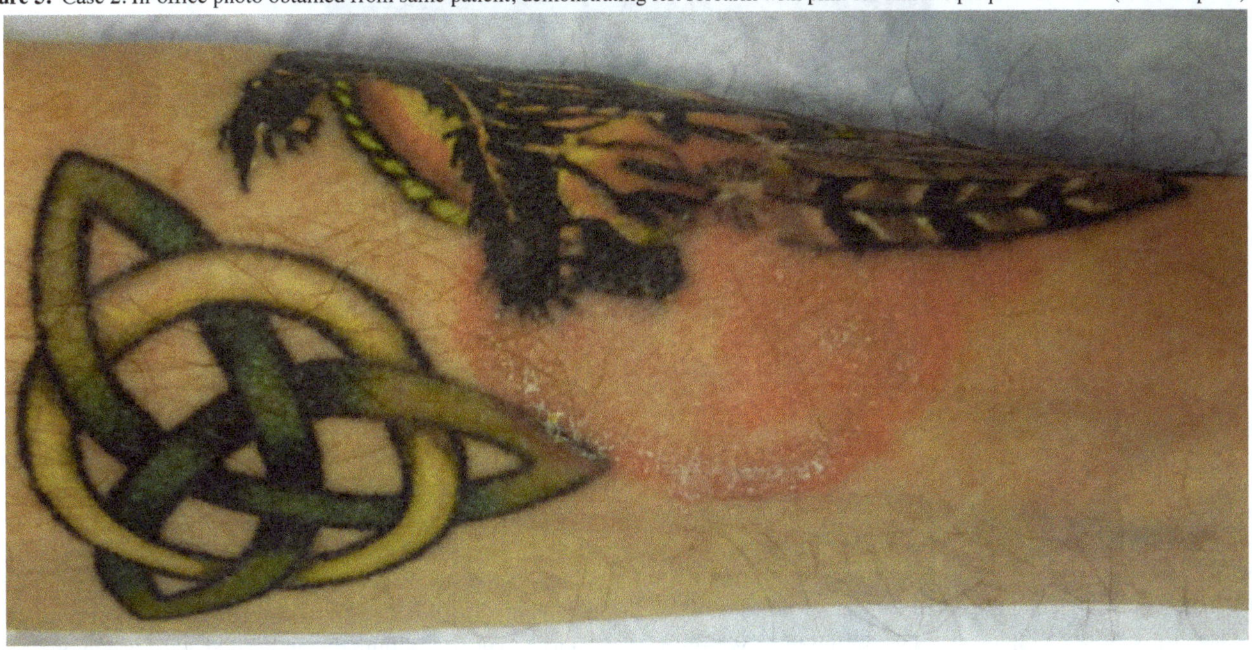

Case 3

A 26-year-old male with a 3-day history of a round pink plaque on the left cheek, within which were papules and erosions, was referred to teledermatology. At the time of his referral, the referring provider had prescribed treatment of this plaque with topical clotrimazole. The patient reported that he had worn a mask and participated in paintball and jiujitsu a few days prior to presentation and that his lesions appeared shortly afterwards. He reported that the lesion started as a pimple or vesicle, and then progressed into a plaque. A single submitted clinical image showed a limited view of the left cheek (Figure 6). The teledermatologist's differential diagnosis included impetigo, tinea faciei, Majocchi granuloma, and contact dermatitis. The teledermatologist advised the referring provider to obtain a superficial bacterial culture of the plaque, continue clotrimazole, and start empiric treatment with doxycycline if the patient was unable to return for the culture. The patient subsequently reported progression of his rash and was scheduled for an in-person visit with the dermatologist 1 week later. At that time, the initial lesions had crusted over, and new lesions on his left upper medial cheek, left nasal bridge, and left nasal ala in a dermatomal distribution were noted (Figure 7). A clinical diagnosis of herpes zoster was made, the patient was prescribed oral acyclovir, and the rash subsequently resolved.

Figure 6. Case 3. Limited view of the face from teledermatologist consult.

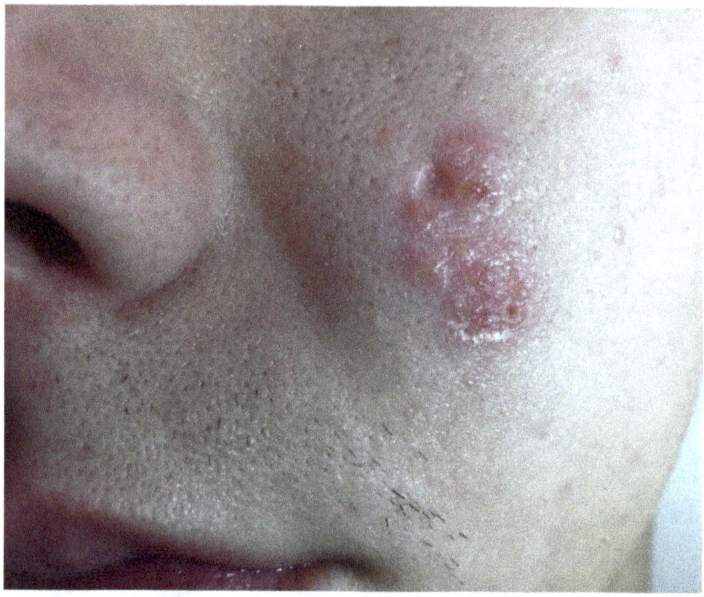

Figure 7. Case 3. Images from clinic 1 week later.

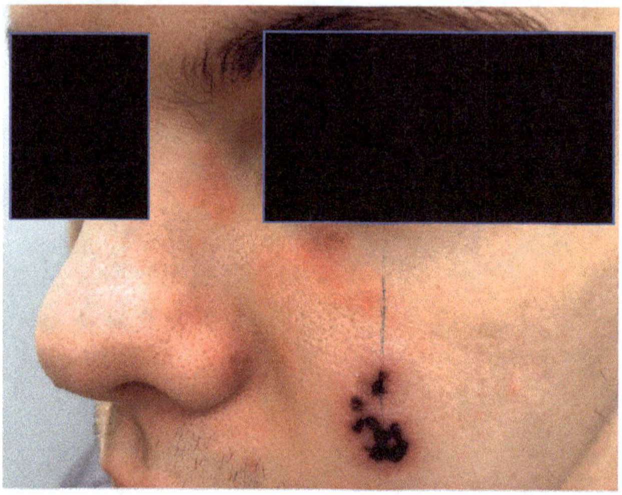

Case 4

A 63-year-old man was referred to teledermatology for evaluation of a 7-month history of an enlarging nasal lesion. The teledermatologist reviewed the image and described erythematous macules that appeared to have scale or crust on the nasal tip and ala (Figure 8). The differential diagnosis provided by the teledermatologist was dependent on textural characteristics and included actinic keratoses if the lesion was rough and excoriated papulopustular rosacea if the texture was not rough. The teledermatologist requested additional textural information. Due to the incomplete information on skin texture, the patient was referred for an in-person visit, where his exam revealed no overlying scale or roughness to suggest actinic keratosis and no features suggestive of squamous cell carcinoma. He denied a history of facial flushing or acneiform or pustular eruptions. He was clinically diagnosed with a telangiectasia, likely due to dermatoheliosis, and no further treatment was recommended.

Figure 8. Case 4. Submitted image to teledermatology showing erythematous macules with apparent scale or crust on the nasal tip and ala.

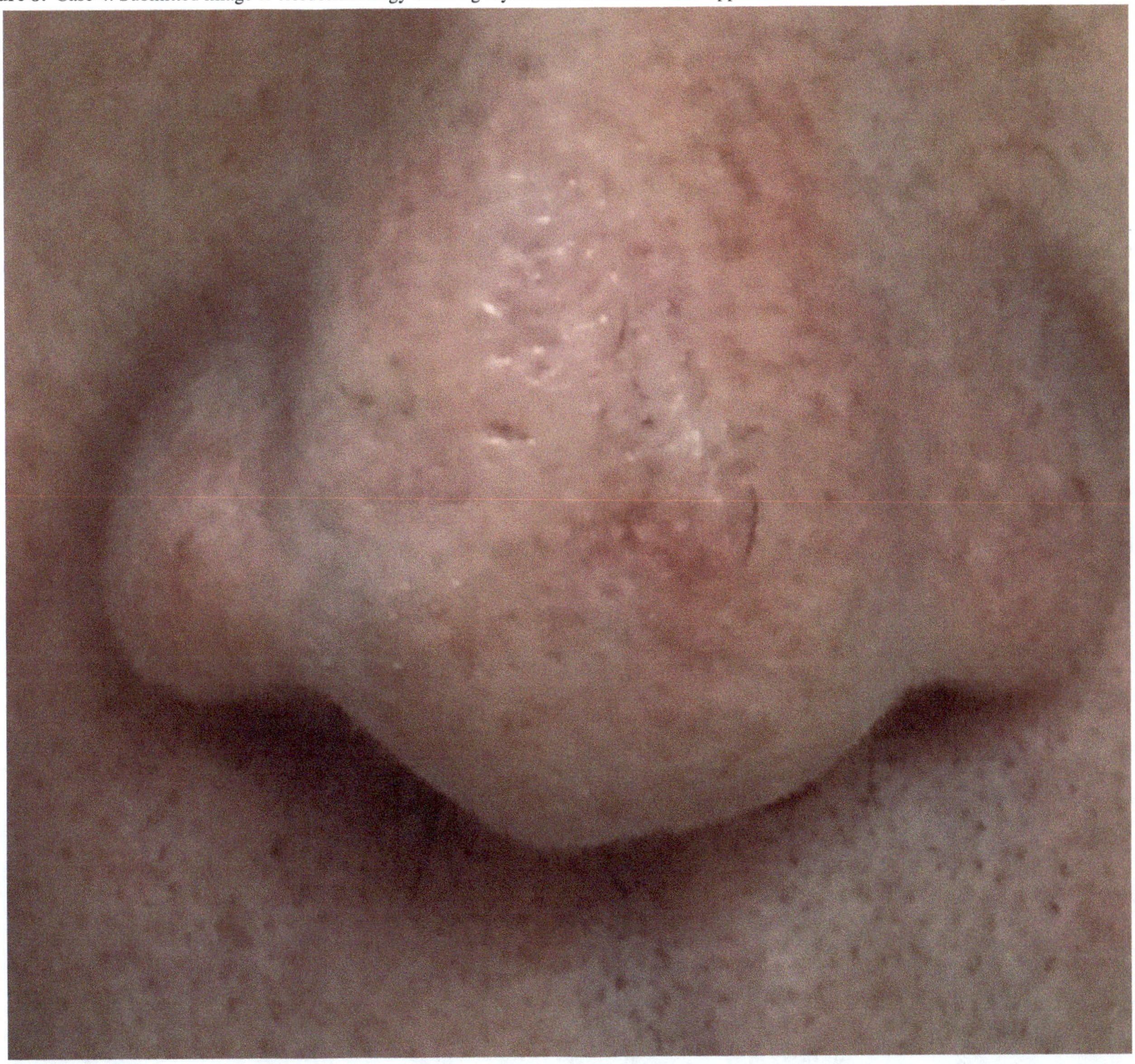

Case 5

A 69-year-old man with a 2-month history of blistering lips with skin peeling and pain unresponsive to Vaseline was referred to teledermatology. The submitted image showed a focal erosion with hemorrhagic crust and vesiculation (Figure 9), and the differential included herpes simplex virus (HSV), erythema multiforme, contact dermatitis, pemphigus vulgaris, and paraneoplastic pemphigus. The teledermatologist pointed out that the patient was not asked about history of similar eruptions, involvement of the oral mucosa, or associated symptoms including pain or burning, which would have aided the diagnosis. The consultant also recommended obtaining HSV/varicella zoster virus viral cultures and applying emollient, and the patient was scheduled for an in-office dermatology appointment. During the first in-person visit, the erosions and vesicles were resolving (Figure 10), and a bacterial culture was taken from a focal erosion which grew methicillin-resistant *Staphylococcus aureus*. He was treated with doxycycline and the fissure healed. The lip erosions subsequently recurred (Figure 11) and were biopsied, with pathology most consistent with a lichenoid dermatitis. He was treated with triamcinolone 0.1% cream and his symptoms resolved.

Figure 9. Case 5. Submitted teledermatology image of focal erosion with hemorrhagic crust and vesiculation on lips.

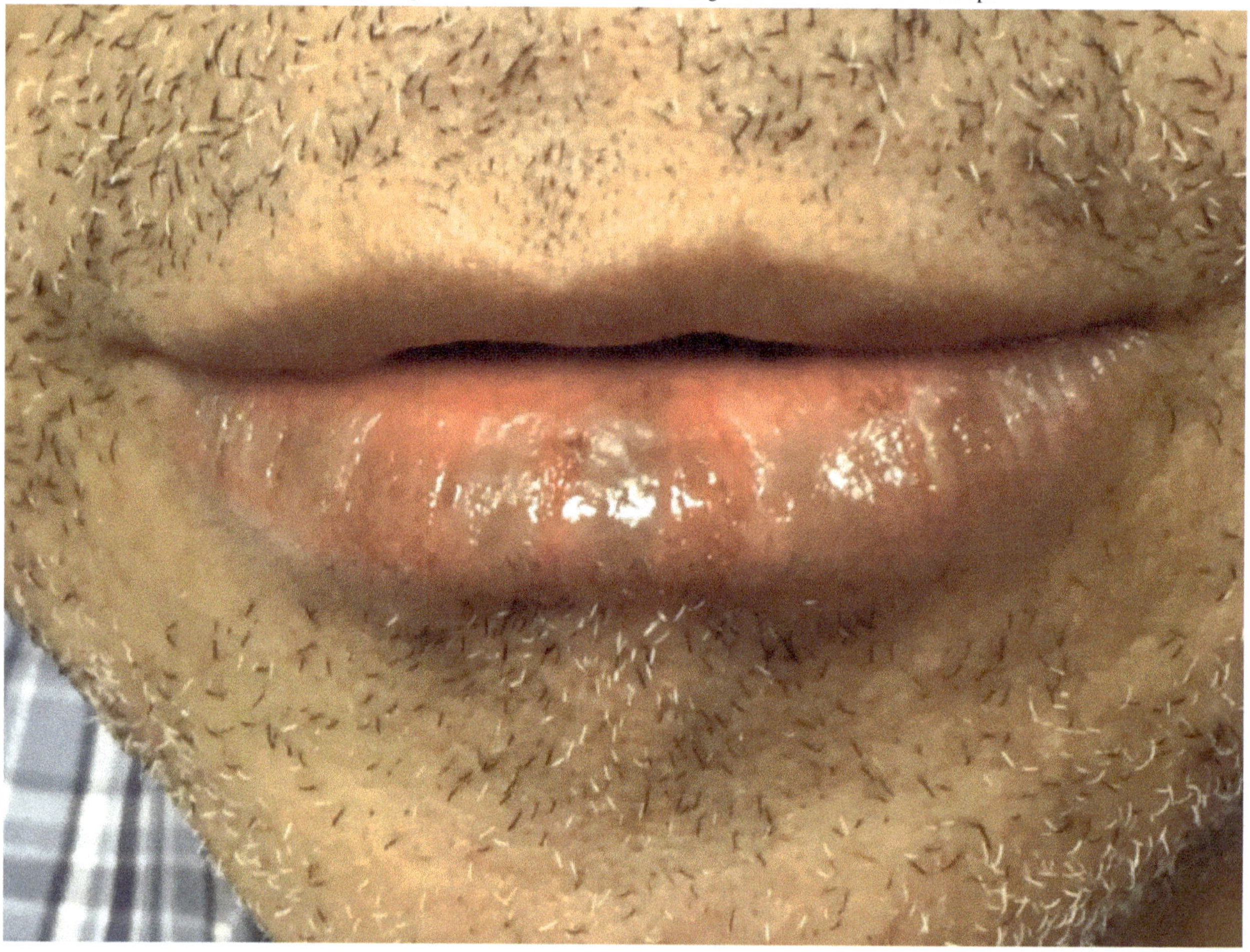

Figure 10. Case 5. Image from first in-person visit showing resolving vesicles and erosions.

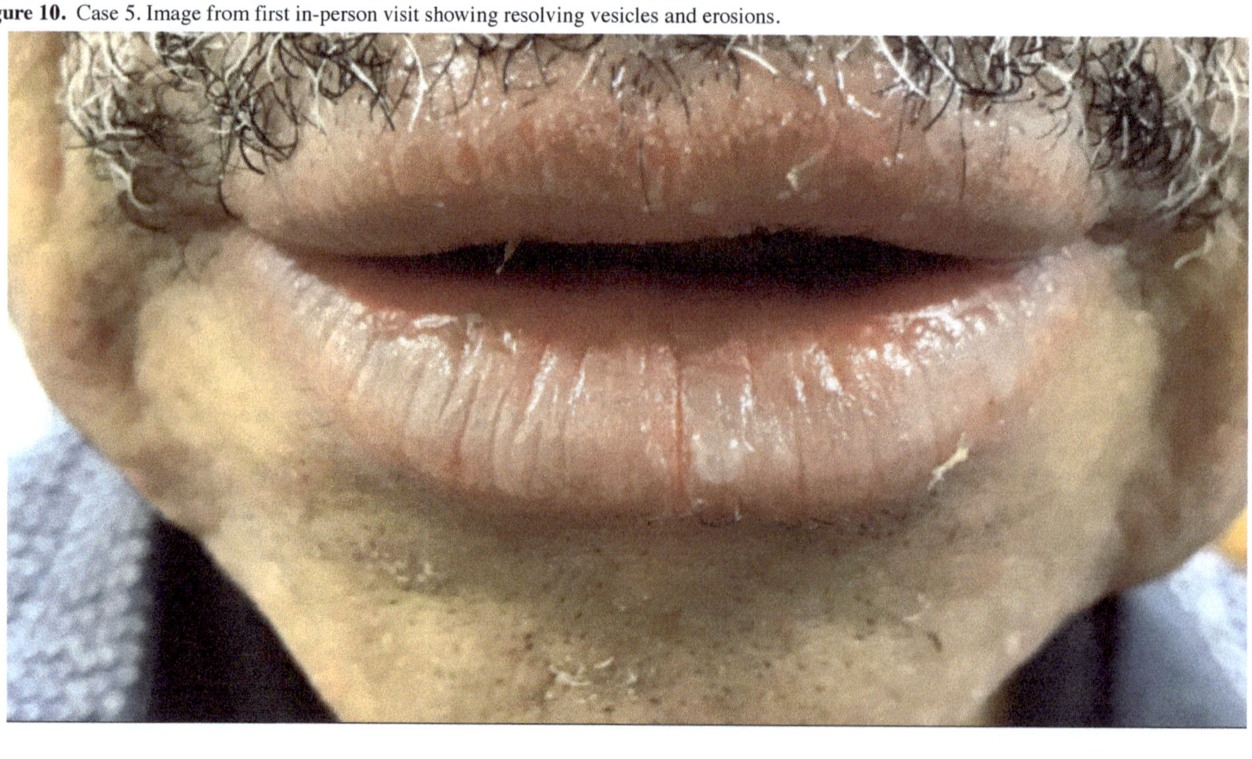

Figure 11. Case 5. Image from second in-person visit, when biopsy was taken.

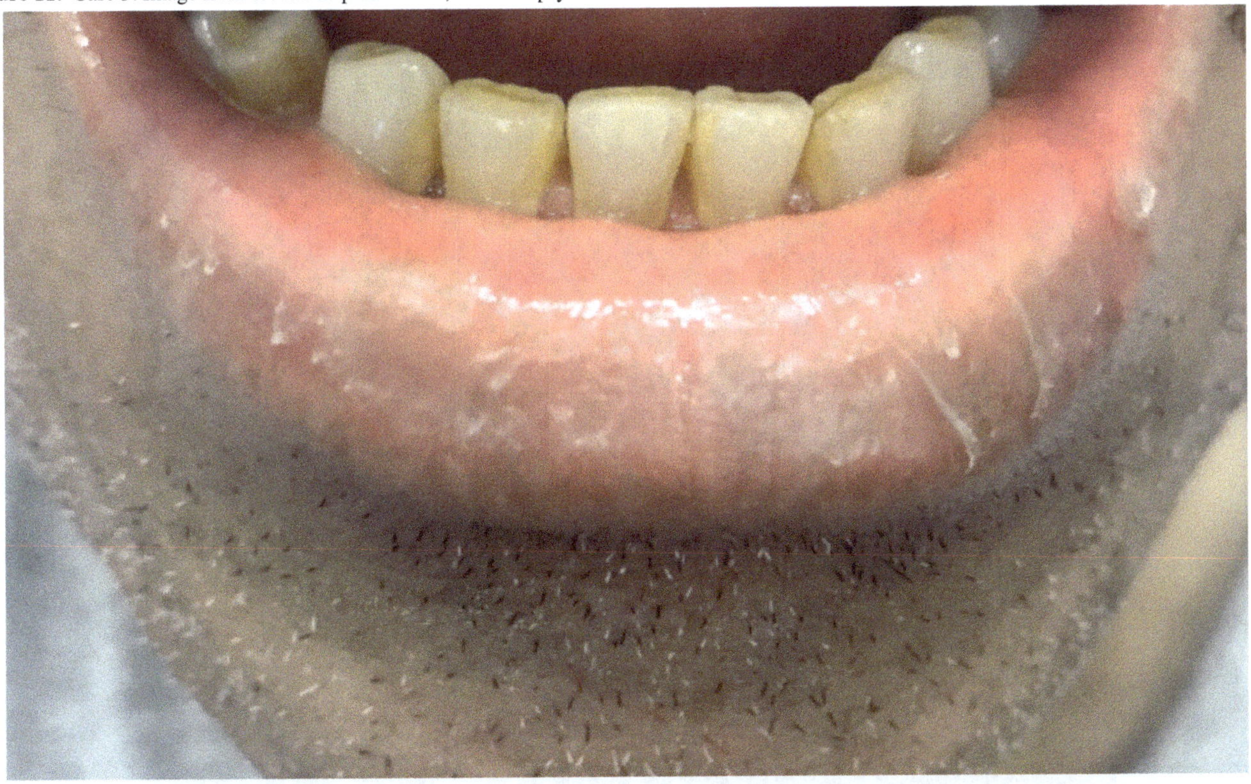

Case 6

A 41-year-old man with no known history of sexually transmitted infections was referred to teledermatology for 1 month of an unchanging nontender penile rash. He was in a monogamous relationship, and his female partner did not have a similar rash. Submitted images demonstrated a cluster of apparent deep-seated vesicles or pustules on the dorsal penile shaft (Figure 12) as well as documented 1.5-2 cm suprapubic lymphadenopathy. The teledermatologist noted difficulty in distinguishing between vesicles and pustules in the images and recommended obtaining a medication history as well as viral and bacterial swab culture for genital vesicles and pustules. The differential included infectious and inflammatory etiologies, including HSV, lymphogranuloma venereum, and a fixed drug eruption. The patient was scheduled for an in-person evaluation (Figure 13), during which a shave biopsy was obtained that demonstrated a foreign body giant cell reaction suggestive of a ruptured epidermal inclusion cyst.

Figure 12. Case 6. Submitted teledermatology image suggestive of vesicles versus pustules on the dorsal penile shaft.

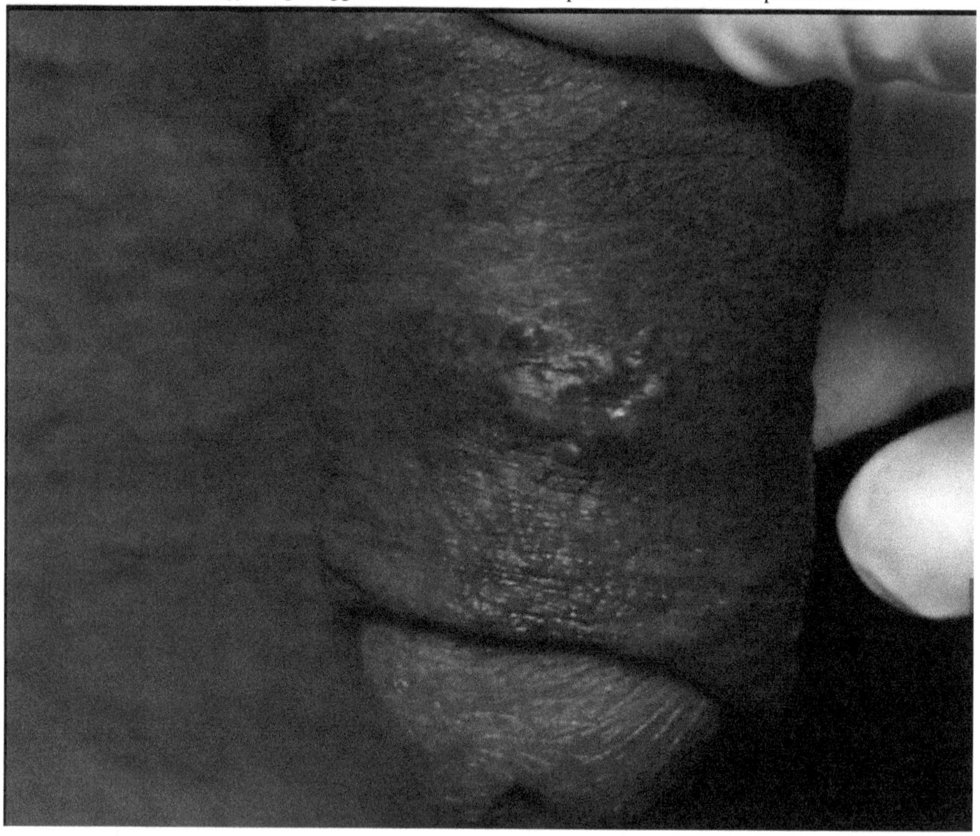

Figure 13. Case 6. Image from in-person visit.

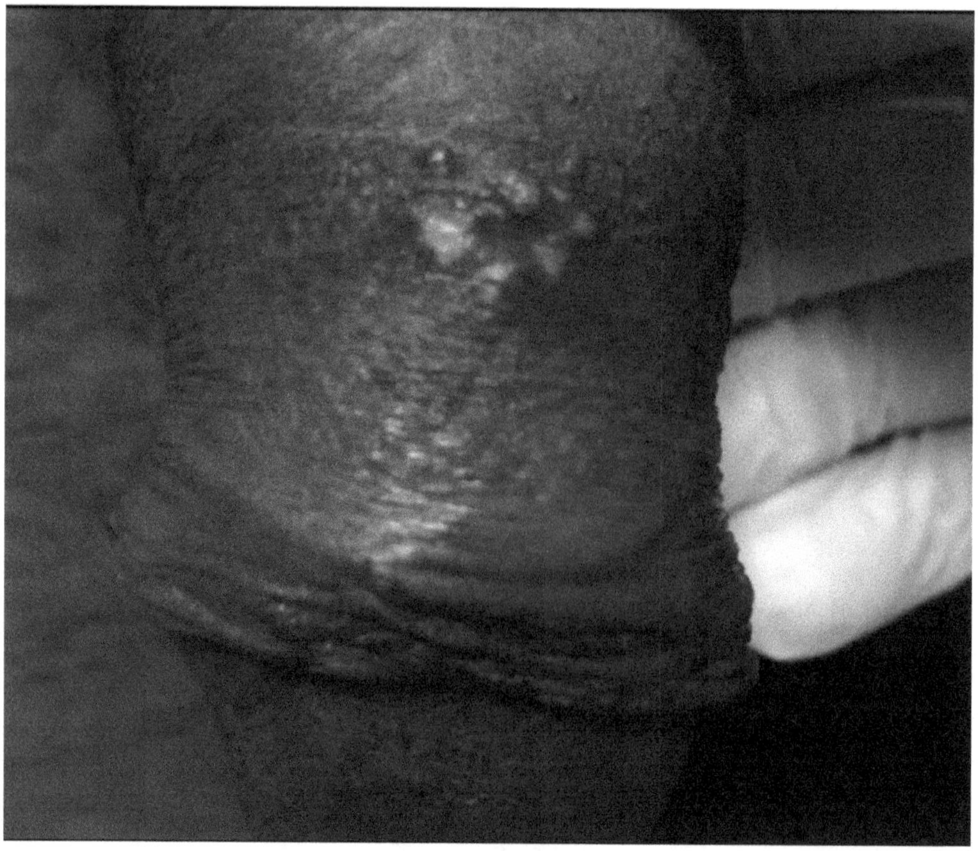

Case 7

A 66-year-old man with a 1- to 2-year history of a hyperpigmented nasal papule was referred for teledermatology consultation. The teledermatologist noted that the two dermatoscopic images provided were poorly focused (Figures 14 and 15), and no gross images were submitted. Thus, the consultant was unable to provide a differential diagnosis with the provided clinical images, and the patient was referred for an in-person visit. During the in-office encounter, exam revealed a 5-6 mm black thin papule with a collarette of scale on the nasal bridge (Figure 16) with a differential of irritated seborrheic keratosis versus melanoma. A shave biopsy was performed of the lesion, which resulted in a diagnosis of pigmented basal cell carcinoma. The patient was referred for Mohs surgery.

Figure 14. Case 7. Submitted image to teledermatologist taken with dermoscopy.

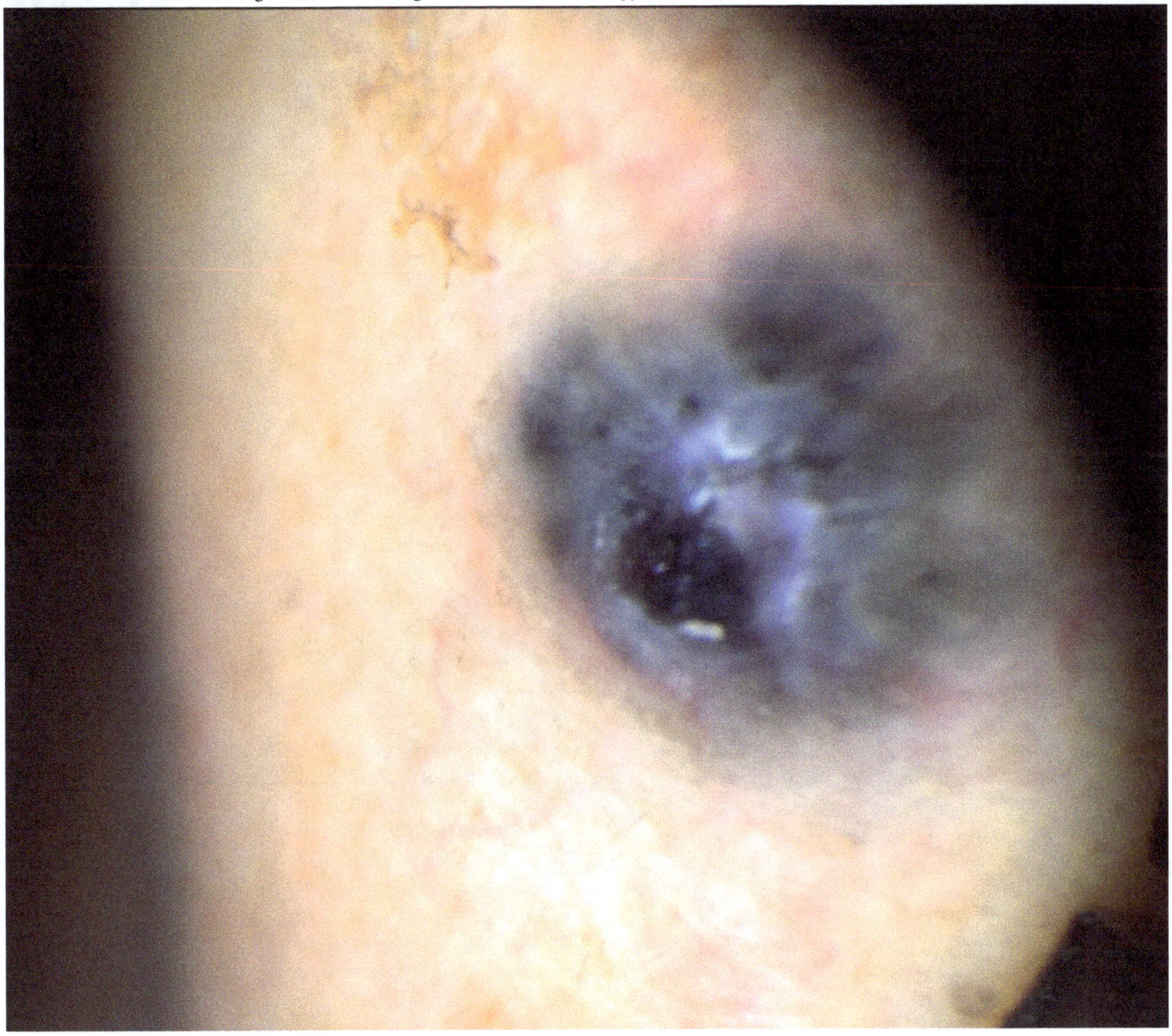

Figure 15. Case 7. Submitted image to teledermatologist taken with dermoscopy.

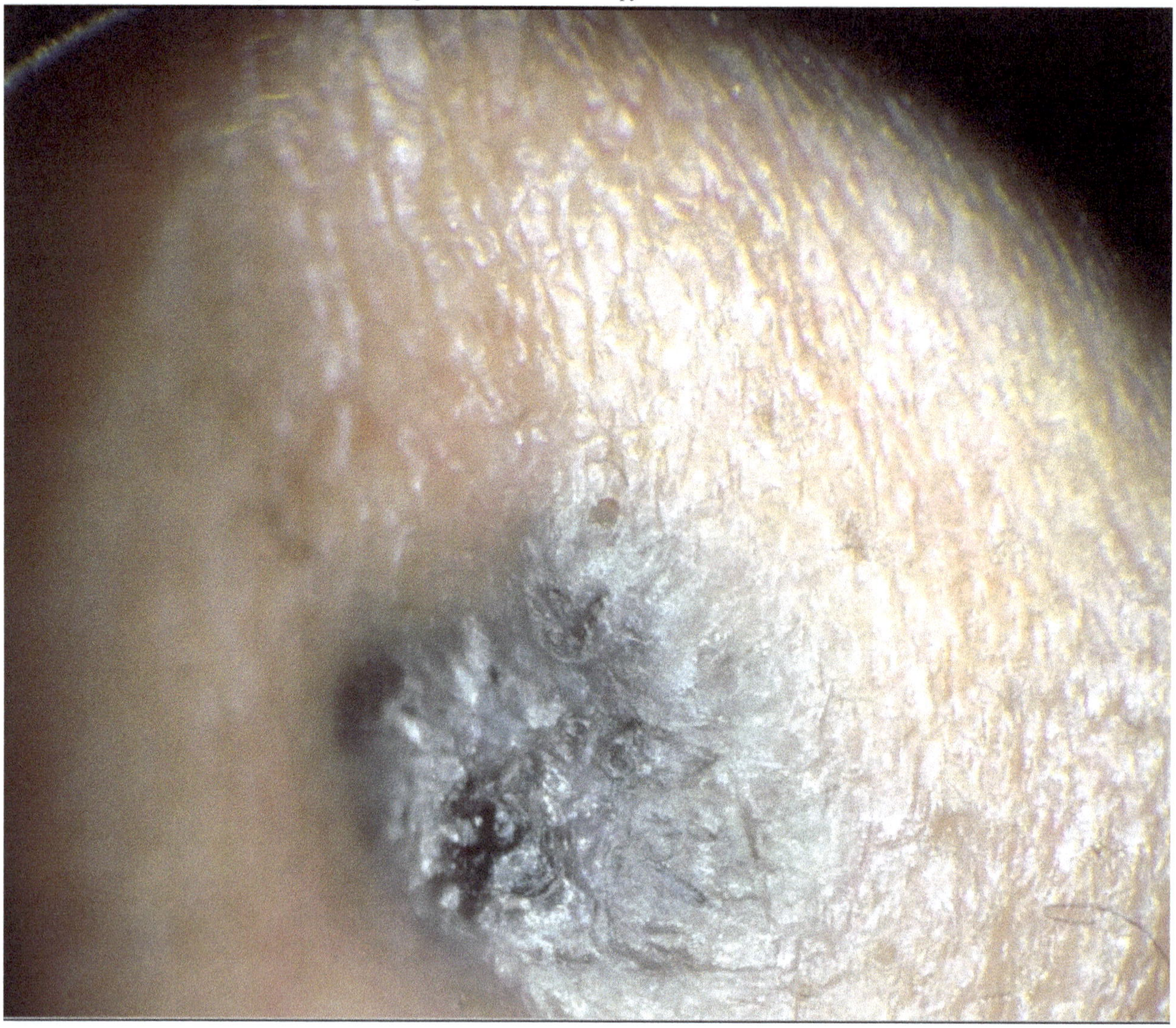

Figure 16. Case 7. In-person image showing 5-6 mm black thin papule with collarette of scale on the nasal bridge.

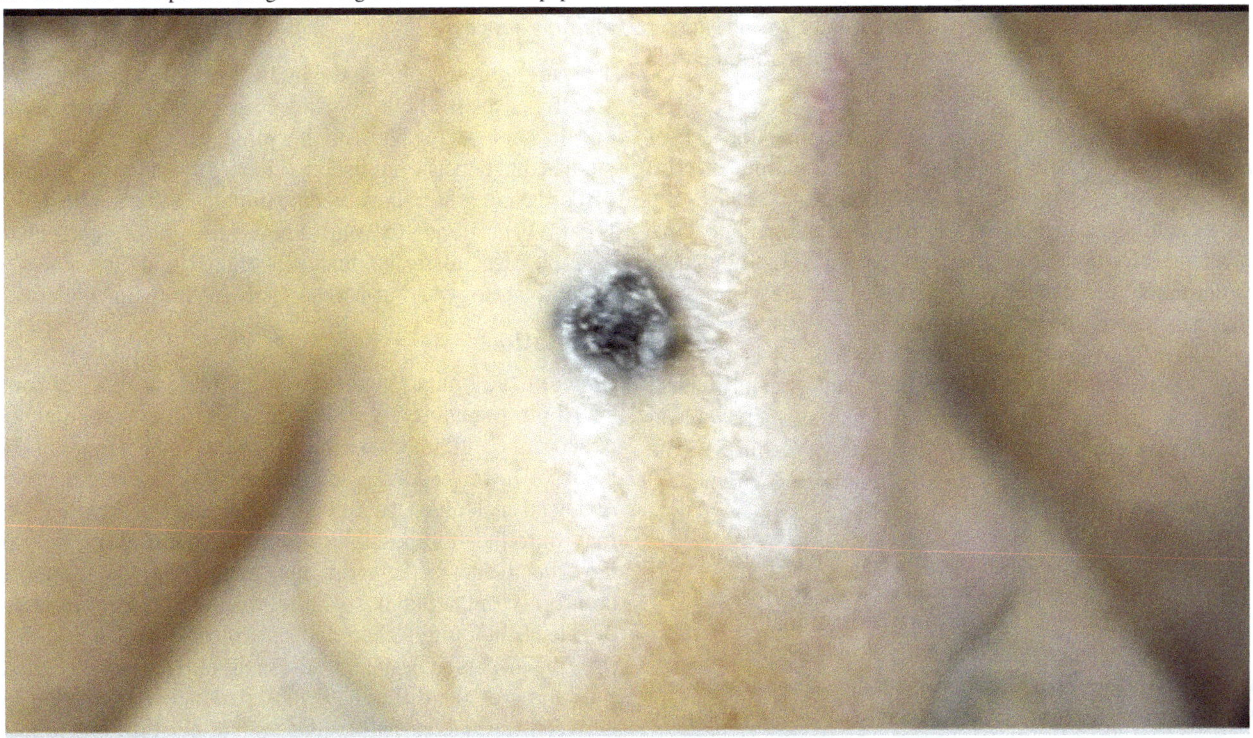

Discussion

Principal Results

From our case analysis, we identified multiple factors that likely contributed to diagnostic discordance between SAF teledermatology consultations and in-person visits in these cases. One contributing factor was poor image quality, including use of bright lighting creating shine artifact (case 1), submission of photos that showed partial views without showing the entire anatomic area involved (cases 1, 2, 3, and 7), and poorly focused images (case 7). These cases demonstrate the importance of education on appropriate image acquisition techniques. Following previously published best practices [21,22] and ongoing feedback to providers submitting photos may facilitate improved photo quality over time.

In some cases, additional clinical history or diagnostic tests provided by the referring clinician would have been helpful in narrowing the differential diagnosis. For example, diagnostic accuracy may have increased if the referring provider had performed bedside diagnostics such as superficial wound cultures, viral cultures, KOH preps (cases 2, 3, and 5), or dermoscopy (case 7). Use of dermoscopy has previously been shown to be a helpful tool in teledermatology programs, particularly in the evaluation of pigmented lesions [12]. Improved training of referring providers in using these diagnostic modalities may be helpful by providing clinical data to the dermatologist that leads to improved diagnostic accuracy. In addition, many cases illustrate the importance of a complete relevant medical history. For example, in case 6, a clinical history of similar vesicular eruptions, involvement of the oral mucosa, new exposures in the affected area, and associated pain or burning would have been helpful in differentiating between HSV, erythema multiforme, contact dermatitis, or pemphigus. Similarly, increased education for referring providers around questions relevant to certain dermatologic presentations (ie, asking about involvement of oral mucosa for bullous eruptions) would help them obtain an optimal history to aid in diagnosis.

Even with high-quality images, some morphologic characteristics may be difficult to appreciate with photos given visual limitations and inability to evaluate textural characteristics. For example, in case 4, palpation for detection of scale and induration may have helped the teledermatologist differentiate actinic damage from telangiectasias, and the teledermatologist interpreted the initial submitted image as a lesion with apparent overlying scale or crust, which was not seen in person. Case 6 also highlights that cystic, pustular, and vesicular structures can sometimes be difficult to distinguish from photos alone, depending on the angle and lighting of the photo taken. These cases highlight inherent diagnostic limitations of teledermatology services.

Finally, some factors such as atypical presentations and evolution of skin lesions over time were not specific to teledermatology and may have occurred in an initial in-person visit as well. For example, multiple cases remained diagnostically challenging even when patients were seen in person due to atypical presentations (cases 1, 5, and 6). Additionally, cases 2 and 3 highlight how morphology and distribution can evolve over time, leading to changes in suspected diagnosis. Teledermatology may have the highest utility for cases with typical presentations as unusual presentations may be difficult for teledermatologists to manage confidently without in-person evaluation and possible skin biopsy. Recognition of these limitations may also help with appropriate selection of patients more likely to benefit from an in-person encounter rather than a teledermatology visit. Even when patients can be managed with teledermatology, it is important for patients and providers to maintain follow-up to ensure appropriate response to management and ongoing support if the patient's condition or morphology changes from the time of original teledermatology consultation.

Our study has important implications given that the use of asynchronous and other types of virtual care continues to rise [9,10], as incorrect diagnosis via teledermatology or lack of a timely referral for an in-person visit may have potential negative consequences for patients. For example, case 2 highlights how a teledermatologist's incorrect diagnosis and prescription of betamethasone for tinea corporis may have contributed to the progression of the rash, although the correct diagnosis also may not have been made at an initial in-person visit given its atypical presentation. In case 7, it was essential that a timely referral was made given the indeterminate images, which allowed the patient to receive a biopsy resulting in a diagnosis of pigmented basal cell carcinoma.

In order to improve the quality of SAF consultations and decrease rates of diagnostic discordance, we advocate for use of a standardized guide to help improve the quality of SAF teledermatology consults, including image quality and appropriate workup. In addition to guidelines already outlined by the American Telemedicine Association [21,22], our study highlights the need for guidelines for proper lighting, examples of dermoscopy images, relevant questions to ask in the patient history for certain morphologic presentations, and certain suggested diagnostic tests to perform before submitting a consult.

In addition, the educational value of SAF consults should continue to be emphasized to both referring and consulting providers in order to help improve the quality of consults and ensure the highest level of diagnostic accuracy. Referring providers' ability to obtain an optimal history and diagnostic testing will also likely improve with increased use of SAF teledermatology and iterative dialogue between providers about patients' medical management. For example, previous studies have highlighted the educational potential of SAF teledermatology systems on improving referring primary care provider knowledge of dermatologic care [23]. Teledermatologists should also be encouraged to engage in education with referring providers to ensure this ongoing learning process.

The strengths of our study include its in-depth analysis of specific cases and side-by-side comparison of teledermatology and in-person consults for the same patients. While several studies have been published on overall rates of diagnostic discordance, which have been estimated at around 39%-67% [12-17,19], none to our knowledge have presented a case-by-case analysis that illustrates and compares the teledermatology and in-person visits for the same patients.

Limitations

Some of the limitations of our study include that our sample size limits our ability to generalize across all cases of diagnostic concordance, although we intend for this to be a more in-depth study of fewer cases. In addition, only one teledermatologist reviewed each image submitted by the referring provider, which may introduce the possibility that diagnostic uncertainty may have been due to the individual teledermatologist's level of comfort with the diagnosis rather than the inherent limitations of teledermatology. The teledermatologist was also different than the in-person dermatologist in all but the second case, and thus some of the differences in experience and comfort level between the teledermatologists and in-person dermatologists may have contributed to the discordant diagnoses.

Conclusions

Collectively, these cases highlight factors that can contribute to diagnostic discordance between teledermatologist and in-person dermatologist and the importance of ensuring that teledermatology services are supported by readily available in-person visits when appropriate to achieve the correct diagnosis in these cases. We also highlight the importance of ongoing education of referring providers to ensure optimal history and diagnostic workup and improve quality of consultations and the development of standardized guidelines for submitting referrals.

Teledermatology can provide substantial benefits to patients, and recognition of its limitations and mitigation of the factors identified in these cases provide opportunities to improve the quality and diagnostic accuracy of SAF teledermatology services.

References

1. Snoswell C, Finnane A, Janda M, Soyer HP, Whitty JA. Cost-effectiveness of Store-and-Forward Teledermatology: A Systematic Review. JAMA Dermatol 2016 Jun 01;152(6):702-708. [doi: 10.1001/jamadermatol.2016.0525] [Medline: 27074289]
2. Rajda J, Seraly MP, Fernandes J, Niejadlik K, Wei H, Fox K, et al. Impact of Direct to Consumer Store-and-Forward Teledermatology on Access to Care, Satisfaction, Utilization, and Costs in a Commercial Health Plan Population. Telemed J E Health 2018 Feb;24(2):166-169. [doi: 10.1089/tmj.2017.0078] [Medline: 28742431]
3. Datta SK, Warshaw EM, Edison KE, Kapur K, Thottapurathu L, Moritz TE, et al. Cost and Utility Analysis of a Store-and-Forward Teledermatology Referral System: A Randomized Clinical Trial. JAMA Dermatol 2015 Dec 01;151(12):1323-1329. [doi: 10.1001/jamadermatol.2015.2362] [Medline: 26375589]
4. Lasierra N, Alesanco A, Gilaberte Y, Magallón R, García J. Lessons learned after a three-year store and forward teledermatology experience using internet: Strengths and limitations. Int J Med Inform 2012 May;81(5):332-343. [doi: 10.1016/j.ijmedinf.2012.02.008] [Medline: 22425394]

5. Chuchu N. Teledermatology for diagnosing skin cancer in adults. Cochrane Database Syst Rev 2018;12. [doi: 10.1002/14651858.cd013193] [Medline: 30521686]
6. Finnane A, Dallest K, Janda M, Soyer HP. Teledermatology for the Diagnosis and Management of Skin Cancer: A Systematic Review. JAMA Dermatol 2017 Mar 01;153(3):319-327. [doi: 10.1001/jamadermatol.2016.4361] [Medline: 27926766]
7. Naka F, Lu J, Porto A, Villagra J, Wu ZH, Anderson D. Impact of dermatology eConsults on access to care and skin cancer screening in underserved populations: A model for teledermatology services in community health centers. J Am Acad Dermatol 2018 Feb;78(2):293-302. [doi: 10.1016/j.jaad.2017.09.017] [Medline: 29061478]
8. G Bianchi M, Santos A, Cordioli E. Benefits of Teledermatology for Geriatric Patients: Population-Based Cross-Sectional Study. J Med Internet Res 2020 Apr 21;22(4):e16700 [FREE Full text] [doi: 10.2196/16700] [Medline: 32314966]
9. Ramaswamy A, Yu M, Drangsholt S, Ng E, Culligan PJ, Schlegel PN, et al. Patient Satisfaction With Telemedicine During the COVID-19 Pandemic: Retrospective Cohort Study. J Med Internet Res 2020 Sep 09;22(9):e20786 [FREE Full text] [doi: 10.2196/20786] [Medline: 32810841]
10. Su MY, Das S. Expansion of asynchronous teledermatology during the COVID-19 pandemic. J Am Acad Dermatol 2020 Dec;83(6):e471-e472 [FREE Full text] [doi: 10.1016/j.jaad.2020.08.054] [Medline: 32822793]
11. Brinker TJ, Hekler A, von Kalle C, Schadendorf D, Esser S, Berking C, et al. Teledermatology: Comparison of Store-and-Forward Versus Live Interactive Video Conferencing. J Med Internet Res 2018 Oct 24;20(10):e11871 [FREE Full text] [doi: 10.2196/11871] [Medline: 30355564]
12. Piccolo D, Smolle J, Argenziano G, Wolf IH, Braun R, Cerroni L, et al. Teledermoscopy--results of a multicentre study on 43 pigmented skin lesions. J Telemed Telecare 2000;6(3):132-137. [doi: 10.1258/1357633001935202] [Medline: 10912329]
13. Warshaw EM, Hillman YJ, Greer NL, Hagel EM, MacDonald R, Rutks IR, et al. Teledermatology for diagnosis and management of skin conditions: a systematic review. J Am Acad Dermatol 2011 Apr;64(4):759-772. [doi: 10.1016/j.jaad.2010.08.026] [Medline: 21036419]
14. Warshaw EM, Gravely AA, Nelson DB. Reliability of store and forward teledermatology for skin neoplasms. J Am Acad Dermatol 2015 Mar;72(3):426-435. [doi: 10.1016/j.jaad.2014.11.001] [Medline: 25599624]
15. Warshaw EM, Gravely AA, Nelson DB. Accuracy of teledermatology/teledermoscopy and clinic-based dermatology for specific categories of skin neoplasms. J Am Acad Dermatol 2010 Aug;63(2):348-352. [doi: 10.1016/j.jaad.2009.10.037] [Medline: 20633809]
16. Piccolo D, Smolle J, Wolf IH, Peris K, Hofmann-Wellenhof R, Dell'Eva G, et al. Face-to-face diagnosis vs telediagnosis of pigmented skin tumors: a teledermoscopic study. Arch Dermatol 1999 Dec;135(12):1467-1471. [doi: 10.1001/archderm.135.12.1467] [Medline: 10606051]
17. Landow SM, Mateus A, Korgavkar K, Nightingale D, Weinstock MA. Teledermatology: key factors associated with reducing face-to-face dermatology visits. J Am Acad Dermatol 2014 Sep;71(3):570-576. [doi: 10.1016/j.jaad.2014.02.021] [Medline: 24704089]
18. Dobry A, Begaj T, Mengistu K, Sinha S, Droms R, Dunlap R, et al. Implementation and Impact of a Store-and-Forward Teledermatology Platform in an Urban Academic Safety-Net Health Care System. Telemed J E Health 2020 Jun 09. [doi: 10.1089/tmj.2020.0069] [Medline: 32522105]
19. Nelson CA, Takeshita J, Wanat KA, Bream KDW, Holmes JH, Koenig HC, et al. Impact of store-and-forward (SAF) teledermatology on outpatient dermatologic care: A prospective study in an underserved urban primary care setting. J Am Acad Dermatol 2016 Mar;74(3):484-90.e1. [doi: 10.1016/j.jaad.2015.09.058] [Medline: 26679528]
20. Barbieri JS, Nelson CA, James WD, Margolis DJ, Littman-Quinn R, Kovarik CL, et al. The reliability of teledermatology to triage inpatient dermatology consultations. JAMA Dermatol 2014 Apr;150(4):419-424. [doi: 10.1001/jamadermatol.2013.9517] [Medline: 24522374]
21. McKoy K, Norton S, Lappan C. Quick Guide to Store-Forward Teledermatology for Referring Providers.: ATA Teledermatology SIG; 2012. URL: http://teledermatology-society.org/wp-content/uploads/2013/08/quick-guide-to-store-forward-and-live-interactive-teledermatology-for-referring-providers.pdf [accessed 2021-01-29]
22. McKoy K, Antoniotti NM, Armstrong A, Bashshur R, Bernard J, Bernstein D, et al. Practice Guidelines for Teledermatology. Telemed J E Health 2016 Dec;22(12):981-990. [doi: 10.1089/tmj.2016.0137] [Medline: 27690203]
23. Mohan GC, Molina GE, Stavert R. Store and forward teledermatology improves dermatology knowledge among referring primary care providers: A survey-based cohort study. J Am Acad Dermatol 2018 Nov;79(5):960-961. [doi: 10.1016/j.jaad.2018.05.006] [Medline: 29753059]

Abbreviations

HSV: herpes simplex virus
KOH prep: potassium hydroxide preparation
SAF: store-and-forward

5

Determinants of the Intention to Use Teledermatology: Evidence from Dermatologists and Primary Care Physicians

Mercedes Sendín-Martín[1*], MD; Ana Jiménez-Zarco[2*], MD, PhD; Francesc Saigí-Rubió[3*], MD, PhD; Julian Conejo-Mir[1*], MD, PhD; Jose Juan Pereyra-Rodriguez[1*], MD, PhD

[1]University Hospital Virgen del Rocio, Sevilla, Spain

[2]Faculty of Economic and Business Sciences, Universitat Oberta de Cataluña, Barcelona, Spain

[3]Faculty of Health Sciences, Universitat Oberta de Cataluña, Barcelona, Spain

[*]all authors contributed equally

Corresponding Author:
Jose Juan Pereyra-Rodriguez, MD, PhD
University Hospital Virgen del Rocio
Avda Manuel Siurot S/N
Sevilla, 41013
Spain

Email: pe3reyra@gmail.com

Abstract

Background: Teledermatology (TD) is one of the applications of electronic health and telemedicine that involves the use of information and communication technologies (ICTs) for the care of skin diseases. Previous studies on TD indicate that it seems to be effective in diagnosing early malignant pathologies, such as melanoma, and in reducing waiting lists by prioritizing urgent cases of pathology. Despite these advantages, the implementation of TD is still low in many areas.

Objective: Most previous studies on TD have focused on analyzing the results of TD use. However, to completely understand TD, it is necessary to consider the determinants of its use. This study analyzes the factors that motivate medical professionals to use TD in their clinical practice.

Methods: A survey that targeted a total population of 743 medical professionals from health care institutions in Andalusia (Spain) was used. The study sample comprised 223 doctors (87 dermatologists and 136 primary care physicians).

Results: Using an extended Technology Acceptance Model and microdata for the 223 physicians, a cluster analysis (of the user's ICT profile) and binary logistic regression analysis were conducted. This analysis demonstrated the presence of 3 clusters in the sample with respect to the use of technology (cluster 1: advanced use of ICTs; cluster 2: moderate use of ICTs; and cluster 3: scarce use of ICTs). The analysis performed confirmed the model's goodness of fit, which allowed 69% of the variable's variance to be explained. The outcomes revealed that the factors that were most important when implementing a TD system were the user's ICT profile (P=.048), system efficiency (P<.001), and preference of the subjects involved (P=.008; P<.005). The quality of the assistance, the difficulties arising from the use of technology (information security and confidentiality), or interests of the administration were not decisive factors for the implementation of TD. Subsequently, we performed a logistic regression analysis, separating primary care doctors from dermatologists. For the former, the determining factors were the ICT profile and the efficiency of the system, whereas, among dermatologists, only the preference of each individual was considered to be a determining factor.

Conclusions: The use of TD should be accompanied by a comprehensive program of validation and evaluation. These results show that determinants of TD implementation differ depending on the subjects involved. Therefore, it is essential to perform studies before the implementation of a TD system to identify and influence the aforementioned predictive factors.

KEYWORDS

telemedicine; dermatology; organizational innovation; health care surveys

Introduction

Background

Information and communication technologies (ICTs) constitute an opportunity for improvement in care quality, both in the effectiveness and efficiency of health services. Incorporating ICTs also contributes to the development of sustainable health systems, justifying its economic and political interest [1,2]. Telemedicine is defined as the use of ICT for the transfer of medical information for diagnostic, therapeutic, and educational purposes [3]. Telemedicine services include assistance applications that aid in the administration and management of patients, as well as provide information and distance training to users and professionals. When this service is used in dermatology, it is referred to as teledermatology (TD), which is probably the most used form of telemedicine.

Despite starting hesitantly, the development and cheapening of information technologies have led to an exponential expansion of TD since the beginning of the 21st century, for example, from having 21 centers that used TD in 2009 to 68 centers in 2014 in Spain [4]. In a recent systematic review, Trettel et al [5] showed that the application of TD increased over the years and is illustrated by the number of countries where digital patient communication is used. Currently, the most used TD model is that of asynchronous TD (one in which clinical data are stored and sent electronically to the dermatologist who responds to the primary care physician with the instructions to follow). This model was the predominant TD modality in 83% of hospitals in 2014 [6].

Previous studies on TD indicate that it seems to be effective when misleading benign or malignant dermatological tumors, improving consultation prioritization by discerning urgent or preferential pathology [5,7]. In addition, TD is also useful as a teaching instrument by facilitating training for primary care physicians and dermatology residents, termed as teletraining [8].

Although most studies have focused on analyzing the results of TD use, to completely understand TD, it is necessary to consider its determinants of use. Despite the advantages of TD and its rapid development, implementation of TD is still low. Only 1% of dermatology consultations are by TD [9], and it has been implemented only in 26% of the hospitals in their reference areas [6]. These data seem to be contradictory, given the good acceptance and the concept of utility regarding TD that both primary care physicians and dermatologists share [6].

Some previous studies have tried to analyze the determinants of TD implementation [10-12]. However, this issue remains unclear, and further research is needed to explain the determinants of TD adoption. In our immediate environment, a study was conducted to analyze the factors associated with the adoption of ICT and its barriers in Andalusia. However, TD itself was not an object of study in this research [13].

Objective

The objective of this work was to identify factors influencing intention to use TD by professionals of the Andalusian Health Service and the typology of the professional according to the use and expectations of the ICT. Subsequently, we proceeded to analyze what factors influence and to what extent these factors can enhance or inhibit the use of telemedicine in the organization where the professionals work.

Methods

Hypothesis and Model

The Technological Acceptance Model (TAM), proposed by Davis in 1989, is the most widely accepted model to assess the acceptance of an information technology within a given organization [11]. The model is based on the theory of reasoned action (TRA) [14]. Since its publication, it has been cited on numerous occasions, being one of the most widely used instruments to assess users' technology acceptance.

This model states that technology acceptance depends mainly on 2 variables: perceived utility (PU) and perceived ease of use (FUP). The PU refers to the belief that a technology system can improve the professional activity. This utility may refer to improving the quality of clinical practice or reducing economic costs, time, or resources. On the other hand, the FUP indicates the perception that the use of a particular system implies less effort to perform their tasks.

From this model, we obtained the following 2 hypotheses:

- H1. The PU of TD influences the professionals' intention to use.
    - H1.1. Improving the quality of care influences the intention to use TD.
    - H1.2. Reduction of costs and resources in the distance influences the intention to use TD.
- H2. The FUP of TD influences professionals' intention to use.

The TAM has been used to predict how the adoption of multiple technologies will behave, including the acceptance of telemedicine by health professionals [15]. It is a model shown to be suitable for both sex, different age groups, and most cultures [16].

Despite the aforementioned advantages, the TAM shows certain limitations. Some authors have pointed out the need to include additional variables to improve model predictions [17,18]. There are a number of variables including social, geographical, economic, and legal context that may influence users when accepting a new technology in our environment. These variables that are summarized in the social influence or *subjective norm* are included in the TRA and the theory of planned behavior. On the basis of these theories, the subjective norm can be included in our model. This rule corresponds to the directors of health care institutions, rest of the doctors, and the patients themselves.

In addition to the subjective norm, a patient's technological profile also determines how they will accept a new telemedicine tool. That profile may be defined according to the patient's use of electronic tools in their daily lives, both for recreational and work-related use. These tools include email, social networks, and the internet. The use of these tools by the subject determines its perception of usefulness and therefore can define a predisposition to accept or reject a new technology. For this reason, for an adequate study of intention to use TD, we consider it necessary to include the user's ICT profile in our variables. There are models, such as the theory of Grewal and Parasuraman on technological preparation [19], that allow variable incorporation relating the user profile of a professional with the intention of using ICTs in their work.

After including these variables (subjective norm and ICT profile) that we thought could influence the model, 2 more hypotheses were obtained:

- H3. The subjective norm (influence exerted by the administration, managers, doctors, and patients) influences the intention to use TD.
  - H3.1. The support of professionals and patients for TD influences the intention to use.
  - H3.2. The institution's support for TD influences its intention to use.
- H4. The ICT profile of a user influences the intention to use TD.

Figure 1 summarizes the TAM for TD, adding the hypotheses that have been discussed in this section.

Questionnaire and Validation

Data Collection

A specific questionnaire based on the TAM and its subsequent derivatives was designed by adapting a general questionnaire on telemedicine acceptance validated by the literature [11]. The final questionnaire is included in Multimedia Appendix 1. Different items that appear in the questionnaire have been formulated to measure variables that we expected to find in the model. In addition, we considered adding questions to these items to get participants' personal characterization (age, sex, professional category, experience, and type of center in which they are currently working). All these data would be used to build participants' technological profile, as described later.

Altogether, 18 questions, divided into 3 blocks, were included in the questionnaire: (1) demographic and professional characterization; (2) adoption of a TD system, and (3) Implementation of a TD system. Questions included in blocks 2 and 3 were based on a Likert scale of 10 points, from 1 (*nothing important /nothing agree*) to 10 (*very important /s* trongly agree).

An electronic version of the questionnaire was constructed and distributed through email using a corporate distribution list of the Andalusian Health System. This distribution list comprised all dermatologists and primary care physicians with a corporate mail in 5 centers with different complexity levels (from county hospitals to third-level centers) from Andalusia. We received answers from professionals (both dermatologists and general practitioners [GPs]) from all of the invited centers.

The questionnaire was addressed to both dermatologists and GPs, whether they were consultants or residents. A total of 574 general medicine physicians and 187 dermatologists were invited to participate (Textbox 1). Between May 25 and June 25, 2018, 2 reminders were sent to participants. Of 761 participants, 223 responses from professionals (29.4% of all invited) were obtained and included in the database leading to this study. Considering the amount of data, the profile of professionals who participated, and the centers involved, the final sample should be considered as representative of the Andalusian Health Service.

Figure 1. Model and hypotheses. H: hypothesis; ICT: information and communication technology.

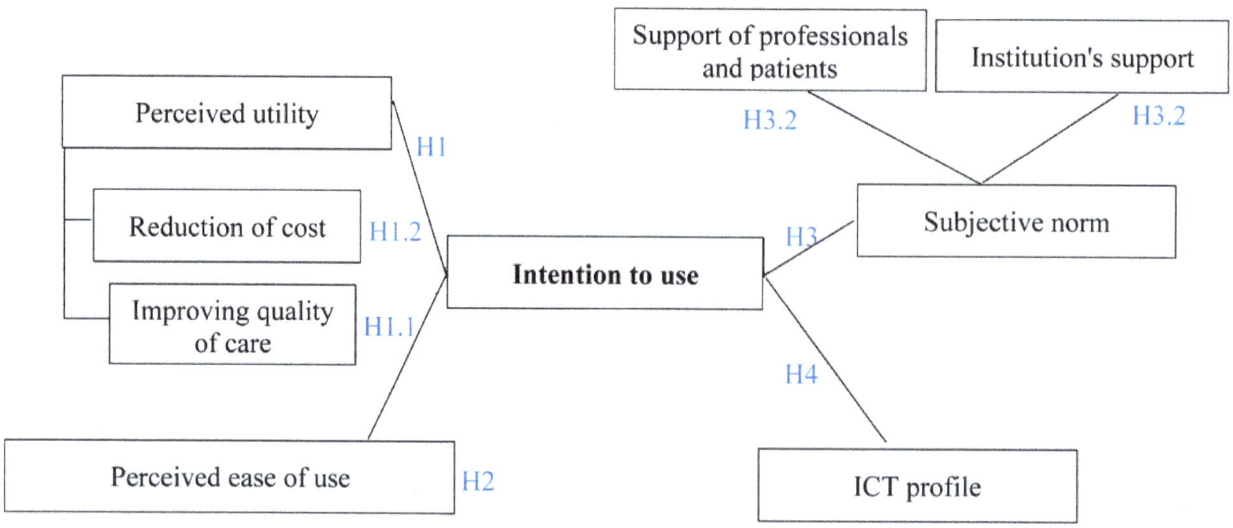

Textbox 1. Study specifications.

Universe:

- 574 general medicine physicians; 187 dermatologists

Sample:

- 138 general medicine physicians; 85 dermatologists

Margin of error:

- 5.52% (p=q) 95% CI

Data collection method:

- Questionnaire

Sampling method:

- Random

Fieldwork:

- Between May 25, 2018, and June 25, 2018

Variables and Statistical Analysis

First, we wanted to analyze the user's ICT profile, owing to several items of the questionnaire measuring the intensity of internet use. A hierarchical cluster analysis was performed for this purpose. Cluster analysis is a multivariate technique that seeks to group objects to form object conglomerates or clusters, with a high degree of internal homogeneity and external heterogeneity. After obtaining 3 clusters in our sample to define 3 levels of the ICT profile, an analysis of variance (ANOVA) test was applied in the obtained clusters.

On the other hand, to test the hypotheses proposed in the model (see hypothesis and model), different contrast tests were used on the variables of the study. Through the questionnaire items, multiple variables could be obtained. First, these variables required an exploratory factorial analysis (EFA) to be defined and calculated. The EFA is a technique that allows to explore the set of latent variables or common factors explaining the answers to the items of a test. Therefore, it is one of the most frequently applied techniques in studies related to the development and validation of tests.

All the variables of the study (the ICT profile and those obtained after the EFA) are summarized in Table 1. All these variables could be framed in the hypotheses we had obtained from the TAM (see point 2.1 hypothesis and model) as is shown in Table 2.

Subsequently, an exploratory factor analysis was carried out, constructing as many metric variables as the EFA had revealed. All these, together with the dependent variable, constituted the final multivariate analysis. A logistic regression was performed to analyze the independent influence in the TD implementation of each factor showed in the EFA. Finally, we wanted to distinguish between factors that were more important for GPs to gain a better acceptance of this technology and those more important for dermatologists.

Table 1. Study variable.

Variable	Explanation
User's ICT[a] profile	Numerical variable obtained from the cluster analysis. This variable measures the use of the internet and social networks at a personal and professional level. The original variables included in the analysis were measured using a 5-point Likert scale
Quality of care	Numerical variable obtained from an exploratory factor analysis. It defines the quality of the medical act as an influencing factor for the implementation of TD[b]. This variable was obtained from questions 15.1-15.4 (see Multimedia Appendix 1) after EFA[c]. The original variables included in the analysis were measured on a 10-point Likert scale
System efficiency	Numerical variable obtained from an exploratory factor analysis. It defines the influence of efficiency (including workload and expenses) on the implementation of TD. This variable was obtained from questions 15.5-15.7 (see Multimedia Appendix 1) after an EFA. The original variables included in the analysis were measured on a 10-point Likert scale
Technological difficulties	Numerical variable obtained from an exploratory factor analysis. It refers to the complications related to technological systems (complexity of the devices, need for training, and security). This variable was obtained from questions 16.1-16.6 (see Multimedia Appendix 1) after an EFA. The original variables included in the analysis were measured on a 10-point Likert scale
Preference of the subjects directly involved	Numerical variable obtained from an exploratory factor analysis. It explains how preferences of professionals and patients influence the implementation of TD. This variable was obtained from questions 17.1-17.3 (see Multimedia Appendix 1) after an EFA. The original variables included in the analysis were measured on a 10-point Likert scale
Interest of the administration	Numerical variable obtained from an exploratory factor analysis. It defines the influence of administrations (including financing capacity or resources that they would have to devote to) on the implementation of TD systems. This variable was obtained from questions 17.4-17.7 (see Multimedia Appendix 1) after an EFA. The original variables included in the analysis were measured on a 10-point Likert scale

[a]ICT: information and communication technology.

[b]TD: teledermatology.

[c]EFA: exploratory factorial analysis.

Table 2. Relationship between the hypotheses based on Davis' Technological Acceptance Model (TAM) and study variables (obtained after an exploratory factorial analysis [EFA] and a cluster analysis [information and communication technology (ICT) profile]).

Variables according to the modified TAM	Study hypothesis according to the modified TAM	Variables obtained after EFA and hierarchical cluster analysis
Perceived utility	H1. The perceived utility of TD[a] influences the professionals' intention to use; H1.1. Improving the quality of care influences the intention to use TD; H1.2. Reduction of costs and resources in the distance influences the intention to use TD	Quality of care (H1.1); System efficiency (H1.2)
Perceived ease of use	H2. The perceived ease of use of TD influences professionals' intention to use	Technological difficulties (H2)
Subjective norm	H3. The subjective norm (influence exerted by the administration, managers, doctors, and patients) influences the intention to use TD; H3.1. The support of professionals and patients for TD influences the intention to use; H3.2. The institution's support for TD influences its intention to use	Preference of the subjects directly involved (H3.1); Interest of the administration (H3.2)
User's ICT profile	H4. The ICT profile of a user influences the intention to use TD.	User's ICT profile (H4)

[a]TD: teledermatology.

Results

Demographic and Professional Characteristics

A total of 223 responses were obtained, including family doctors and dermatologists (29.3% rate of response). In addition, 135 (61%) were women. The professionals' average age was 43.7 years. In our sample, 38% comprised dermatologists (among them, 6% dermatology residents and the rest dermatology specialists). In addition, 61% corresponded to GPs, 14% of these being general medicine residents. The remaining 1.34% corresponded to other professional categories, such as occupational physicians or aesthetic doctors. Moreover, 54.71% of the participants were TD users (60.87% of GPs and 44.71% of dermatologists), and 40.36% of them had been TD users for more than 2 years. Demographic and social characteristics of the sample are summarized in Table 3.

Table 3. Demographic factors.

Variable	Value, n (%)
Age (years)	
25-34	80 (35.9)
35-44	39 (17.5)
45-54	48 (21.5)
>54	56 (25.1)
Sex	
Male	88 (39.5)
Female	135 (60.5)
Professional category	
Dermatology resident	14 (6.23)
Dermatologist (eventual or interim)	39 (17.5)
Dermatologist (owner)	31 (13.9)
General practitioner resident	32 (14)
General practitioner (temporary or interim)	35 (15.7)
General practitioner (owner)	69 (30.9)
Others	3 (1.3)
Working time in sanitary field (years)	
≤1	22 (9.9)
2-10	73 (32.7)
11-20	52 (23.3)
21-30	51 (11.2)
>30	25 (11.2)
Working time in the same center (years)	
≤1	54 (24.2)
2-10	106 (47.5)
11-20	47 (21.2)
21-30	14 (6.3)
>30	2 (0.9)

Information and Communication Technology Profile

To define the user's ICT profile, we used a hierarchical clustering analysis. This analysis showed the presence of 3 clusters in the sample with respect to the use of technology (cluster 1: advanced use of ICTs; cluster 2: moderate use of ICTs; and cluster 3: scarce use of ICTs). The result was compared with an ANOVA test that was statistically significant ($P<.001$). Advanced ICT users had a slightly lower average age (41.86 years) compared with intermediate users (45.65 years) and beginners (42.99 years). However, these findings were not statistically significant ($P=.21$). The number of components in each cluster was well balanced, as shown in Tables 4 and 5.

Table 4. Hierarchical clustering analysis (information and communication technology user's profile).

Cluster number	Distances between clusters		
	1	2	3
1	—[a]	3.419	3.306
2	3.419	—	4.777
3	3.306	4.777	—

[a]Data not aplicable.

Table 5. Number of cases in each cluster.

Cluster	Frequency (n)
Cluster 1 (high use)	98
Cluster 2 (moderate use)	52
Cluster 3 (scarce use)	73
Valid	223
Lost	0

Determinants of Teledermatology Use

After the EFA, 5 independent variables were obtained (see Table 1) to which a numerical value was assigned. The factors obtained were classified as quality of care, system efficiency, technological difficulties, preference of the subjects directly involved (which included patients and professionals), and interest of the administration. All variables of the correlation matrix showed high correlation, with a determinant value of .000005989. The value of Kaiser-Meyer-Olkin was 0.843 and that of Bartlett's spherical test was 2575.479 with a significance of <.001 This analysis explained 69.238% of the variance (see Table 6). The values of Cronbach alpha in the factors between 0.782 and 0.894 confirmed the reliability of the results obtained.

After extracting the factors involved in the implementation of TD through the EFA, a multivariate analysis was performed, specifically, a logistic regression to obtain variables showing an independent impact. The results of this analysis are shown in Table 7, which provided the following statistics: χ^2_6=25.1; *P*<.001; Hosmer-Lemeshow test=9.481; *P*=.30; R^2 of Nagelkerke=0.155.

The ICT profile of the users (*P*=.048), the efficiency of the system (*P*<.001), and the preferences were found to be influential factors when implementing a TD system (*P*=.008). The remaining factors obtained after the EFA (assistance quality, the possible technological difficulties, and the administration interest) did not show an independent influence in the multivariate analysis.

In this way, based on our results, we were able to accept hypotheses H1.2, H3.1, and H4, whereas H1.1, H2, and H3.2 could not be accepted.

Subsequently, the same analysis was carried out by separating the sample into 2 different groups: GPs (both residents and consultants) and dermatologists (both residents and consultants). A logistic regression was performed including only GPs (the results are shown in Table 8), which provided the following statistics: χ^2_6=4.8; *P*=.57; Hosmer-Lemeshow test=6.562; *P*=.59; R^2 of Nagelkerke=0.054.

In this subgroup, the ICT profile was influenced by the TD implementation implantation (*P*=.03) and system efficiency (*P*=.002). The same analysis was then carried out in the subgroup of dermatologists, finding that only the preference of the subjects directly involved was a significant variable (Table 9). It provided the following statistics: χ^2_6=16.2; *P*=.012; Hosmer-Lemeshow test=7.402; *P*=.39; R^2 of Nagelkerke=0.238.

Table 6. Exploratory factor analysis results.

Item	Quality of care	System efficiency	Technological difficulties	Preference of the subjects directly involved	Interest of the administration
How important are they in the implementation of teledermatology?					
15.1. Quality of care	0.864	—[a]	—	—	—
15.2. Patient health	0.877	—	—	—	—
15.3. Therapeutic compliance	0.844	—	—	—	—
15.4. Frequency of face-to-face consultation	0.712	—	—	—	—
15.5. The workload of professionals	—	0.742	—	—	—
15.6. Health expenditure	—	0.787	—	—	—
15.7. Paperwork/bureaucracy	—	0.790	—	—	—
How much do you worry about the following problems related to teledermatology?					
16.1. Security and confidentiality of patient data	—	—	0.674	—	—
16.2. Complexity of the devices to carry out teledermatology	—	—	0.803	—	—
16.3. Registration of professional's actions	—	—	0.745	—	—
16.4. The need for specific formation	—	—	0.703	—	—
16.5. Technical difficulties related to the use of ICT	—	—	0.783	—	—
16.6. The time required to perform a teledermatology consultation	—	—	0.714	—	—
How do you think the following factors affect the implementation of teledermatology in usual clinical practice?					
17.1. Patients' preference for face-to-face consultations	—	—	—	0.836	—
17.2. Professionals' preference for face-to-face consultations	—	—	—	0.759	—
17.3. Technological skills of patients	—	—	—	0.763	—
17.4. Technological skills of professionals	—	—	—	—	0.720
17.5. Time dedicated to each patient	—	—	—	—	0.692
17.6. Technological equipment suitable for the teledermatology project	—	—	—	—	0.855
17.7. Financing of the teledermatology program	—	—	—	—	0.723
Variance explained by each factor (%)	17.636	16.458	12.997	11.318	10.889
Cumulative variance (%)	17.636	34.094	47.091	58.409	69.298
Cronbach alpha	.801	.894	.801	.858	.782

[a]Values lower than 0.5 have been suppressed to facilitate reading.

Table 7. Results of the logistic regression (global sample).

Variable	B	Standard error	Wald	df	*P* value	Exp (B)
User's ICT[a] profile	0.430	0.234	3.926	1	*.048* [b]	1.589
Quality of care	0.021	0.194	0.012	1	.91	1.021
System efficiency	0.858	0.197	19.047	1	*<.001*	0.986
Technological difficulties	−0.14	0.199	0.005	1	.95	0.986
Preference of the subjects directly involved	−0.557	0.211	6.982	1	*.008*	0.573
Interest of the administration	0.148	0.195	0.579	1	.45	1.160
Constant	0.928	0.442	4.400	1	.04	2.529

[a]ICT: information and communication technology.

[b]Italicized values mean statistical significance.

Table 8. Results of the general practitioners' subgroup of the logistic regression.

Variable	B	Standard error	Wald	df	*P* value	Exp (B)
User's ICT[a] profile	1.160	0.535	4.708	1	*.03* [b]	3.191
Quality of care	−0.212	0.455	0.216	1	.64	0.809
System efficiency	1.356	0.447	9.202	1	*.002*	3.883
Technological difficulties	0.002	0.330	0.000	1	.995	1.002
Preference of the subjects directly involved	−0.394	0.387	1.038	1	.31	0.674
Interest of the administration	0.090	0.376	0.057	1	.81	1.094
Constant	283	0.804	0.124	1	.73	1.327

[a]ICT: information and communication technology.

[b]Italicized values mean statistical significance.

Table 9. Results of the dermatologists' subgroup of the logistic regression between the factors obtained after an exploratory factorial analysis.

Variable	B	Standard error	Wald	df	*P* value	Exp (B)
User's ICT[a] profile	0.350	0.282	1.324	1	.25	1.384
Quality of care	0.098	0.233	0.178	1	.67	1.103
System efficiency	0.202	0.277	0.531	1	.47	1.224
Technological difficulties	0.040	0.271	0.021	1	.88	1.041
Preference of the subjects directly involved	−0.807	0.353	5.226	1	*.02* [b]	0.446
Interest of the administration	0.167	0.257	0.421	1	.52	1.182
Constant	0.579	0.639	0.819	1	.37	1.784

[a]ICT: information and communication technology.

[b]Italicized values mean statistical significance.

Discussion

Principal Findings

The objective of this study was to identify factors influencing the intention to use TD in a group of GPs and dermatologists. The influence of the typology of the professional (based on the use and expectations of the use of ICT) was also analyzed. To this end, an expanded TAM containing 5 scales that were previously validated [11,12,20] was used. To our knowledge, there are few previous studies regarding the use of TD in a health institution. The study evaluating influencing factors in the intention to use telemedicine by a group of professionals of the Andalusian Health Service deserves special mention. In this study, Villalba-Mora et al [13] concluded that telemedicine was fully adopted. According to these authors, utility perceived by professionals was the main factor related to telemedicine adoption. However, they did not focus on TD implementation, but in all forms of telemedicine in this region, it was found that financial issues remain as a major barrier even with a strong policy commitment from the government. In 2018, Romero et al [6] published a study analyzing TD models in Spanish real practice, focusing on the organization, the technical aspects, and the perceived advantages/disadvantages of Spanish dermatologists but were not able to establish variables influencing their implementation. In their study, TD is being described as implanted in 26% of Spanish hospitals and their health areas. Dermatologists' overall satisfaction with TD is good, scoring a 6.9 on a scale up to 10 [6].

Furthermore, 3 variables of the study showed an influence on the intention to use TD in the global analysis with statistical significance: the user's ICT profile, system efficiency, and preferences of the subjects involved. Regarding the first, as expected, the personal and professional level of use of the internet and social networks of the user makes them prone to the use of telemedicine methods. This result is concordant with that of Pereyra et al [10], where the user's ICT profile was also considered to be a significant factor to established telemedicine use. In addition, another study [13] on the factors associated with the adoption of ICT in Andalusia concluded that the doctor's PU was related to telemedicine adoption. The preferences of the subjects involved have also been a determining variable so that the acceptance and support of professionals and patients is one of the factors that would most influence the implementation of the TD system.

In terms of efficiency, understood as cost reduction, the doctor's PU also showed significance as a determining variable for the implementation of TD. These results overlap those of the acceptance of telemedicine in Malaysia's public hospitals [21]. Cost-effectiveness of TD has been analyzed widely [7]. In 2018, Vidal-Alaball et al [22] carried out a cost-saving analysis comparing TD with dermatology face-to-face visits in Bages, Spain. They demonstrated how TD could save money from administrations, improving the efficiency of the system.

It is important to highlight the lack of significance in terms of the administrations' interest in TD system implementation. In most previous studies [11,21,23], this was a determining factor Pereyra et al established the administrations' interest as the most related factor in the use of telemedicine through the studied institution [10].

Regarding the analysis by subgroups, it is highlighted that the only significant variable in the group of dermatologists was the preference of the subjects involved. Perhaps, the efficiency was not very decisive in this subgroup because it is not the dermatologist who makes the referral (the efficiency was significantly variable in the group of GPs). On the other hand, the ICT profile was only significant in the group of GPs probably because they perform most activities involved at this level, such as taking photographs, editing them, sending the teleconsultation, receiving the answer, and acting accordingly. However, there are several limitations to consider in this study. First, the questionnaire distribution method consisted mainly of a Web-based tool that may have facilitated the response among users with greater familiarity in the use of ICTs, therefore implying a selection bias. Although paper questionnaires were also delivered, the answers through this format were scarce in number (32 vs 201). In addition, some user subgroups were underrepresented in our sample, such as dermatology residents (only 14 participants).

However, even considering the previously mentioned limitations, we could establish some recommendations to implement a TD system. Priority should be given to projects associating efficient, agile, and easy-to-use systems, resulting in a reduction of both economic and temporary costs in the medical practice. Projects that implement the ICT profile of users adapting to them to facilitate the implementation of the TD should also be encouraged.

Given the large differences expected in each population or health system (economic, social, cultural factors, and use of ICT), the determining variables to implement a TD or telemedicine system are likely to show great variability. It is therefore necessary to carry out more studies before the implementation of these systems. This will allow better adaptability to different target populations, thus multiplying acceptance and usefulness possibilities.

Conclusions

Despite its many advantages, the implementation of teledermatology (TD) is still low in some areas. To better understand this phenomenon, it is necessary for a comprehensive program of TD determinants of use. On the basis of an extended TAM, we obtained the following after an EFA of 3 determinants of TD use: user's information and communication technology profile, system efficiency, and preference of the subjects involved. According to our results, the quality of assistance, the difficulties because of the use of technology, and the interest of the administration were not decisive factors for the implementation of TD. Given the large differences expected in each population or health system, the determining variables to implement a TD show great variability. As a consequence, further studies are needed to better adapt TD to target populations.

References

1. Chaudhry B, Wang J, Wu S, Maglione M, Mojica W, Roth E, et al. Systematic review: impact of health information technology on quality, efficiency, and costs of medical care. Ann Intern Med 2006 May 16;144(10):742-752. [Medline: 16702590]
2. Schwamm LH, Holloway RG, Amarenco P, Audebert HJ, Bakas T, Chumbler NR, American Heart Association Stroke Council, Interdisciplinary Council on Peripheral Vascular Disease. A review of the evidence for the use of telemedicine within stroke systems of care: a scientific statement from the American Heart Association/American Stroke Association. Stroke 2009 Jul;40(7):2616-2634. [doi: 10.1161/STROKEAHA.109.192360] [Medline: 19423852]
3. Norris AC. Essentials of telemedicine and telecare. Chichester: J Wiley; 2001.

4. Moreno-Ramírez D, Romero-Aguilera G. Teledermatology: From the Tempest of Debate to Calmer Waters. Actas Dermosifiliogr 2016 Jun;107(5):366-368. [doi: 10.1016/j.ad.2016.01.006] [Medline: 26956401]
5. Trettel A, Eissing L, Augustin M. Telemedicine in dermatology: findings and experiences worldwide - a systematic literature review. J Eur Acad Dermatol Venereol 2018 Feb;32(2):215-224. [doi: 10.1111/jdv.14341] [Medline: 28516492]
6. Romero G, de Argila D, Ferrandiz L, Sánchez MP, Vañó S, Taberner R, et al. Practice models in teledermatology in Spain: longitudinal study, 2009-2014. Actas Dermosifiliogr 2018 Sep;109(7):624-630. [doi: 10.1016/j.ad.2018.03.015] [Medline: 29807618]
7. Snoswell C, Finnane A, Janda M, Soyer HP, Whitty JA. Cost-effectiveness of store-and-forward teledermatology: a systematic review. JAMA Dermatol 2016 Jun 01;152(6):702-708. [doi: 10.1001/jamadermatol.2016.0525] [Medline: 27074289]
8. Gimeno Carpio E. Teledermatology: a useful tool for physicians, patients, and administrators? Actas Dermosifiliogr 2018 Sep;109(7):577-578. [doi: 10.1016/j.ad.2018.07.001] [Medline: 30031487]
9. Buendía-Eisman A, Arias-Santiago S, Molina-Leyva A, Gilaberte Y, Fernández-Crehuet P, Husein-ElAhmed H, et al. Outpatient dermatological diagnoses in Spain: results from the national DIADERM random sampling project. Actas Dermosifiliogr 2018 Jun;109(5):416-423. [doi: 10.1016/j.ad.2018.02.003] [Medline: 29571521]
10. Pereyra-Rodriguez JJ, Jiménez-Zarco AI, Saigí-Rubió F. [Factors that determine the intention to use telemedicine in a healthcare organisation]. J Healthc Qual Res 2018;33(6):319-328. [doi: 10.1016/j.jhqr.2018.08.004] [Medline: 30482649]
11. Saigi-Rubió F, Jiménez-Zarco A, Torrent-Sellens J. Determinants of the intention to use telemedicine: evidence from primary care physicians. Int J Technol Assess Health Care 2016 Jan;32(1-2):29-36. [doi: 10.1017/S0266462316000015] [Medline: 27472158]
12. Saigí-Rubió F, Torrent-Sellens J, Jiménez-Zarco A. Drivers of telemedicine use: comparative evidence from samples of Spanish, Colombian and Bolivian physicians. Implement Sci 2014 Oct 08;9:128 [FREE Full text] [doi: 10.1186/s13012-014-0128-6] [Medline: 25293651]
13. Villalba-Mora E, Casas I, Lupiañez-Villanueva F, Maghiros I. Adoption of health information technologies by physicians for clinical practice: the Andalusian case. Int J Med Inform 2015 Jul;84(7):477-485. [doi: 10.1016/j.ijmedinf.2015.03.002] [Medline: 25823578]
14. Davis FD. Perceived usefulness, perceived ease of use, and user acceptance of information technology. MIS Q 1989 Sep;13(3):319. [doi: 10.2307/249008]
15. Hu P, Chau P, Sheng O, Tam K. Examining the technology acceptance model using physician acceptance of telemedicine technology. J Manag 1999;16(2):91-112. [doi: 10.1080/07421222.1999.11518247]
16. Yarbrough AK, Smith TB. Technology acceptance among physicians: a new take on TAM. Med Care Res Rev 2007 Dec;64(6):650-672. [doi: 10.1177/1077558707305942] [Medline: 17717378]
17. Bagozzi R. The legacy of the technology acceptance model and a proposal for a paradigm shift. J Assoc Inf Syst 2007 Apr;8(4):244-254. [doi: 10.17705/1jais.00122]
18. Venkatesh V, Morris MG, Davis G, Davis FD. User acceptance of information technology: toward a unified view. MIS Q 2003;27(3):425-478. [doi: 10.2307/30036540]
19. Parasuraman A, Grewal D. The impact of technology on the quality-value-loyalty chain: a research agenda. J Acad Mark Sci 2000 Jan 01;28(1):168-174. [doi: 10.1177/0092070300281015]
20. Orruño E, Gagnon MP, Asua J, Ben Abdeljelil A. Evaluation of teledermatology adoption by health-care professionals using a modified Technology Acceptance Model. J Telemed Telecare 2011;17(6):303-307. [doi: 10.1258/jtt.2011.101101] [Medline: 21844171]
21. Zailani S, Gilani MS, Nikbin D, Iranmanesh M. Determinants of telemedicine acceptance in selected public hospitals in Malaysia: clinical perspective. J Med Syst 2014 Sep;38(9):111. [doi: 10.1007/s10916-014-0111-4] [Medline: 25038891]
22. Vidal-Alaball J, Garcia Domingo JL, Garcia Cuyàs F, Mendioroz Peña J, Flores Mateo G, Deniel Rosanas J, et al. A cost savings analysis of asynchronous teledermatology compared to face-to-face dermatology in Catalonia. BMC Health Serv Res 2018 Aug 22;18(1):650 [FREE Full text] [doi: 10.1186/s12913-018-3464-4] [Medline: 30134891]
23. Keshvari H, Haddadpoor A, Taheri B, Nasri M, Aghdak P. Survey determinant factors of telemedicine strategic planning from the managers and experts perspective in the health department, isfahan university of medical sciences. Acta Inform Med 2014 Oct;22(5):320-324 [FREE Full text] [doi: 10.5455/aim.2014.22.320-324] [Medline: 25568581]

Abbreviations

ANOVA: analysis of variance
EFA: exploratory factorial analysis
GP: general practitioner
ICT: information and communication technology
PU: perceived utility
TAM: Technological Acceptance Model
TD: teledermatology
TRA: theory of reasoned action

6

Evaluating the Experiences of New and Existing Teledermatology Patients During the COVID-19 Pandemic

Judy Hamad[1], MPH; Amy Fox[1], MD; Maria Suzanne Kammire[1], BS; Alison Nancy Hollis[1], BS; Saif Khairat[2,3], MPH, PhD

[1]Department of Dermatology, School of Medicine, University of North Carolina at Chapel Hill, Chapel Hill, NC, United States

[2]Carolina Health Informatics Program, University of North Carolina at Chapel Hill, Chapel Hill, NC, United States

[3]Healthcare Systems, School of Nursing, University of North Carolina at Chapel Hill, Chapel Hill, NC, United States

Corresponding Author:
Saif Khairat, MPH, PhD
Carolina Health Informatics Program
University of North Carolina at Chapel Hill
428 Carrington Hall
Chapel Hill, NC, 27514
United States

Email: saif@unc.edu

Abstract

Background: As teledermatology has been widely adopted during the COVID-19 pandemic, it is essential to examine patients' experiences and satisfaction with teledermatology.

Objective: We aimed to assess the teledermatology experiences of new and existing clinic patients in the context of the rapid shift toward teledermatology practices during the COVID-19 pandemic.

Methods: We conducted a cross-sectional study of 184 teledermatology patients who were assessed during the COVID-19 pandemic at a major southeastern medical center from May 13 to June 5, 2020. The primary outcome was patient satisfaction levels among new and existing patients. The secondary outcome was patients' willingness to use teledermatology in the future.

Results: Of the 288 teledermatology patients who were assessed during the study period, 184 (63.9%) completed the survey. Patients reported high overall satisfaction with teledermatology, with 86.4% (159/184) of participants reporting positive overall satisfaction and experiences with teledermatology. New patients had significantly higher Likert scores for overall satisfaction with teledermatology than those of follow-up patients (new patients: mean 4.70; existing patients: mean 4.43; *P*=.03). Overall, patients' satisfaction with teledermatology did not significantly differ based on age (*P*=.36), race and ethnicity (*P*=.46), education level (*P*=.11), residence (*P*=.74), or insurance status (*P*=.74). There were no significant differences in overall satisfaction between patients with and without prior telehealth experience (*P*=.53), between the video and telephone visit types (*P*=.17), and among platform types (*P*=.22). Prior telehealth experience was associated with higher odds of being willing to use telehealth in the future (odds ratio 2.39, 95% CI 1.31-4.35; *P*=.004).

Conclusions: This cross-sectional survey study demonstrates that during the rapid expansion of teledermatology, new clinic patients had significantly higher scores for overall satisfaction with their teledermatology experience compared to those of established clinic patients (*P*=.03). Prior telehealth experience was associated with higher odds of being willing to use teledermatology in the future. Overall, teledermatology expansion was met with high levels of patient satisfaction during the COVID-19 pandemic.

KEYWORDS

teledermatology; telehealth; patient satisfaction; patient-centered outcomes; COVID-19; dermatology; implementation; virtual health; digital health; cross-sectional

Introduction

With the rapid shift toward converting office-based dermatology clinics into web-based clinics during the COVID-19 pandemic [1,2], teledermatology has been increasingly used in clinical practice and has been a common subject of scientific literature in the past year [3]. Prior to the continuation of widespread teledermatology implementation, it is imperative that dermatologists examine patients' experiences with teledermatology. The exchange of information through video, audio, and imagery has made it possible for dermatologists to visualize, diagnose, and communicate with patients throughout the pandemic. This rapid evolution has also resulted in the recognition of web-based services by most health insurance organizations [4,5] and the recording of telemedicine encounters in electronic health records. These changes will allow teledermatology to remain a prominent communication method in the future of the field.

Patients' experiences likely differ based on patient-provider relationships and whether patients are new clinic patients or established clinic patients. Although some studies have reported high patient satisfaction after the use of teledermatology for new referrals or consults [6-9], to our knowledge there are no studies that examine new and existing patients' satisfaction with teledermatology. Our objective was to assess new and existing patients' satisfaction with teledermatology in the context of the COVID-19 pandemic–related rapid shift toward teledermatology practices.

Methods

Study Design

We conducted a cross-sectional study of teledermatology patients' satisfaction during the COVID-19 pandemic at a major southeastern medical center. The rationale for this quality improvement initiative was to characterize patients' experiences with teledermatology in order to improve our delivery of this mode of care. We reported this study per the Standards for Quality Improvement Report Excellence 2.0 guidelines [10]. This study was exempt from institutional review board approval due to its quality improvement objectives.

Study Materials and Participants

Eligible participants were new and existing patients who attended teledermatology visits for acute and chronic conditions. Patients were invited to complete a postvisit survey, which was a voluntary survey that was adapted from a validated telehealth satisfaction study [11]. We recorded survey responses by using the web-based survey tool Qualtrics. We piloted the survey among 22 patients and made iterative survey changes based on patients' and service providers' feedback. We included responses from the piloted survey in the analysis, as there were minimal survey changes. We administered the survey from May 13 to June 5, 2020, to the patients of 8 dermatologists who delivered adult and pediatric teledermatology services. All patients who used adult and pediatric teledermatology services during the study period were eligible for inclusion in this study; however, the parents or guardians of pediatric patients completed the survey.

Survey Questions

The survey instrument was adapted from the Telehealth Satisfaction Scale and modified by a telehealth domain expert so that the survey met the needs of this study. The survey consisted of 25 questions that addressed demographics, visit characteristics, and satisfaction measures (Multimedia Appendix 1). Patients reported whether they were new or existing patients of the clinic, whether they were telehealth-experienced patients or telehealth-naïve patients (no prior telehealth experience), and whether they were willing to use telehealth in the future (answered "yes" or "no"). Patients rated their satisfaction with 12 items on a Likert scale (1=poor; 2=fair; 3=good; 4=very good; 5=excellent). Satisfaction-related items included patients' overall satisfaction with teledermatology, patient-related outcomes (personal comfort with teledermatology, the ease of using teledermatology, and respect for patients' privacy), the voice and visual quality of the visit, time characteristics (the length of wait time and the length of time with the service provider), and service provider–related outcomes (treatment explanations, thoroughness, and the courtesy of the provider).

Outcomes

The primary outcome was satisfaction levels among new and existing patients. The secondary outcome was patients' willingness to use teledermatology in the future.

Statistical Analysis

Satisfaction ratings of very good and excellent were considered positive ratings. Continuous measures were reported as means with SDs. Categorical variables were reported as numbers and percentages. Fisher exact tests were used for categorical variables, and *t* tests and one-way analysis of covariance tests were used to determine differences in the means of continuous variables. Univariable logistic regression was conducted to identify predictors of willingness to use teledermatology in the future. Statistical analyses were performed using Stata 16 (StataCorp LLC). A *P* value of <.05 was considered statistically significant.

Results

Study Population Characteristics

Of the 288 teledermatology patients assessed, 184 (63.9%) completed the survey (Table 1). The mean age of participants was 37.8 years, and 72.8% (134/184) of participants were females. Most teledermatology visits were conducted for existing patients (123/184; 66.8%) and telehealth-naïve patients (107/184; 58.2%). Most respondents were White (114/184; 62.0%) and had a Bachelor's degree or other higher education degree (92/184; 50%). The majority of the respondents were privately insured (109/184; 59.2%), a large subset of patients had public insurance (69/184; 37.5%), and a minority of patients were uninsured (6/184; 3.3%).

Table 1. Participants' characteristics (N=184).

Characteristic	Value
Age (years), mean (SD)	37.8 (18.3)
Sex, n (%)	
Male	50 (27.2)
Female	134 (72.8)
Race, n (%)	
White	114 (62)
Black/African American	44 (23.9)
Hispanic/Latino	12 (6.5)
Asian/Pacific Islander	10 (5.4)
Other	4 (2.2)
Education level, n (%)	
Less than high school	21 (11.4)
High school or equivalent	32 (17.4)
Some college	28 (15.2)
Associate degree	11 (6)
Bachelor's degree	46 (25)
Graduate, doctorate, or professional degree	46 (25)
Residence, n (%)	
Urban	47 (25.5)
Suburban	87 (47.3)
Rural	50 (27.2)
Unique patient zip codes reached, n	84
Insurance status, n (%)	
Uninsured	6 (3.3)
Private insurance	109 (59.2)
Medicare, Medicaid, or Tricare	69 (37.5)
Impairments, n (%)	
Visual	29 (15.8)
Auditory	5 (2.7)
Both	3 (1.6)
None	147 (79.9)
Patient type, n (%)	
New	61 (33.1)
Existing	123 (66.8)
Prior telehealth experience, n (%)	
Yes (telehealth-experienced patient)	77 (41.8)
No (telehealth-naïve patient)	107 (58.2)
Visit type, n (%)	
Video	171 (92.9)
Telephone	13 (7.1)

Patient-Reported Satisfaction

Patients reported high overall satisfaction with teledermatology (Figure 1), with 86.4% (159/184) of participants reporting a positive teledermatology experience. New patients had significantly higher Likert scores for overall satisfaction with teledermatology than those of follow-up patients (new patients: mean 4.70; follow-up patients: mean 4.43; P=.03). Patients' satisfaction with teledermatology did not significantly differ based on age (P=.36), race and ethnicity (P=.46), education level (P=.11), residence (P=.74), or insurance status (P=.74). There were no significant differences in overall satisfaction between patients with and without prior telehealth experience (P=.53) and between the video and telephone visit types (P=.17). In terms of all of the satisfaction measures, new patients reported higher satisfaction scores compared to those reported by existing patients; however, these differences were not statistically significant (Figure 2).

Figure 1. Patient-centered satisfaction outcomes following the completion of teledermatology visits.

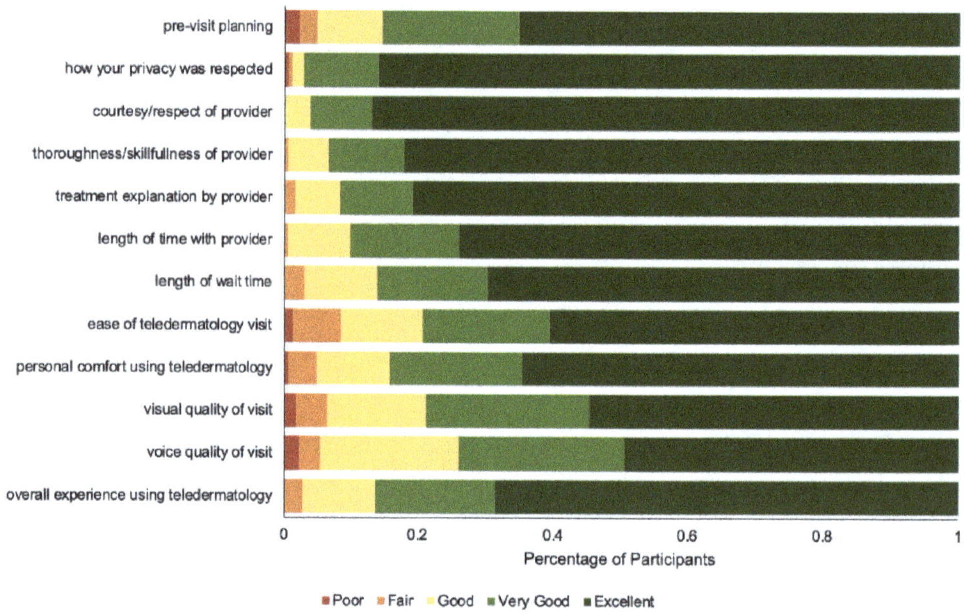

Figure 2. New and follow-up patients' overall satisfaction with teledermatology.

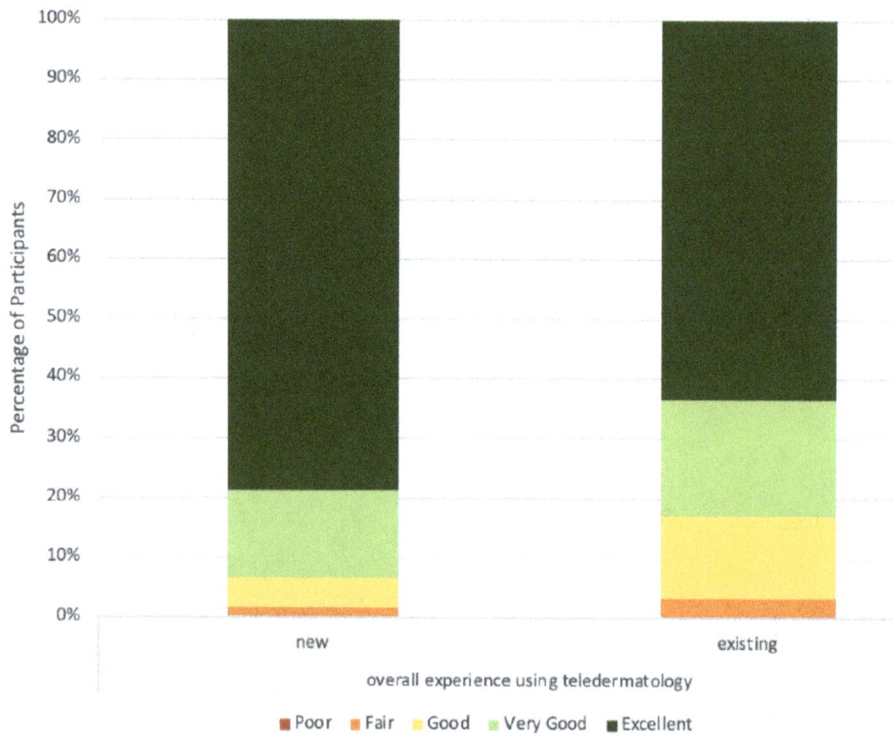

Patients' personal comfort with using telehealth and the ease of using telehealth were similar between new and follow-up patients (Figure 3). Participants reported high satisfaction with the privacy of telehealth visits, with 85.2% (52/61) of new patients and 82% (100/122) of follow-up patients rating their satisfaction as "excellent" (Figure 3). Patients' satisfaction with previsit planning was different between the two groups (*P*=.15); follow-up patients reported lower levels of satisfaction (excellent: 75/123, 61%; very good: 28/123, 22.8%; good: 11/123, 8.9%; fair: 5/123, 4.1%; poor: 4/123, 3.3%), while new patients reported slightly higher levels of satisfaction with the teledermatology process (excellent: 45/61, 73.7%; very good: 9/61, 14.8%; good: 7/61, 11.5%; fair and poor: 0/61, 0%; Figure 3). Participants' overall satisfaction with the voice quality of visits was low, and follow-up patients' satisfaction with voice quality was lower than new patients' satisfaction. Patients' satisfaction with visual quality was slightly higher than their satisfaction with voice quality and similar between follow-up patients and new patients. The length of wait time, length of time with the service provider, and provider-related satisfaction were highly rated among participants.

Figure 3. New and follow-up patients' satisfaction with the following patient-related outcomes: comfort, ease, privacy, and previsit planning experiences.

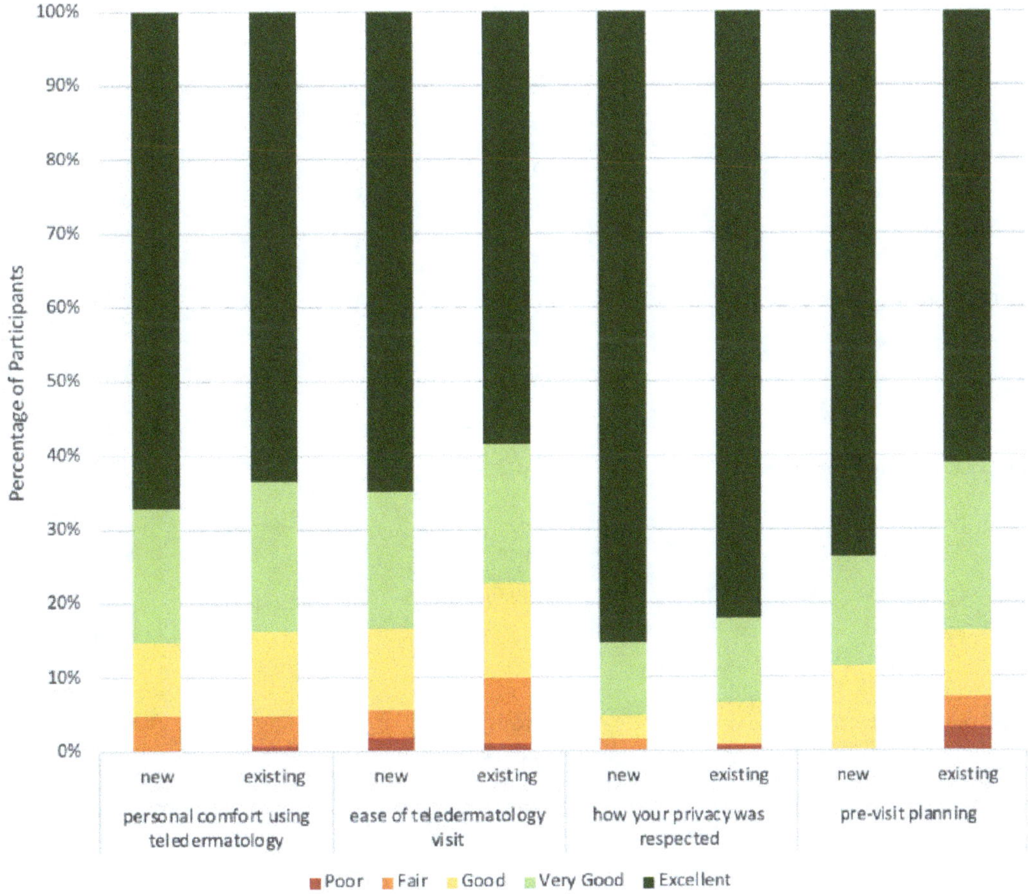

Willingness to Use Teledermatology in the Future

Our univariable logistic regression showed that prior telehealth experience was associated with higher odds of being willing to use teledermatology in the future (odds ratio [OR] 2.39, 95% CI 1.31-4.35; *P*=.004). Age, sex, race, education, residence, and insurance status were not associated with significant odds of preferring teledermatology (Table 2). Compared to new patients, existing patients had nonsignificantly higher odds of using of telehealth in the future (OR 1.46, 95% CI 0.79-2.72; *P*=.23).

Table 2. Univariate logistic regression results for predicting patient's willingness to use teledermatology in the future.

Predictor	Preferred telehealth, odds ratio (95% CI)	*P* value
Age (years)		
<18	Referent	N/A[a]
18-34	1.51 (0.54-4.24)	.44
35-64	1.14 (0.40-3.25)	.80
≥65	0.42 (0.11-1.55)	.11
Sex		
Female	Referent	N/A
Male	1.16 (0.61-2.23)	.65
Race		
White	Referent	N/A
Black/African American	1.19 (0.59-2.39)	.62
Other	1.19 (0.51-2.80)	.69
Education level		
Less than high school	Referent	N/A
High school or equivalent	0.62 (0.21-1.89)	.40
Some college	0.43 (0.13-1.38)	.16
Associate degree	0.20 (0.03-1.17)	.08
Bachelor's degree	1.41 (0.50-4.01)	.51
Graduate, doctorate, or professional degree	0.99 (0.35-2.79)	.99
Residence		
Rural	Referent	N/A
Suburban	1.23 (0.61-2.48)	.56
Urban	1.57 (0.70-3.50)	.70
Insurance status		
Medicare, Medicaid, or Tricare	Referent	N/A
Private insurance	1.2 (0.66-2.20)	.55
Uninsured	0.61 (0.11-3.57)	.59
Patient type		
New	Referent	N/A
Follow-up	1.46 (0.79-2.72)	.23
Prior telehealth experience		
No	Referent	N/A
Yes	2.39 (1.31-4.35)	.004

[a]N/A: not applicable.

Discussion

Principal Findings

We conducted an evaluation of teledermatology implementation as a response to the COVID-19 crisis. Although there is a limited number of prior teledermatology studies that evaluate patients' satisfaction, this study found that patients' satisfaction was high across numerous key measures. We found that 97.3% (179/184) of patients reported a positive overall experience with teledermatology (ratings of good, very good, or excellent). These findings are consistent with those of prior teledermatology studies in related literature [7-9]. Additionally, we found that patients' overall satisfaction with telehealth did not vary significantly based on patients' demographic characteristics, locations of residence, education, or insurance status.

Our results demonstrated that new patients had significantly higher overall scores for satisfaction with teledermatology than those of existing patients (*P*=.03). Furthermore, new patients reported higher satisfaction for all satisfaction metrics. This may be due to the fact that new patients did not have prior in-person experiences with the dermatologist that they were seeing; therefore, they could not compare different teledermatology experiences. Furthermore, existing patients may have been more inclined to compare their teledermatology visit to those they experienced in person. This high satisfaction among new patients could also be related to the fact that we reached out to geographically diverse patients across 84 zip codes who were enthusiastic about having increased access to dermatology services.

Interestingly, over half of our participants (107/184, 58.2%) never used telehealth services prior to their teledermatology visit during the COVID-19 pandemic. In an Italian study of teledermatology patients of an acne center that was conducted during the COVID-19 pandemic, patients reported favorable experiences, and 92% of patients appreciated their visits [12]. This was similar to our study. However, the Italian study's patient population entirely consisted of existing patients. In contrast, we observed various conditions among the new and existing patients, especially among telehealth-naïve patients. We found that prior telehealth experience was associated with a willingness to use teledermatology in the future. The increasing awareness of telehealth benefits, such as time and cost savings, among patients with no telehealth experience may help mitigate people's resistance to future telehealth use [13]. Additionally, because people compare prior in-person visits to teledermatology visits, our patients may have considered in-person visits to be more thorough than video visits. The deployment of teledermatology during our study period likely reflected the broader use of telehealth for conditions other than those that would be present after the COVID-19 pandemic and the need for disease-specific scheduling algorithms, which can ensure that the telehealth modality suits the target condition. However, the overall satisfaction of both new and follow-up patients was extremely positive, and the expansion of teledermatology services seemed to be well received by patients.

The impacts of the national health crisis have undoubtedly influenced patients' perception of care and have likely influenced patients' willingness to engage in teledermatology in a way that is unprecedented in prior studies. We suspect that at least a portion of the highly positive responses to teledermatology visits from our surveyed patients was due to teledermatology providing patients with the ability to avoid high-risk settings and continue to practice social distancing by staying at their homes [14]. In addition, many patients travel long distances to be seen by specialists at the clinic and are pleased to save time, money, and energy by not having to physically appear at clinics. It is for these reasons that the amplification of the role of telehealth has been regarded as a silver lining or "bright spot" of the pandemic [15-18]. Although the Centers for Medicare & Medicaid Services have provided payment parity for telehealth visits and service providers can bill patients for telehealth visits at the same rates as in-person visit rates, patients have likely saved money by taking less time off of work and not having to consider gas costs for trips to clinics.

Limitations

The findings of our research are limited by the nature of our study. First, this study reported findings from a single cross-sectional sample of patients who were treated by 8 participating dermatologists. Although patients were recruited consecutively at the end of telehealth visits, several patients did not stay on the phone or video call to immediately complete the survey. It is possible that patients who did not complete the survey had characteristics that considerably differed from the characteristics of those who did complete the survey, given that we had a nonresponse rate of 36%. Participants in this study were more likely to be White; educated; insured; and, on average, younger than the general population. Although we did not find statistical differences in satisfaction based on the many demographic characteristics we analyzed, it is possible that a larger sample size would have resulted in the observation of important differences in satisfaction. One study reported a potential disparity—the decreased amount of video visit use among older adults [19]. This highlighted the following key questions: (1) which populations do or do not have access to telehealth, and (2) how does this impact disparities in care? Second, this study took place at a single dermatology department at an academic institution. Thus, we cannot generalize our results to the larger dermatology patient population. Third, we did not collect information regarding diagnosis; it is plausible that patients' satisfaction with telehealth may differ based on dermatologic conditions that require more or less complicated management. Finally, we observed a ceiling effect in our data. Since satisfaction scores were rated on a Likert scale of 1-5, the ratings tended to be grouped at the higher end of the scale. This ceiling effect likely resulted in less variability among the data and limited our ability to test associations or build multivariable regression models.

Conclusion

We report that the rapid expansion of teledermatology resulted in new patients reporting higher satisfaction with their teledermatology experiences compared to the satisfaction of existing patients of the clinic. Prior telehealth experience was associated with higher odds of being willing to use teledermatology in the future. The rapid adoption of teledermatology during the study period was met with high overall levels of patient satisfaction during the COVID-19 pandemic. The deployment of teledermatology during our study period likely reflected the broader use of telehealth for conditions other than those that would be present after the COVID-19 pandemic and highlighted the need for disease-specific scheduling algorithms, which can ensure that the telehealth modality suits the target condition.

Authors' Contributions

JH was responsible for data collection and analysis. AF was the domain expert who assisted with the study design and data collection. ANH was responsible for manuscript preparation. MSK was responsible for manuscript preparation and data analysis. SK was responsible for study design and analysis.

References

1. Perkins S, Cohen JM, Nelson CA, Bunick CG. Teledermatology in the era of COVID-19: Experience of an academic department of dermatology. J Am Acad Dermatol 2020 Jul;83(1):e43-e44 [FREE Full text] [doi: 10.1016/j.jaad.2020.04.048] [Medline: 32305442]
2. Price KN, Thiede R, Shi VY, Curiel-Lewandrowski C. Strategic dermatology clinical operations during the coronavirus disease 2019 (COVID-19) pandemic. J Am Acad Dermatol 2020 Jun;82(6):e207-e209 [FREE Full text] [doi: 10.1016/j.jaad.2020.03.089] [Medline: 32277972]
3. Doraiswamy S, Abraham A, Mamtani R, Cheema S. Use of telehealth during the COVID-19 pandemic: Scoping review. J Med Internet Res 2020 Dec 01;22(12):e24087. [doi: 10.2196/24087] [Medline: 33147166]
4. Medicare telemedicine health care provider fact sheet. Centers for Medicare & Medicaid Services. URL: https://www.cms.gov/newsroom/fact-sheets/medicare-telemedicine-health-care-provider-fact-sheet [accessed 2021-04-28]
5. Notification of enforcement discretion for telehealth remote communications during the COVID-19 nationwide public health emergency. Health & Human Services Health Information Privacy. URL: https://www.hhs.gov/hipaa/for-professionals/special-topics/emergency-preparedness/notification-enforcement-discretion-telehealth/index.html [accessed 2021-04-28]
6. Marchell R, Locatis C, Burgess G, Maisiak R, Liu W, Ackerman M. Patient and provider satisfaction with teledermatology. Telemed J E Health 2017 Aug;23(8):684-690 [FREE Full text] [doi: 10.1089/tmj.2016.0192] [Medline: 28375822]
7. Mounessa JS, Chapman S, Braunberger T, Qin R, Lipoff JB, Dellavalle RP, et al. A systematic review of satisfaction with teledermatology. J Telemed Telecare 2018 May;24(4):263-270. [doi: 10.1177/1357633X17696587] [Medline: 28350281]
8. Mair F, Whitten P. Systematic review of studies of patient satisfaction with telemedicine. BMJ 2000 Jun 03;320(7248):1517-1520 [FREE Full text] [doi: 10.1136/bmj.320.7248.1517] [Medline: 10834899]
9. Hills Z, Khairat S. Teledermatology: Using collaborative technologies to enhance public health awareness. 2014 Presented at: 2014 International Conference on Collaboration Technologies and Systems (CTS); May 19-23, 2014; Minneapolis, MN, USA. [doi: 10.1109/cts.2014.6867599]
10. Ogrinc G, Davies L, Goodman D, Batalden P, Davidoff F, Stevens D. SQUIRE 2.0 (Standards for QUality Improvement Reporting Excellence): revised publication guidelines from a detailed consensus process. BMJ Qual Saf 2016 Dec;25(12):986-992 [FREE Full text] [doi: 10.1136/bmjqs-2015-004411] [Medline: 26369893]
11. Morgan DG, Kosteniuk J, Stewart N, O'Connell ME, Karunanayake C, Beever R. The telehealth satisfaction scale: reliability, validity, and satisfaction with telehealth in a rural memory clinic population. Telemed J E Health 2014 Nov;20(11):997-1003 [FREE Full text] [doi: 10.1089/tmj.2014.0002] [Medline: 25272141]
12. Ruggiero A, Megna M, Annunziata MC, Abategiovanni L, Scalvenzi M, Tajani A, et al. Teledermatology for acne during COVID-19: high patients' satisfaction in spite of the emergency. J Eur Acad Dermatol Venereol 2020 Nov;34(11):e662-e663 [FREE Full text] [doi: 10.1111/jdv.16746] [Medline: 32534472]
13. Al Quran HA, Khader YS, Ellauzi ZM, Shdaifat A. Effect of real-time teledermatology on diagnosis, treatment and clinical improvement. J Telemed Telecare 2015 Mar;21(2):93-99. [doi: 10.1177/1357633X14566572] [Medline: 25589469]
14. Fisk M, Livingstone A, Pit SW. Telehealth in the context of COVID-19: Changing perspectives in Australia, the United Kingdom, and the United States. J Med Internet Res 2020 Jun 09;22(6):e19264 [FREE Full text] [doi: 10.2196/19264] [Medline: 32463377]
15. Sharma A, Jindal V, Singla P, Goldust M, Mhatre M. Will teledermatology be the silver lining during and after COVID-19? Dermatol Ther 2020 Jul;33(4):e13643 [FREE Full text] [doi: 10.1111/dth.13643] [Medline: 32441373]
16. Olayiwola JN, Magaña C, Harmon A, Nair S, Esposito E, Harsh C, et al. Telehealth as a bright spot of the COVID-19 pandemic: Recommendations from the virtual frontlines ("Frontweb"). JMIR Public Health Surveill 2020 Jun 25;6(2):e19045 [FREE Full text] [doi: 10.2196/19045] [Medline: 32479413]
17. Khairat S, Haithcoat T, Liu S, Zaman T, Edson B, Gianforcaro R, et al. Advancing health equity and access using telemedicine: a geospatial assessment. J Am Med Inform Assoc 2019 Aug 01;26(8-9):796-805 [FREE Full text] [doi: 10.1093/jamia/ocz108] [Medline: 31340022]
18. Khairat S, Lin X, Liu S, Man Z, Zaman T, Edson B, et al. Evaluation of patient experience during virtual and in-person urgent care visits: Time and cost analysis. J Patient Exp 2021 Jan 12;8:1-8 [FREE Full text] [doi: 10.1177/2374373520981487]
19. Schifeling CH, Shanbhag P, Johnson A, Atwater RC, Koljack C, Parnes BL, et al. Disparities in video and telephone visits among older adults during the COVID-19 pandemic: Cross-sectional analysis. JMIR Aging 2020 Nov 10;3(2):e23176 [FREE Full text] [doi: 10.2196/23176] [Medline: 33048821]

Abbreviations

OR: odds ratio

7

Impact of an Intrainstitutional Teledermatology Service: Mixed-Methods Case Study

Trevor Champagne[1], BSc, BMath (Hons), MD, FRCP; Peter G Rossos[2,3,4], MD, MBA, FRCP, FACP; Veronica Kirk[2], BSc; Emily Seto[2,3], PEng, PhD

[1]Division of Dermatology, Women's College Hospital, University of Toronto, Toronto, ON, Canada

[2]Institute of Health Policy, Management and Evaluation, Dalla Lana School of Public Health, University of Toronto, Toronto, ON, Canada

[3]Centre for Global eHealth Innovation, University Health Network and Techna Institute, Toronto, ON, Canada

[4]Department of Medicine, Dalla Lana School of Public Health, University of Toronto, Toronto, ON, Canada

Corresponding Author:
Trevor Champagne, BSc, BMath (Hons), MD, FRCP
Division of Dermatology
Women's College Hospital
University of Toronto
76 Grenville Street, Room 3415
Toronto, ON, M5S 1B2
Canada

Email: trevor.champagne@wchospital.ca

Abstract

Background: Teledermatology provides timely access to consultative dermatology services while reducing the need for travel among patients in rural and underserviced areas. However, knowledge about the potential benefits of such a service in urban areas is limited.

Objective: This study aimed to determine the impact of a geographically unrestricted, intrainstitutional, secure, email teledermatology service for dermatology.

Methods: We employed a mixed-methods approach using chart review, surveys, and semistructured interviews from the Canada Health Infoway Benefits Evaluation Framework. Patient charts were reviewed for demographics, clinical characteristics, and outcomes. Electronic and paper surveys were sent to patients and providers to quantify aspects of the service, such as satisfaction and usability, on a Likert scale. Semistructured interviews of referring providers and a convenience sample of academic consultant dermatologists who were considering teledermatology for their practice were conducted. Interviews were transcribed and analyzed using manual coding and thematic analysis by both the primary author and a second independent reviewer. All results were concurrently triangulated in an overarching analysis.

Results: A total of 76 consultations were reviewed over a period of 18 months, of which 84% were completely managed without an in-person visit. Only 6% of rashes required a subsequent in-person visit to a dermatologist for management, compared to 41% of lesions. In addition, 28% (21/76) of patients responded to the survey. Patients "strongly agreed" to use the service again, were satisfied with the management of their skin issue, and thought the service saved them time. In general, providers who answered the electronic survey "strongly agreed" that the service demonstrated quality, timeliness, and an educational benefit, but increased their administrative time. A total of 9 interviews of 5 referring providers and 4 dermatologists were completed. Triangulation of all study components supported the hypothesis that teledermatology benefits providers, patients, and the health care system.

Conclusions: Intrainstitutional teledermatology has high satisfaction among patients and providers and saves patients time, even when there are no geographic or systemic barriers to access. This service may be most effective when targeted at rashes rather than lesions. Additional research on the cost-effectiveness and educational benefits of this service is warranted.

KEYWORDS

dermatology; e-health; teledermatology

Introduction

Teledermatology allows dermatologists to manage patients with generally equivalent clinical outcomes and requires less resources and less time with the consultant than in-person visits [1]. Its impact is evident in geographic areas that do not have timely access to dermatology, which is the most-studied aspect of teledermatology; for example, in the United States, 80% of dermatologists are clustered in 3 large metropolitan areas [2]. There is a similar disproportionate clustering of dermatologists in metropolitan areas in Canada [3]. These substantial disparities in the geographic distribution of dermatologists have been increasing [4].

Knowledge of the potential of *intrainstitutional* teledermatology, wherein geographic access is not a factor of the net benefit assessment of the value of teledermatology, is limited. Other pilot studies have assessed the feasibility and diagnostic concordance of these implementations [5], but formal assessments of their impact are lacking.

We hypothesize that teledermatology will have value beyond geographic access if implemented by the consultants and referring physicians intrainstitutionally. We designed this study to investigate the potential benefits, barriers, and impact of teledermatology in such an intrainstitutional setting, where the traditional geographic barriers to access do not exist. We further hoped to identify specific characteristics of the teledermatology service that would be useful for implementing the service at other institutions. Studies have reported the usefulness of teledermatology in only a few specific scenarios, and there is disagreement about the clinical conditions that are suitable for teledermatology in the literature; for example, several studies have reported the potential of teledermatology for identifying any suspicious skin lesions [6,7]; in contrast, the American Telemedicine Association guidelines for teledermatology [8] state that it is difficult to assess pigmented lesions and special sites such as the scalp with teledermatology.

Methods

Overview

We performed a mixed-methods evaluation using broad categories of the Canada Health Infoway (CHI) Benefits Evaluation Framework [9] to include at least one aspect of qualitative and quantitative analyses for each category as well as case studies, surveys, and semistructured interviews. The key results were triangulated in a final, overarching analysis. This study was approved by the research ethics boards of Women's College Hospital and the University of Toronto in Toronto, Ontario, Canada.

Design of the Intrainstitutional Teledermatology Service

Parameters were chosen to balance convenience (encourage use) and pragmatic considerations of the practice guidelines for teledermatology [8]. We selected a store-and-forward design with secondary teledermatology, as it is a funded model in our region, and secure institutional email as a common, accessible technology. Clinically, the referring providers were informed that they could send any request they deemed appropriate and a response would be guaranteed within 1 week. The primary author was the sole consultant providing responses. The details of the implementation are described in Table 1.

Table 1. Components of the intrainstitutional teledermatology service and the rationale for choosing the components.

Component	Rationale
Modality	
Asynchronous	Most-convenient method for the consultant dermatologist and requires the least amount of coordination or additional technology
Secondary teledermatology (referring a health care provider to a consultant dermatologist)	Meets identity and privacy guideline requirements, and secondary teledermatology is a regionally insured service by the provincial government
Technology	
Secure intrainstitutional email	A convenient, ubiquitous technology that is secure; limited to institutional use, with no barrier to entry; and shared across clinics
Photography	Referring providers were requested to provide in-focus images; at least one close-up image; and if widespread, photos representing the overall distribution
Clinical	
One-week response time	A four-fold improvement over existing wait times at our institution, and enough time to discourage urgent consultations through this service, which would be better provided at an emergency care institution
Free-form text permitted (no template)	To permit benefit evaluation, we did not restrict the clinical use of the system or make implicit suggestions about what conditions would be appropriate

Data Collection

Chart Review

Stored medical records for each consultation were reviewed from service initiation in late 2016 through 2017. All patients were previously registered in the hospital electronic medical record system, as they were a part of the referring family-practice unit. Contact information was collected for emailing or mailing surveys. Demographic information including age and gender was collated. Each chart was reviewed for clinical characteristics including diagnosis and management. For each patient, the hospital-wide electronic medical record was additionally reviewed for evidence of treatment failure, symptom recurrence of the treated dermatosis, or any other pertinent follow-up information.

Referring Provider Survey

Emails for each referring attending provider who submitted at least one consultation request were collated, and an email invitation from SurveyMonkey [10] was sent to request their participation in an electronic survey assessing satisfaction, time expenditure, educational value, and adverse events, which ranked these parameters on a Likert scale. If the provider did not complete the survey, invitations were resent 2 weeks and 1 month after the initial invitation. Health care providers rated each question on a scale of 1-7, where 1 was "Strongly disagree," 7 was "Strongly agree," and 4 was "Neutral."

Patient Survey

Patients were invited to participate in a survey assessing satisfaction with the service, potential benefits, and attitudes toward teledermatology. Email invitations were sent to the subset of patients who had provided an email address for hospital registration. An email was resent a month after the initial invitation if a survey was not received by the patient. For all patients, a paper survey with a self-addressed, stamped return envelope was mailed. Patients rated each question on a scale of 1-7, where 1 was "Strongly disagree," 7 was "Strongly agree," and 4 was "Neutral." The responses were averaged and interpreted according to the final score.

Participants were offered the opportunity to submit their email at the end of the study to be entered in a draw to receive a Can $100 gift card.

Referring Provider and Potential Consultant Semistructured Interviews

In the email invitations mentioned above (see Patient Survey section), referring providers were invited to participate in a semistructured interview exploring the perceived impact, current use, and attitudes and opinions toward teledermatology. Similarly, potential consultant dermatologists identified from a convenience sample of dermatologists in academic practice in the same hospital setting, who could potentially participate in a teledermatology service, were recruited via email for the semistructured interviews. Interview guidelines were prepared using the categories of the CHI Benefits Evaluation Framework to complement other data-collection strategies assessing satisfaction, use, educational benefits, and experience and attitudes toward teledermatology. The primary author conducted interviews over a 3-month period after study initiation, with no other parties present. The interviews were audio-recorded and subsequently transcribed verbatim from the recordings by a professional transcription service.

Data Analysis

Chart Review

Demographic and clinical information including complaints and diagnoses was collected. The primary author characterized complaints as "lesion," "rash," or "other," depending on whether the consultation was consistent with multiple or progressive skin findings over a generalized area (rash) or a single, stable skin finding in a localized area (lesion). We recorded the immediate follow-up plan including recommendation for subsequent in-person consultation, optional in-person consultation if the issue was not resolved by the prescribed method, and the proposed timing.

Referring Provider and Patient Surveys

Results from the Likert scales were collated, and the scores averaged with standard deviation. Free-form text answers were collated and reviewed using word cloud analysis and manual inspection for incorporation of the patterns or pertinent feedback into the final triangulation.

Referring Provider and Potential Consultant Interviews

For each set of interviews, the primary author and a secondary independent reviewer conducted independent qualitative analyses according to the interpretive description [11]. The transcripts were sequentially reviewed and evaluated with reference to categories from the CHI Benefits Evaluation Framework. Thematic analysis was used to identify unique emerging concepts potentially beyond the scope of the interview guide. The independent reviewers submitted their qualitative analyses to the primary author for review. Identified themes from both sets of analyses were included in the final mixed-methods analysis. No discordant themes required dispute management by a third party.

Mixed-Methods Concurrent Triangulation

For the final overarching analysis, we used the CHI Benefits Evaluation Framework to organize a mixed-methods concurrent triangulation strategy that used both qualitative and quantitative assessment methods. We added the evaluative components of potential educational benefits to this strategy. Emergent themes derived from any component were triangulated with other data analyses to support the conclusions.

Results

Chart Review

A total of 76 participants used the service between November 2016 and December 2017, including 17 (22%) pediatric patients, 3 pregnant patients, 28 men (37%), and 48 women (63%). Consultation data for all patients were subjected to chart review. The average age of patients using the service was 39.3 years, and the average response time was 23.5 h, with a minimum response time of 0.5 h and a maximum time of 142.6 h (6 days).

Clinical characteristics were grouped into diagnostic dermatology categories, similar to previous teledermatology evaluations [12], and are presented in Table 2. Each case was broadly categorized into an easily recognizable presenting complaint: a "rash," which presents in multiple areas of the skin with the same general appearance, most typically represented by eczematous dermatoses, infections, or reactive skin conditions; a "lesion," which is a focal, persistent eruption on the skin, typified by benign and malignant growths; or a "question" about a treatment (Table 3). Of all cases, 12 (16%) required a subsequent in-person visit.

We assumed that clinicians would use photographs from a patient visit to their office; however, in 14% of all consultations, parent- or patient-initiated photographs were used. In 6 (35%) of the pediatric cases, photographs for analysis were provided by the parents, and 5 adult patients provided their own photographs to the clinician. None of these patients required additional photographs or in-person follow-up, and cases wherein the data were available, the conditions were appropriately resolved. In one case, the parent-initiated photograph showed evidence of a rare condition that occurs only under specific conditions.

Our results showed that it was possible to manage 94% of "rashes" by teledermatology alone, but only 59% of "lesions" could be managed by this method. Additionally, in 21 cases (27%), the primary management aimed to increase the prescribed potency of or choose a more-effective vehicle for the topical steroid used. Finally, in at least one case, a response time of 24 h permitted initiation of therapy to prevent postherpetic neuralgia complications of herpes zoster; however, the recommended 72-h time window for treatment [13] would have been exceeded if the maximum response time of the service (1 week) was applied in this case.

Referring Provider Survey

Of the 14 invitations sent, we received 11 responses for the online survey (79% response rate). Responses were averaged and interpreted according to the final score. The results of the survey and the Likert interpretation of the average score are presented in Table 4. Feedback was generally very positive for satisfaction and educational value. The clinicians reported that the service did not save any time, but increased the administrative time. However, they indicated that the benefits of the service outweighed the lost time and the service had educational value. No adverse events were reported.

Patient Survey

A total of 76 patients were sent paper surveys and 26 patients, who had provided an email address for provider registration at the institution, were sent a duplicate email invitation.

We received 22 responses (29%). Patients were generally satisfied with the service and reported that it saved time and money and prevented them from missing work. However, their views were divided when they were asked if they "prefer to use this system instead of going to see a specialist in-person." Their responses were instructive: Some patients indicated that they generally prefer in-person consultations, as they provide a greater opportunity to ask questions and clarify the rationale for therapeutic choices. These results are summarized in Table 5.

Table 2. Clinical characteristics of the consultations grouped by diagnostic categories in dermatology.

Diagnosis	Cases (N=76), n (%)[a]	Patients transitioned to in-person consultation (N=76), n (%)[b]
Eczematous or inflammatory (eczema or contact dermatitis)	30 (39)	1 (1)
Infection requiring Intervention (fungal, viral, or bacterial)	10 (13)	0 (0)
Urticarial or self-limited (morbilliform eruptions or pediatric urticaria)	7 (9)	1 (1)
Lesion (malignant, premalignant, indeterminate, or benign)	21 (28)	9 (43)
Other (genetic, acneiform, etc)	8 (11)	1 (1)
Total	76 (100)	12 (16)

[a]Total number of cases seen within the category.

[b]Cases where the primary and only recommendation was that the patient visit a dermatologist in-person.

Table 3. Clinical characteristics of the consultations grouped by the presenting complaint.

Presenting complaint	Cases (N=76), n (%)	Patients transitioned to in-person consultation (N=76), n (%)
Rash	53 (70)	3 (6)
Lesion	22 (29)	9 (41)
Question	1 (1)	0 (0)
Total	76 (100)	12 (16)

Table 4. Health care providers' responses to the survey (N=11).

Question	Mean (SD)	Interpretation
The responses from the dermatologist were complete.	6.6 (0.6)	Strongly agree
The responses from the dermatologist were timely.	6.8 (0.4)	Strongly agree
The service was reliable.	6.5 (0.8)	Strongly agree
I was satisfied with the answers to the clinical questions.	6.5 (0.7)	Strongly agree
I was satisfied with the educational value of the system.	6.4 (0.9)	Strongly agree
The service was easy to use.	6.6 (0.5)	Strongly agree
The educational value of the e-consults was generally superior to that of in-person consult letters.	5.5 (1.2)	Agree
This service saves me time.	4.9 (1.2)	Neither
This service provides advantages to me that outweigh any lost time.	5.8 (1.0)	Agree
This service saves patients time.	6.8 (0.4)	Strongly agree
This service saves the health care system resources.[a]	6.5 (0.7)	Strongly agree

[a]n=10.

Table 5. Patients' responses to the surveys.

Question	n (%)	Mean (SD)	Interpretation
I would want to use this service again.	22 (100)	6.7 (0.6)	Strongly agree
I would recommend this service to a friend or family member.	21 (95)	6.6 (0.7)	Strongly agree
I was satisfied with how my skin issue was managed.	21 (95)	6.4 (1.0)	Strongly agree
I am comfortable with the idea of a physician I have never met evaluating my skin condition based on pictures.	22 (100)	6.2 (0.7)	Strongly agree
I would prefer to use this system instead of going to see a specialist in-person.	20 (91)	4.9 (1.8)	Neutral
I would recommend this type of medical care to a friend or family member.	22 (100)	5.8 (1.1)	Agree
I think that the government should pay for me to talk to the dermatologist online directly.	21 (95)	5.4 (1.8)	Agree
I would personally pay to talk to the dermatologist online directly if it was not paid for by the government.	20 (91)	3.7 (2.0)	Disagree
I would have liked to see what was said between my family doctor and the dermatologist.	22 (100)	5.2 (1.8)	Agree
Overall, this service saved me time.	22 (100)	6.6 (0.6)	Strongly agree
Overall, this service saved me money.	15 (68)	5.7 (1.8)	Agree
Because of this service, I missed less work for my health appointments.	16 (73)	5.9 (1.3)	Agree

Referring Provider and Potential Consultant Interviews

A total of 8 interviews of 4 referring providers who had experience with the system and 4 consultant dermatologists who had experience with other implementations of teledermatology or were open to participating in the service were analyzed.

Efficiency of care emerged as a theme. For referring providers…

> *...the option to send a photo with a quick email and get a response really quickly is actually a huge asset...[The patients are] really happy not to go and see another physician for the same matter because some things are easily treatable or diagnosed through that service.* [Interview F2]

Although dermatologists were open to email communication, they expressed concern that additional administrative overhead may prevent uptake; for example, one dermatologist felt that,

> *[In some systems,] the platform is not efficient, it doesn't keep track of cases seen, billing codes, billing numbers, the kind of information that we need in the logistics of how we provide care...a proper kind of charting system or billing system.* [Interview D3]

Interviews supported the data from patient surveys that both providers and patients were satisfied with the service. One provider stated,

> *The patients are absolutely thrilled because...You can get back to them so quickly with such an informed opinion.* [Interview F4]

Table 6. Summary and interpretation of the unified mixed-methods evaluation using the Canada Health Infoway Benefits Evaluation Framework [9].

Component	Chart review	Quantitative (surveys)	Qualitative (interviews)	Interpretation
System quality: functionality, performance, and security	The technology demonstrated robustness with no lost messages	Providers "strongly agreed" that the service was reliable and easy to use	Referring providers and dermatologists found the institutional email to be an appropriate medium, despite the increased administrative burden	Institutional email facilitated a functional service with adequate performance and security
Information quality: content and availability	All consultations were generally completed with one question and one response	Providers "strongly agreed" that the responses were complete, provided satisfactory answers to the clinical questions, and had educational value	Interviewees spoke positively about the structure of the consultations; one interviewee commented, "What I like to have the best is a plan that has multiple steps if the first doesn't work" (Interview F1)	A consultation format that incorporates morphology, diagnosis, reasoning used, and a treatment ladder was satisfactory and educational to providers
Service quality: responsiveness	The average response time was consistent with that of other systems in the literature [14], and in at least one case, potentially prevented morbidity	Providers "strongly agreed" that the responses were timely. Patients also commented positively on the rapid response	"It works because your notes are good and your turnaround time is fast" (Interview F5)	A 24-h average response rate was appropriate for most outpatient clinical situations
Use: behavior, self-reported use, and intention to use	Unexpectedly, parent- and patient-initiated photos were used. Recent research suggests they can be used accurately for diagnosis while saving additional visits [15]	Although the service did not generally save providers time, they "agreed" that the benefits outweighed the increased administrative burden	In interviews, dermatologists expressed that they would be more likely to offer the service if it represented an integrated workflow with medical records and billing	Although the evident benefits to patients and the educational value ameliorates the burden to providers, a more integrated workflow may have increased utilization by referees and potential consultants
User satisfaction: competency, satisfaction, and ease of use	A total of 92.8% (13 of 14) providers used the service more than once	Providers and patients "strongly agreed" that they were satisfied with the outcomes of the system	"Most patients that I follow up with afterwards are really happy that they didn't have to go to any more measures (to be treated)" (Interview F2)	The service demonstrated satisfaction for providers and patients
Quality: safety and outcomes	In cases of independent follow-up, the results supported the diagnosis and management plan of the teledermatology consultant	No adverse events were reported in the survey. Patients "strongly agreed" that they would use this service again or recommend its use. Patient comments supported the idea that the correct management plan was identified	No adverse events or areas for improvement were reported in interviews	Intrainstitutional teledermatology (concordant with existing literature) was safe and effective
Access: ability to access services, and patient and caregiver participation	The service was used for a broad demographic of patients and complaints, suggesting no barriers to access	Patients "strongly agreed" that they were comfortable if a physician they had never met evaluated their skin. However, they also "agreed" they would like to know what was communicated between the consultant and referring physician; this idea was supported by patient comments	Interviewees cited several patient factors (anxiety, sensitive locations, etc) that could theoretically prevent use, but no barriers noted in interviews actually prevented use	Although easy to access, further integration of the patient into the physician-physician communication channel may have been beneficial
Productivity: efficiency, care coordination, and net cost	For the Ontario billing codes, managing 84% of the consultations by teledermatology results in 30% savings overall for visits to consultant dermatologists[a]	Providers "strongly agreed" that the service saved health care system resources. Patients "agreed" that the service saved them time and money and resulted in less work missed	Both potential dermatologists and referring providers characterized institutional email as an efficient tool for consultations. This efficiency increased when email communication was used between the provider and the patients	Intrainstitutional teledermatology increased productivity and efficiency even when geography was not a barrier to care

[a]A dermatology consultation is billed at Can $72.15; a teleconsultation, at Can $44.45; and a subsequent visit required after teledermatology, at Can $38.70. The calculation on savings from billing of services was performed as follows: 1-(0.16*[44.45+38.70]+0.84*44.45)/72.15=0.298 [16].

In addition, providers expressed satisfaction for the educational value of the system with regard to the speed of access; for example, one provider commented,

> *When you get a referral back a month later or a few weeks later, sometimes you can't relate the two things and remember exactly, but when you get it back in*

> *real time or very promptly, it's a better learning experience for me and I can do a better job.* [Interview F4]

Finally, referring providers noted that the service was very useful in situations when they identified the diagnosis but wanted to be up to date on management. One provider stated,

> *Next time that I see a similar presentation I know how to treat it and then if it doesn't work then I know where I should go.* [Interview F2]

Dermatologists agreed that they were more comfortable answering management questions than diagnostic questions in telemedicine or remote situations; one dermatologist said,

> *I like questions about disease entities and management, as long as the diagnosis has already been established.* [Interview D4]

Mixed-Methods Analysis

Triangulation Using the CHI Benefits Evaluation Framework

In the concurrent triangulation evaluation, we correlated the categories of the CHI Benefits Evaluation Framework with our multiple lines of inquiry (Table 6). The hypothesis of net benefit was supported by both qualitative and quantitative evidence.

Discussion

Principal Findings

The concurrent triangulation analysis was consistent with our hypothesis: The intrainstitutional teledermatology service was effective and satisfying to providers and patients even when geographic access was not a barrier. Store-and-forward teledermatology demonstrated diagnostic concordance [17]. In addition, a previous systematic review supported the idea that teledermatology is associated with high satisfaction [18]. Prior work has suggested that cost-effectiveness is not a universal feature of teledermatology [19] and would be highly dependent on regional factors. In our study, the service demonstrated 30% savings in visitation fees [16], and according to the patients, the service saved time and money and prevented them from missing work, which are important components of social cost.

To our knowledge, this is one of the first few studies to investigate the educational potential of teledermatology for referring providers embedded in a consultation service. Other studies have reported the value of incorporating trainees into the teleconsultation process [20] or initiatives such as project ECHO [21] that explore virtual education separate from the service. In our initiative, we found that an appropriately structured consultation note that explains clinical reasoning and offers a treatment ladder was educational and helpful to the referring provider. Furthermore, both dermatologists and referring providers suggested that the greatest educational value of this service was management, not diagnosis. This is supported by the chart review, which showed that 27% of all recommendations involved only alteration of the existing topical treatment. A dermatologist noted, "We all know that the challenge with skin diseases; people don't think about it from a morphology point of view. They think about it as; that person I saw with psoriasis three years ago, this looks like that, right? And so that educated piece, in terms of diagnostics, I think would be lost." (Interview D4). Incorporating formal management and educational initiatives into teleconsultation is an area of potential expansion and study in the future.

In our chart review, 41% of lesions required a subsequent in-person visit compared to only 6% of rashes. Therefore, in the future, such a service would be most productive and efficient if it targeted the management of "rashes" alone. This finding is in line with the view of dermatologists who expressed concern about their comfort with regard to managing lesions by traditional teledermatology and the abovementioned educational findings: There are fewer management options for lesions and therefore potentially less educational value in the discussion of those consultations.

Future services should consider a 24-h consultation response time to manage the most-serious outpatient clinical scenarios. Other pilot services in the literature meet or surpass this response time [22,23]. Important clinical conditions that are time sensitive, meaning that they need ≤24 h for diagnosis and rapid management in dermatology, are infections requiring intervention and serious drug rashes [24] because of the risk of significant morbidity and mortality. In our study, there was only one case of a treatable infection where identification within the period prevented morbidity; however, this may be because referring providers would less likely consider using teledermatology for high-acuity dermatoses if the "maximum" response time allotted was 1 week. However, setting the response time too low may decrease the number of potential dermatologists willing to participate in the service, unless adequately remunerated or alternatively structured (eg, shared "on-call" responsibilities or triage responsibilities delegated to trainees or other health care professionals).

Limitations

One limitation of this study is that this was a small case study at a single institution in a region that is supportive of virtual care. Therefore, the results may not be generalizable. As the primary author is currently the only consulting teledermatologist in our institution, there may be a better way to provide improved care and faster response times than a "usual case" scenario, which could lead to potential bias towards positivity. In addition, follow-ups or "second opinion" consultations may not have been accounted for if they were referred to other care clinics in the city outside the circle of care of the institution.

Conclusion

This is the first reported study on intrainstitutional teledermatology using a mixed-methods approach to explore the benefits of teledermatology, namely, rapid access, high satisfaction, safe and effective clinical outcomes, and increased efficiency and productivity in the health care system. The integration of teledermatology into a routine clinical workflow has remarkable potential value, irrespective of existing access to consultative dermatology. Specifically, by reducing healthcare visits, patients can save time and money and avoid missing work. Additionally, this study provides evidence that management of rashes is ideal via teledermatology, which may lead to better outcomes because of the rapid response and high proportion of cases that can be managed through teledermatology alone. This finding is concordant with the expressed opinions of dermatologists in our study who did not want to assess lesions with traditional teledermatology. The impact and satisfaction of an intrainstitutional teledermatology service that primarily targets rashes and, according to our study, ideally provides responses within 24 h to maximize safety, is worth evaluating in future studies. Further research is necessary to elucidate the educational value of intrainstitutional teledermatology for referring providers and its potential for saving costs.

References

1. Russo L, Campagna I, Ferretti B, Agricola E, Pandolfi E, Carloni E, et al. What drives attitude towards telemedicine among families of pediatric patients? A survey. BMC Pediatr 2017 Dec 17;17(1):21 [FREE Full text] [doi: 10.1186/s12887-016-0756-x] [Medline: 28095894]
2. Yoo J, Rigel DS. Trends in dermatology: geographic density of US dermatologists. Arch Dermatol 2010 Jul;146(7):779. [doi: 10.1001/archdermatol.2010.127] [Medline: 20644040]
3. Canadian Dermatology Association. 2018. Find a dermatologist URL: https://dermatology.ca/public-patients/about-dermatology/find-a-dermatologist/ [accessed 2018-09-01] [WebCite Cache ID 71a6rtiq7]
4. Feng H, Berk-Krauss J, Feng PW, Stein JA. Comparison of Dermatologist Density Between Urban and Rural Counties in the United States. JAMA Dermatology 2018 Nov 01;154(11):1265-1271. [doi: 10.1001/jamadermatol.2018.3022] [Medline: 30193349]
5. Carter Z, Goldman S, Anderson K, Li X, Hynan LS, Chong BF, et al. Creation of an Internal Teledermatology Store-and-Forward System in an Existing Electronic Health Record: A Pilot Study in a Safety-Net Public Health and Hospital System. JAMA Dermatol 2017 Jul 01;153(7):644-650 [FREE Full text] [doi: 10.1001/jamadermatol.2017.0204] [Medline: 28423156]
6. Fabbrocini G, De Vita V, Pastore F, D'Arco V, Mazzella C, Annunziata MC, et al. Teledermatology: from prevention to diagnosis of nonmelanoma and melanoma skin cancer. Int J Telemed Appl 2011;2011:125762 [FREE Full text] [doi: 10.1155/2011/125762] [Medline: 21776252]
7. Naka F, Lu J, Porto A, Villagra J, Wu ZH, Anderson D. Impact of dermatology eConsults on access to care and skin cancer screening in underserved populations: A model for teledermatology services in community health centers. J Am Acad Dermatol 2018 Dec;78(2):293-302. [doi: 10.1016/j.jaad.2017.09.017] [Medline: 29061478]
8. Krupinski E, Burdick A, Pak H, Bocachica J, Earles L, Edison K, et al. American Telemedicine Association's Practice Guidelines for Teledermatology. Telemed J E Health 2008 Apr;14(3):289-302. [doi: 10.1089/tmj.2007.0129] [Medline: 18570555]
9. Canada Health Infoway. 2018. Benefits Evaluation Framework URL: https://www.infoway-inforoute.ca/en/what-we-do/research-and-insights/benefits-evaluation/benefits-evaluation-framework [accessed 2018-09-01] [WebCite Cache ID 71a7q6GWZ]
10. Survey Monkey. URL: https://www.surveymonkey.com/ [accessed 2018-11-02]
11. Thorne S. Interpretive Description: Qualitative Research for Applied Practice. New York, NY: Routledge; Mar 21, 2016.
12. Nelson C, Takeshita J, Wanat KA, Bream KDW, Holmes JH, Koenig HC, et al. Impact of store-and-forward (SAF) teledermatology on outpatient dermatologic care: A prospective study in an underserved urban primary care setting. J Am Acad Dermatol 2016 Mar;74(3):484-90.e1. [doi: 10.1016/j.jaad.2015.09.058] [Medline: 26679528]
13. Whitley R, Volpi A, McKendrick M, Wijck A, Oaklander A. Management of herpes zoster and post-herpetic neuralgia now and in the future. Journal of Clinical Virology 2010 May;48:S20-S28. [doi: 10.1016/S1386-6532(10)70005-6]
14. Callahan CW, Malone F, Estroff D, Person DA. Effectiveness of an Internet-based store-and-forward telemedicine system for pediatric subspecialty consultation. Arch Pediatr Adolesc Med 2005 Apr;159(4):389-393. [doi: 10.1001/archpedi.159.4.389] [Medline: 15809396]
15. O'Connor DM, Jew OS, Perman MJ, Castelo-Soccio LA, Winston FK, McMahon PJ. Diagnostic Accuracy of Pediatric Teledermatology Using Parent-Submitted Photographs: A Randomized Clinical Trial. JAMA Dermatol 2017 Dec 01;153(12):1243-1248. [doi: 10.1001/jamadermatol.2017.4280] [Medline: 29141082]
16. Ministry of Health and Long Term Care. Ontario Schedule of Benefits: Physician Services Under the Health Insurance Act URL: http://www.health.gov.on.ca/en/pro/programs/ohip/sob/physserv/sob_master11062015.pdf [accessed 2018-09-01] [WebCite Cache ID 72BL7Jgxc]
17. Du Moulin MF, Bullens-Goessens YI, Henquet CJ, Brunenberg DE, de Bruyn-Geraerds DP, Winkens RA, et al. The reliability of diagnosis using store-and-forward teledermatology. J Telemed Telecare 2003 Jun;9(5):249-252. [doi: 10.1258/135763303769211247] [Medline: 14599326]

18. Mounessa JS, Chapman S, Braunberger T, Qin R, Lipoff JB, Dellavalle RP, et al. A systematic review of satisfaction with teledermatology. J Telemed Telecare 2018 May;24(4):263-270. [doi: 10.1177/1357633X17696587] [Medline: 28350281]
19. Snoswell C, Finnane A, Janda M, Soyer HP, Whitty JA. Cost-effectiveness of Store-and-Forward Teledermatology: A Systematic Review. JAMA Dermatol 2016 Jun 01;152(6):702-708. [doi: 10.1001/jamadermatol.2016.0525] [Medline: 27074289]
20. Patel J, Parr K, Buehler-Bota T, Hood AF. Integrating Outpatient Teledermatology Education Into the Dermatology Resident Curriculum. J Grad Med Educ 2016 Jul;8(3):468-469 [FREE Full text] [doi: 10.4300/JGME-D-15-00792.1] [Medline: 27413472]
21. Katzman J, Comerci G, Boyle JF, Duhigg D, Shelley B, Olivas C, et al. Innovative telementoring for pain management: project ECHO pain. J Contin Educ Health Prof 2014;34(1):68-75. [doi: 10.1002/chp.21210] [Medline: 24648365]
22. McGoey S, Oakley A, Rademaker M. Waikato Teledermatology: a pilot project for improving access in New Zealand. J Telemed Telecare 2015 Oct;21(7):414-419. [doi: 10.1177/1357633X15583216] [Medline: 26033844]
23. Nami N, Massone C, Rubegni P, Cevenini G, Fimiani M, Hofmann-Wellenhof R. Concordance and time estimation of store-and-forward mobile teledermatology compared to classical face-to-face consultation. Acta Derm Venereol 2015 Jan;95(1):35-39 [FREE Full text] [doi: 10.2340/00015555-1876] [Medline: 24889827]
24. Usatine RP, Sandy N. Dermatologic emergencies. Am Fam Physician 2010 Oct 01;82(7):773-780 [FREE Full text] [Medline: 20879700]

Abbreviations

CHI: Canada Health Infoway

8

Skin Lesion Classification with Deep Convolutional Neural Network: Process Development and Validation

Arnab Ray, BTech; Aman Gupta, BTech; Amutha Al, MEng

SRM Institute of Science and Technology, Chennai, India

Corresponding Author:
Arnab Ray, BTech
SRM Institute of Science and Technology
SRM Nagar, Kattankulathur
Chennai, 603203
India

Email: ad733943@gmail.com

Abstract

Background: Skin cancer is the most common cancer and is often ignored by people at an early stage. There are 5.4 million new cases of skin cancer worldwide every year. Deaths due to skin cancer could be prevented by early detection of the mole.

Objective: We propose a skin lesion classification system that has the ability to detect such moles at an early stage and is able to easily differentiate between a cancerous and noncancerous mole. Using this system, we would be able to save time and resources for both patients and practitioners.

Methods: We created a deep convolutional neural network using an Inceptionv3 and DenseNet-201 pretrained model.

Results: We found that using the concepts of fine-tuning and the ensemble learning model yielded superior results. Furthermore, fine-tuning the whole model helped models converge faster compared to fine-tuning only the top layers, giving better accuracy overall.

Conclusions: Based on our research, we conclude that deep learning algorithms are highly suitable for classifying skin cancer images.

KEYWORDS

deep convolutional neural network; VGG16, Inceptionv3; Inception ResNet V2; DenseNet; skin cancer; cancer; neural network; machine learning; melanoma

Introduction

Skin Cancer

One in every three cancers diagnosed is skin cancer. Although melanomas represent fewer than 5% of all skin cancers, they account for approximately 75% of all skin cancer–related deaths and are responsible for over 10,000 deaths annually. Early detection of the mole would decrease the number of skin cancer deaths.

Skin cancer is significantly lower in India due to the presence of eumelanin in India's dark-skinned population, which provides some protection against the development of skin cancer. Still, skin cancer constituted 3.18% of all patients with cancer in India. Of this, 54.76% were basal cell carcinomas, while 36.91% were squamous cell carcinoma and malignant melanoma was only 8.33%. The majority of patients were from rural areas (88%) and many were involved in agriculture (92%) [1].

Neural Networks in the Context of Skin Cancer

We searched for research papers that used neural networks in the context of skin cancer from Google Scholar, PubMed, Research Gate, and the ISIC (International Skin Imaging Collaboration) archive. We included the results in the literature survey. Deep learning has solved many complex modern problems. The increasing amount of data on the internet helps in this process. There is a huge improvement in image classification using convolutional neural networks (CNN). The first few layers of deep CNN (DCNN) can learn the general features of an image, which can be used for different models. Using fine-tuning, DCNN models trained on one data set can be reused for image classification of other data sets. By fine-tuning Inceptionv3, Esteva et al [2] proposed that, "CNN achieves performance on par with all tested experts, demonstrating an artificial intelligence capable of classifying skin cancer with a level of competence comparable to dermatologists". Esteva and colleagues used their own obtained dermatologist-labelled data set consisting of 129,450 clinical images, including 3374 dermoscopy images. This data set includes 2032 skin diseases, belonging to 9 skin disease partitions. By fine-tuning Inceptionv3 on this data set, Esteva and colleagues achieved up to 66% accuracy classification on these 9 classes.

Another previously published study that used DCNN used AlexNet [3]. The data set consisted of 200 pictures. However, by image augmentation (ie, rotating all the pictures), 4400 images were made. This study used the transfer learning model, in which the AlexNet model was trained on ImageNet data, and the last layer was replaced with the softmax layer that is classified into melanoma, seborrheic keratosis, and nevus. For the change of weights, they used the stochastic gradient descent (SGD) algorithmic program. They were able to achieve an accuracy of 98%.

In another study, the authors planned a mechanized strategy for malignant melanoma determination connected to an arrangement of dermoscopy photos [4]. Highlights removed relied upon using a multilayer perceptron (MLP) classifier and coevent network to distinguish between melanocytic nevi and melanoma. The authors proposed two different procedures for MLP: programmed MLP and conventional MLP. Both techniques were useful for the separation of melanocytic carcinoma with a high accuracy. Following this, the arrangement procedure was executed with an MLP classifier that involved two strategies: automatic MLP and traditional MLP. The MLP classifier displayed distinctive grouping accuracy. The programmed MLP planned 93.4% and 76% training and testing accuracy, respectively.

A different study used a model that uses support vector machine (SVM) learning algorithms [5]. Their model did not use annotated information. The feature transfer that they used allowed the system to draw similarities between observations of dermoscopic pictures and that of the natural world. It mimics the method specialists use to explain patterns in skin lesions. Two-fold cross-validation was performed 20 times for analysis (40 experiments in total), and two discrimination tasks were examined: malignant melanoma versus atypical lesions, and malignant melanoma versus all nonmelanoma lesions. This approach achieved an accuracy of 93.1% for the primary task and 73.9% accuracy for the second task.

In another study, authors designed and modelled a system that can collect and combine past pigmented skin lesion (PSL) image results, their analysis, and corresponding observations and conclusions by medical experts, using a prototyping methodology [6]. One area of the system used computational intelligence techniques to research, process, and classify the images and their probable morphology. Trained medical personnel in remote locations can use mobile knowledge acquisition devices to take pictures of PSL and input the pictures into the planned system, which would classify the imaged PSL as malignant or benign.

Another group used a similar concept using DCNN. They trained their model on a data set of 129,450 images. They used the Inceptionv3 architecture model and classified images among 757 different melanoma classes. The accuracy achieved was 72%; this value was relatively low due to the high number of classes in this data set [2].

Another study used lesion segmentation as the first step of processing [7]. They identified morphological features specific to certain lesions. Preprocessing steps included changing the color channel, smoothing the image, removing hairs, etc. They modelled the algorithm as a binary classification model (ie, benign or malignant). Lesion-related morphological features (including diameter, color, and magnification) were used as the input to a number of classifiers. The best accuracy (79%) was found with the k-nearest neighbors (KNN) algorithm.

In this project, we used the HAM10000 data set obtained by ViDIR Group, Department of Dermatology, Medical University of Vienna. Figure 1 shows example images from the data set that was used for this study.

In this study, we fine-tuned DCNNs and compared the performance of 4 DCNNs: VGG16, Inception-ResNet V2, Inceptionv3, and DenseNet-201. Each DCNN was fine-tuned from the top layers. Fine-tuning of all layers was performed with Inceptionv3 and DenseNet-201. Finally, we created an ensemble of Inceptionv3 and DenseNet-201 with all layers fine-tuned.

Figure 1. Example lesion photos from the HAM10000 data set (ViDIR Group, Department of Dermatology, Medical University of Vienna).

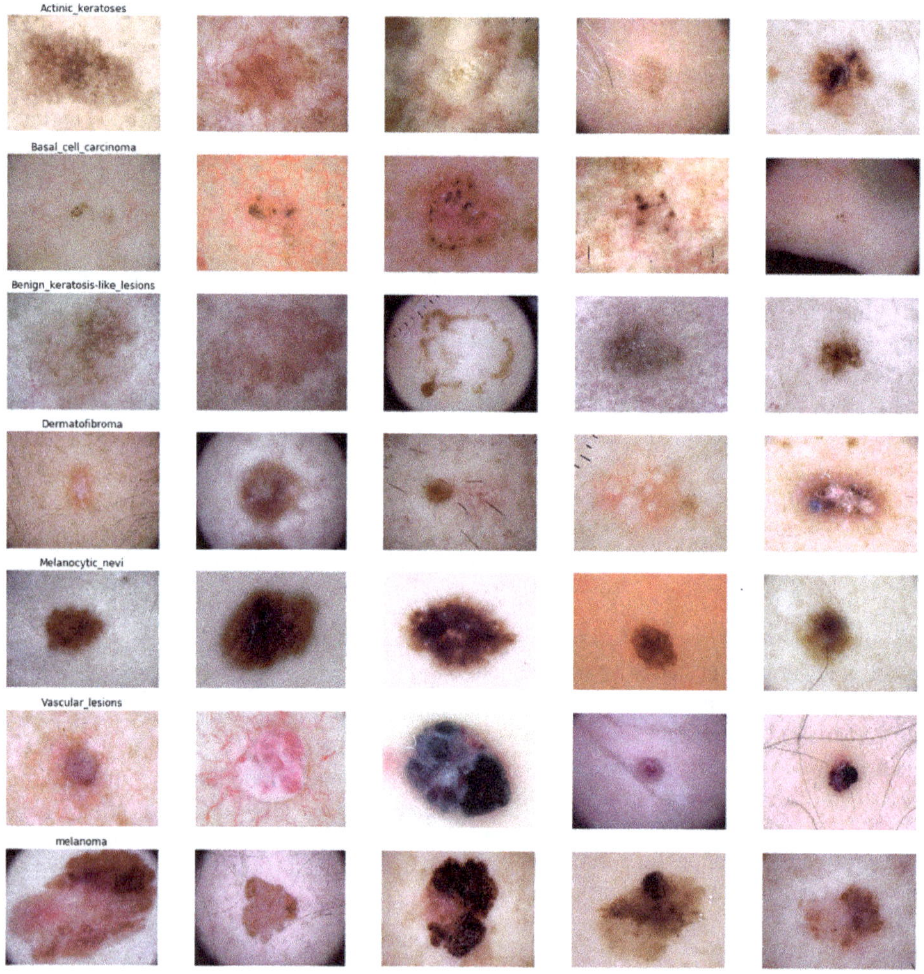

Methods

Exploratory Data Analysis

This step was performed to better understand the data and prepare the data for neural networks. In this project, we used the HAM10000 data set obtained by ViDIR Group, Department of Dermatology, Medical University of Vienna. The diagnostic accuracy for melanoma was significantly higher with dermoscopy compared to unaided eye diagnosis (respectively, log OR 4.0 [95% CI 3.0-5.1] versus log OR 2.7 [95% CI 1.9-3.4], an improvement of 49%, $P<.001$) [8]. The diagnostic accuracy solely depended on the experience and knowledge of the examiner.

We observed that this data set is biased toward melanocytic nevi, as seen in Table 1. Hence, in the worst-case scenario, our neural network model will have an accuracy higher than 60%.

All the original images (450□600 pixels) were resized to 64□4-pixel RGB images for the baseline model and 192□256 pixels for fine-tuning models. The data set was split into 7210 training examples, 1803 validation examples, and 1002 test examples.

Table 1. Counts for each type of lesion in the data set

Type of lesion	Number of images
Melanocytic nevi	6705
Melanoma	1113
Benign keratosis	1099
Basal cell carcinoma	514
Actinic keratoses	325
Vascular lesions	142
Dermatofibroma	115

Baseline Model

We built a baseline CNN to estimate the difficulty of the problem. Our architecture consisted of 6 layers: (1) a convolutional layer with 16 kernels each of size 3 and padding such that the size of the image is maintained, (2) a max-pooling layer with 2□2 window, (3) a convolutional layer with 32 kernels each of size 3 and padding to maintain size, (4) a max-pooling layer with 2□2 window, (5) a convolutional layer with 64 kernels each of size 3 and padding to maintain size, and (6) a max-pooling layer with 2□2 window.

To train the model, data augmentation was required. The learning rate was initialized at 0.01 and Adam Optimizer was used. The baseline model was trained for a total of 35 epochs.

VGG16 Model

VGG16 is a convolutional neural net architecture (Figure 2 [9]) that won the ImageNet competition in 2014 and is generally regarded as one of the best current vision models architecture. Even though it is an old model, we chose VGG16 because of its simplicity.

Figure 2. VGG16 architecture.

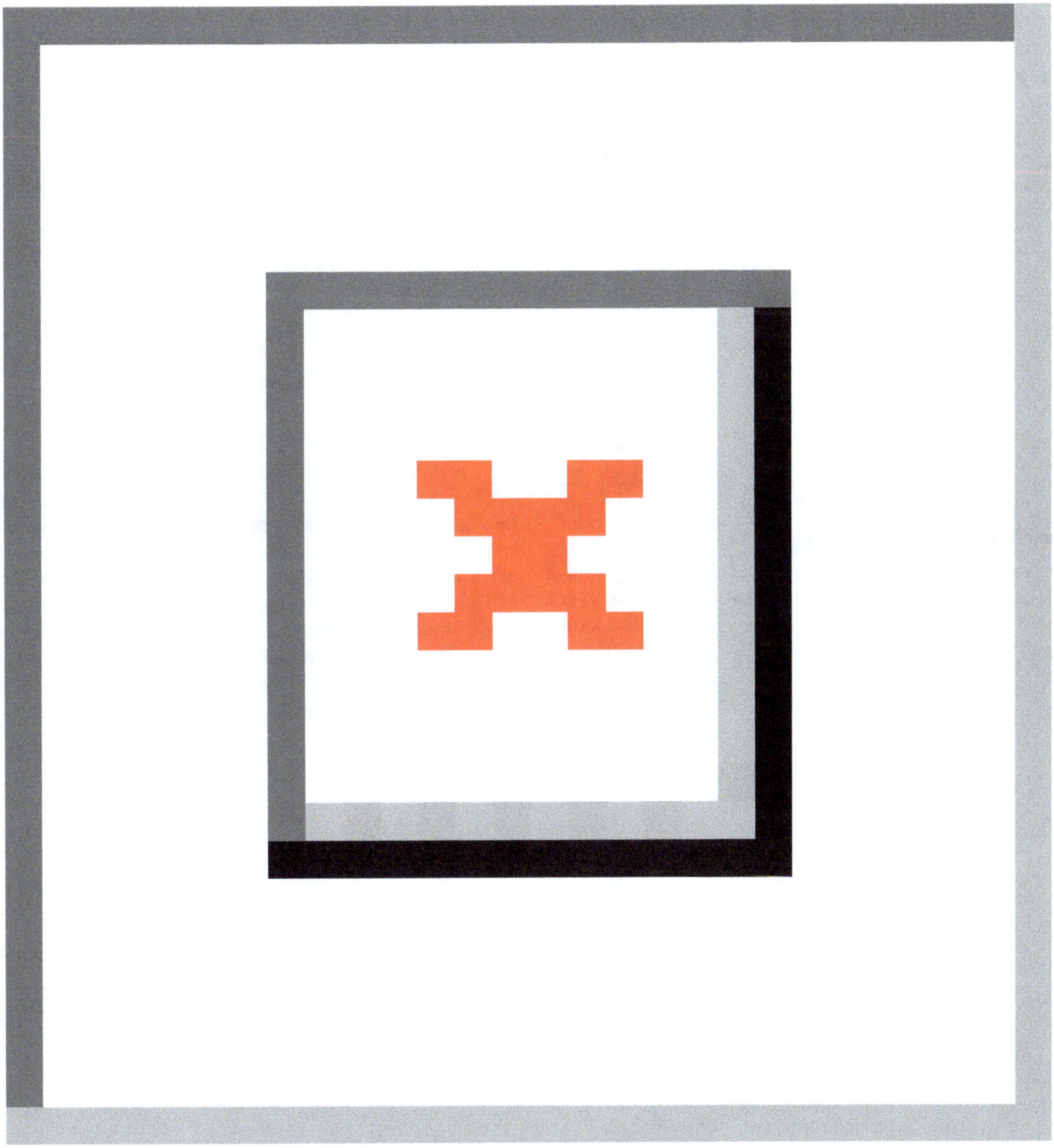

On the ImageNet data set, VGG16 achieved an accuracy of 90.1% for top-5 and 71.3% for top-1.

Data augmentation was performed to increase the data set image count. Fine-tuning was performed on the model by removing the top, fully-connected layers that were then replaced with following: (1) a max-pooling layer, (2) a fully connected layer with 512 units, (3) a dropout layer with 0.5 rate, and (4) a softmax activation layer for 7 types of skin lesions.

The first step included freezing all layers in VGG16 and performing feature extraction for newly added layers. After 3 epochs, we unfroze the final convolutional block of VGG16 and started fine-tuning a model for 20 epochs. The learning rate was set to 0.001 and Adam Optimizer was used. VGG16 was fine-tuned for a total of 30 epochs.

Inception Model

Inceptionv3 produced an accuracy of 93.7% for top-5 and 77.9% for top-1 on the ImageNet data set. The Inception module has 1□1, 3□3, and 5□5 convolutions, all in parallel (Figure 3 [10]). The intention was to let the network decide, through training, what information would be learned and used. It also allows for multi-scale processing; the model can recover low-level features via small convolutional layers and high-level features with large convolutional layers.

We fine-tuned all layers of Inceptionv3 and the top two inception blocks with batch normalization layers. Inceptionv3 was fine-tuned for 20 epochs.

Additionally, we tried Inception-ResNet, a variant of Inception. It uses a residual connection, which has become necessary for training very deep convolutional models. The same training strategy used for Inceptionv3 was used for Inception-ResNet.

Figure 3. Inceptionv3 architecture. Published with permission.

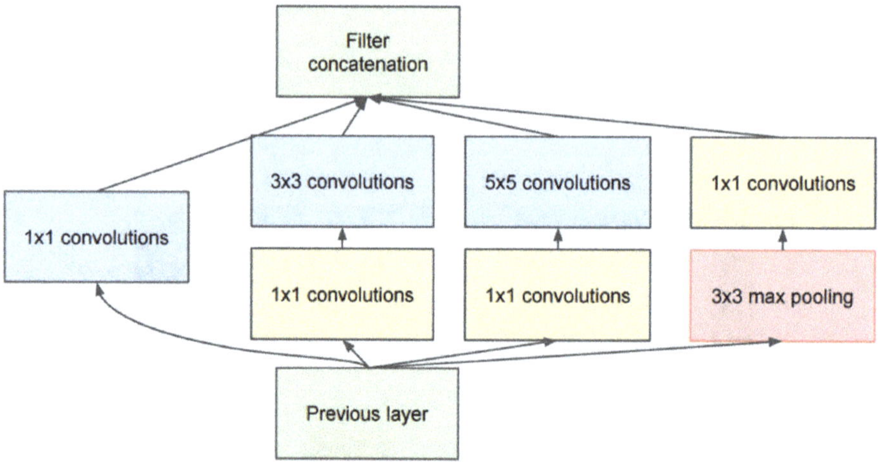

DenseNet Model

This is a new architecture that performed exceptionally well in the ImageNet data set competition, giving an accuracy of 93.6% in top-5 and 77.3% on top-1. DenseNet has 4 dense blocks and uses approximately 20 million parameters (Figure 4 [11]).

In a dense block, one layer generates feature maps through a composite function, consisting of three consecutive operations: batch normalization, ReLU (rectified linear activation unit), and a 3□3 convolution. We used DenseNet-201, which uses 4 dense blocks, and we performed two types of fine-tuning on it: (1) fine-tuning on the last dense block (32 layers; Part A), and (2) fine-tuning on the whole network (Part B). Part A was trained for 27 epochs and Part B was trained for 20 epochs.

Figure 4. DenseNet architecture. Published with permission.

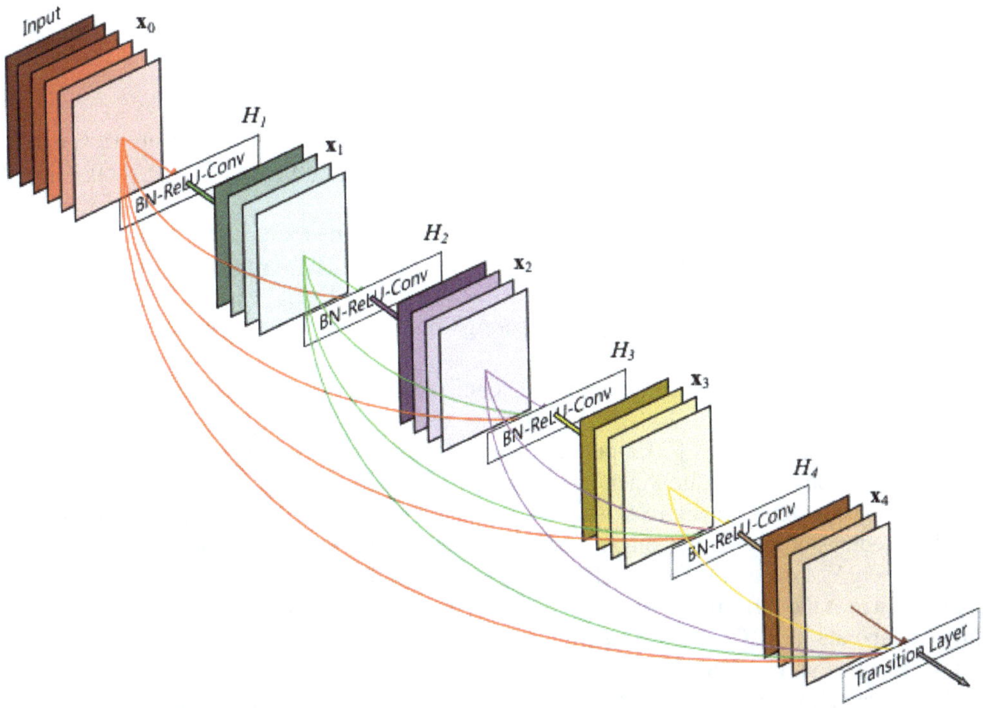

Results

Table 2 shows the classification results from each model when the top layers were fine-tuned (Part A). Table 3 displays the classification results for each model when all layers were fine-tuned. All experiments were performed on a laptop with GPU NVIDIA 1050Ti. To speed up processing times, Google Colab (P100 GPU) was used.

From training a custom model, it was clear that the problem cannot be solved by a simple CNN model with a few layers. Therefore, we incorporated fine-tuning of the pretrained model. By hypertuning the pretrained model that had over 100 layers, we achieved better results. Fine-tuning all layers (Part B) gave us better results than fine-tuning only the top layers (Part A). Crucially, Part B was trained for fewer epochs, which helped the model converge faster. However, in both cases, DenseNet gave us better results than Inceptionv3. Using the concepts of ensemble learning, we created an ensemble of Inceptionv3 and DenseNet-201. This combination achieved a further improved accuracy of 88.8% on the validation set and 88.5% on the test set.

Table 2. Fine-tuning the top layers.

Model	Validation (%)	Test (%)	Test loss	Depth (layers)
Custom model	77.48	76.54	0.646671	11
VGG16	79.82	79.64	0.708	23
Inceptionv3	79.935	79.94	0.7482	315
Inception-ResNet V2	80.82	82.53	0.6691	784
DenseNet-201	85.8	83.9	0.691	711

Table 3. Fine-tuning all layers.

Model	Validation (%)	Test (%)	Test loss
Inceptionv3	86.92	86.826	0.6241
DenseNet-201	86.696	87.725	0.5587
Ensemble (Inceptionv3 and DenseNet-201)	88.8	88.52	0.41156

Discussion

Our results indicate that deep learning algorithms are highly suitable for classifying skin cancer images. Additionally, by using the concepts of fine-tuning and the ensemble learning model, improved results were achieved. Finally, we found that fine-tuning the whole model helped the model converge faster compared with fine-tuning only the top layers, giving an overall better accuracy.

References

1. Lal ST, Banipal RP, Bhatti DJ, Yadav HP. Changing Trends of Skin Cancer: A Tertiary Care Hospital Study in Malwa Region of Punjab. J Clin Diagn Res 2016 Jun;10(6):PC12-PC15 [FREE Full text] [doi: 10.7860/JCDR/2016/18487.8051] [Medline: 27504344]
2. Esteva A, Kuprel B, Novoa RA, Ko J, Swetter SM, Blau HM, et al. Dermatologist-level classification of skin cancer with deep neural networks. Nature 2017 Jan 25;542(7639):115-118. [doi: 10.1038/nature21056]
3. Hosny KM, Kassem MA, Foaud MM. Skin Cancer Classification using Deep Learning and Transfer Learning. 2018 Presented at: 9th Cairo International Biomedical Engineering Conference (CIBEC); December 20-22; Cairo, Egypt p. 90-93. [doi: 10.1109/CIBEC.2018.8641762]
4. S.Mabrouk M, A.Sheha M, Sharawy A. Automatic Detection of Melanoma Skin Cancer using Texture Analysis. IJCA 2012 Mar 31;42(20):22-26. [doi: 10.5120/5817-8129]
5. Codella N, Cai J, Abedini M, Garnavi R, Halpern A, Smith JR. Deep Learning, Sparse Coding, and SVM for Melanoma Recognition in Dermoscopy Images. In: Machine Learning In Medical Imaging. Cham: Springer; 2015:118-126.
6. Okuboyejo DA, Olugbara OO, Odunaike SA. Automating Skin Disease Diagnosis Using Image Classification. 2013 Presented at: Proceedings of the World Congress on Engineering and Computer Science; October 23-25; San Francisco.
7. Codella N, Rotemberg V, Tschandl P, Celebi ME, Dusza S, Gutman D, et al. Skin lesion analysis toward melanoma detection: A challenge at the 2017 International Symposium on Biomedical Imaging (ISBI), hosted by the International Skin Imaging Collaboration (ISIC). 2018 Presented at: IEEE 15th International Symposium on Biomedical Imaging (ISBI 2018); April 4; Washington, DC, USA.
8. Kittler H, Pehamberger H, Wolff K, Binder M. Diagnostic accuracy of dermoscopy. Lancet Oncol 2002 Mar;3(3):159-165. [doi: 10.1016/s1470-2045(02)00679-4] [Medline: 11902502]
9. VGG16 architecture. 2020 Jun 02. Classez et segmentez des données visuelles URL: https://tinyurl.com/ya49hbpk
10. Szegedy C, Liu W, Jia Y, Sermanet P, Reed S, Anguelov D, et al. Going deeper with convolutions. 2015 IEEE Conference on Computer Vision and Pattern Recognition (CVPR) 2015 Jun [FREE Full text]
11. Huang G, Liu Z, van der Maaten L, Weinberger KQ. Densely connected convolutional networks. arXiv 2016 Aug 25 [FREE Full text]

Abbreviations

CNN: convolutional neural network
DCNN: deep convolutional neural network
ISIC: International Skin Imaging Collaboration
KNN: k-nearest neighbor
MLP: multilayer perceptron
PSL: pigmented skin lesion

9

Patients' Experiences of Using Skin Self-Monitoring Apps with People at Higher Risk of Melanoma

Emily Habgood[1], BSc; Christopher McCormack[2], MBBS; Fiona M Walter[1,3,4], MA, MD, MB BCh; Jon D Emery[1,3], MA, MB BCh, DPhil

[1]Department of General Practice and Centre for Cancer Research, University of Melbourne, Melbourne, Australia

[2]Department of Surgical Oncology, Peter MacCallum Cancer Centre, Melbourne, Australia

[3]Primary Care Unit, Department of Public Health and Primary Care, University of Cambridge, Cambridge, United Kingdom

[4]Wolfson Institute of Population Health, Queen Mary University of London, London, United Kingdom

Corresponding Author:
Emily Habgood, BSc
Department of General Practice and Centre for Cancer Research
University of Melbourne
Level 10 Grattan Street
Melbourne, 3000
Australia

Email: emily.habgood@unimelb.edu.au

Abstract

Background: Melanoma is the fourth most commonly diagnosed cancer in Australia. Up to 75% of melanomas are first detected by patients or their family or friends. Many mobile apps for melanoma exist, including apps to encourage skin self-monitoring to improve the likelihood of early detection. Previous research in this area has focused on their development, diagnostic accuracy, or validation. Little is known about patients' views and experiences of using these apps.

Objective: This study aims to understand patients' views and experiences of using commercially available melanoma skin self-monitoring mobile apps for a period of 3 months.

Methods: This qualitative study was conducted in two populations: primary care (where the MelatoolsQ tool was used to identify patients who were at increased risk of melanoma) and secondary care (where patients had a previous diagnosis of melanoma, stages T0-T3a). Participants downloaded 2 of the 4 mobile apps for skin self-monitoring (SkinVision, UMSkinCheck, Mole Monitor, or MySkinPal) and were encouraged to use them for 3 months. After 3 months, a semistructured interview was conducted with participants to discuss their experiences of using the skin self-monitoring mobile apps.

Results: A total of 54 participants were recruited in the study, with 37% (20) of participants from primary care and 62% (34) from secondary care. Interviews were conducted with 34 participants when data saturation was reached. Most participants did not use the apps at all (n=12) or tried them once but did not continue (n=14). Only 8 participants used the apps to assist with skin self-monitoring for the entire duration of the study. Patients discussed the apps in the context of the importance of early detection and their current skin self-monitoring behaviors. A range of features of *perceived quality* of each app affected engagement to support skin self-monitoring. Participants described their skin self-monitoring routines and potential mismatches with the app reminders. They also described the technical and practical difficulties experienced when using the apps for skin self-monitoring. The app's positioning within existing relationships with health care providers was crucial to understand the use of the apps.

Conclusions: This study of patients at increased risk of melanoma highlights several barriers to engagement with apps to support skin self-monitoring. The results highlight the wide-ranging and dynamic influences on engagement with mobile apps, which extend beyond app design and relate to broader contextual factors about skin self-monitoring routines and relationships with health care providers.

KEYWORDS

melanoma; skin cancer; early detection; mobile apps; qualitative; mHealth; mobile phone

Introduction

Skin cancers account for 80% of all newly diagnosed cancers in Australia, with melanoma being the most harmful [1]. Early detection is key, as it provides a better chance of receiving timely treatment. More than 91% of Australians survive if their melanomas are detected early [1]. Up to 75% of melanomas are first detected by patients or their family or friends [2]. Encouraging people to self-monitor their skin for suspicious moles on their bodies could encourage early diagnosis [2]. Current guidelines already recommend Australians at increased risk of melanoma to monitor their own skin in between appointments [3,4]. However, there is currently little information on how patients are recommended to do this, and many patients are completing this insufficiently [5].

Mobile apps for melanomas are becoming increasingly popular. There is an abundance of commercially available mobile apps for melanoma across the different mobile app stores [6,7]. The purpose of these apps varies from prevention (UV exposure apps) to treatment management (drug and side effect management). Apps that encourage skin self-monitoring are designed to support the early detection of melanoma by identifying changes in moles. Most research into these mobile apps for skin self-monitoring for melanoma has focused on their development or diagnostic accuracy [8-11], but there have been limited studies on the actual use of these apps outside controlled *laboratory* settings. Qualitative research provides a deeper understanding of people's experiences, thoughts, and opinions to explore what determines the effective implementation of digital interventions [12,13]. Recent research has shed light on patients' perceptions of the use of mobile health apps for melanoma. Specifically, Koh et al [14] found that patients had positive views about apps for skin self-monitoring and thought they would benefit from using them, but this was based on the intended use of a hypothetical app. We suggest that allowing participants to experience using these types of apps over a period of time provides greater ecological validity. In this study, we aim to understand users' experiences and use of skin self-monitoring mobile apps for melanoma over a 3-month period, focusing on people who were at increased risk of melanoma, as this is consistent with the current Australian guidelines [3,4].

More specifically, we aim to understand participants' experiences of actually using these mobile apps and the reasons they chose whether to use and engage with the apps. We also wanted to determine if this was a potentially feasible way to recruit people at risk of melanoma in future studies of skin self-monitoring apps.

Methods

Study Design and Ethics Approval

This study used a qualitative design with a 3-month follow-up period using a baseline questionnaire and semistructured interviews. A 3-month period was considered to be sufficient to understand participants' interest and patterns of use of the mobile apps and understand their experiences. Participants downloaded the apps on their own phones, were provided with a brief demonstration of both apps, and received automated reminders once per month via each app. Semistructured interviews were used to understand participants' thoughts and experiences after the 3-month period of ad libitum use of 2 of the 4 apps allocated to them on the basis of their phone's operating system (iOS or Android). This study was reviewed and approved by the University of Melbourne Health Sciences Human Ethics Committee (1749081) and the Peter MacCallum Cancer Centre Human Research Ethics Committee (HREC/17/PMCC/214).

Recruitment

Study Setting

Participants were recruited from two different populations: Melbourne general practices, where participants were identified as at increased risk of melanoma on the basis of risk factors; and the Melanoma Outpatient Clinic at Peter MacCallum Cancer Centre (Melbourne, Australia), where participants had a previous diagnosis of melanoma. The study was conducted between October 2018 and February 2019.

Primary Care

In primary care, recruitment was undertaken across 3 busy Melbourne general practices. All patients in the waiting room of the practices were consecutively approached and invited to complete the MelatoolsQ tool [15] to determine if they were eligible. Patients were excluded if they were aged <18 years, unable to understand English, or acutely unwell.

The MelatoolsQ tool is a self-completed survey, which is delivered on an iPad. It contains a modified version of the Williams melanoma risk prediction model [16], which includes the following risk factors: sex, age, natural hair color at the age of 15 years, number of raised moles on both arms, the density of freckles on both arms before the age of 20 years, number of severe sunburns up to the age of 18 years, and previous nonmelanoma skin cancer (basal cell carcinoma and squamous cell carcinoma). A melanoma risk score was calculated from the patients' responses; if they scored 25 or more, they were categorized as increased risk of melanoma and invited to participate in the study [15,16].

Secondary Care

In secondary care, all patients attending an outpatient appointment for their current or previous early-stage melanoma (stages T0-T3a) and aged 18 years or older were approached and invited to participate in the study. Patients were ineligible if they had suspicion or evidence of metastatic disease or were receiving palliative treatment.

Procedure

All participants who were eligible from either primary or secondary care were invited to participate. The aims of the study were discussed, and all participants were provided with a plain English statement explaining the details of participation. Participants recruited to the study had to own a compatible smartphone (Android or iOS operating system) and have sufficient data storage on their phone to download and store photographs (approximately 130 MB). Written consent was obtained from all participants before completing a short baseline survey.

Consented participants were assisted in downloading 2 study apps onto their own phones, which were dependent on their phone's operating system. They were provided with a short booklet and demonstration of how to use each app. Participants were asked to use the apps at least once a month for the 3 months of the study, with a monthly SMS text reminder to check their moles through the app.

Data Collection

A baseline questionnaire collected data on demographics and patterns of mobile phone use. All participants were invited to participate in a telephonic semistructured interview at the end of the 3-month time point, which was audio recorded. The interview guide was designed to explore participants' experiences and preferences for using the apps and their skin monitoring behaviors (Multimedia Appendix 1).

App Selection

The melanoma skin self-monitoring mobile apps identified for the study were SkinVision, UMSkinCheck, Mole Monitor, and MySkinPal. The researchers have no association with the development or marketing of these apps. Inclusion criteria for app selection were apps that were designed for patient use, allowed users to take photographs of their skin within the app, compare photographs over time, and had built-in reminder notifications and information on skin self-monitoring.

The selected apps were identified through a previous review of available mobile apps designed for early detection of melanoma [7]. Kassianos et al [7] identified 39 apps available at that time on app stores for melanoma, and we selected 4 apps on the basis of their functionality. The apps varied by the operating system they were compatible with (either Android or iOS) and the level of assistance provided to determine changes between photos. The Mole Monitor and UMSkinCheck apps were only available on iOS at the time of the study. During the study period, there were no updates to 3 of the apps and minor bug fixes to SkinVision. The apps were allocated to participants depending on their phone's operating system. We wanted to understand participants' experiences of using a melanoma skin self-monitoring mobile app per se rather than the specific apps selected. Therefore, we decided to provide participants with 2 apps each (depending on their phone operating system) to allow comparison of app features and content but to minimize participant burden. We believed that this more closely reflected the usual consumer approaches to trialing new apps while studying those that had similar functionality to support skin self-monitoring.

Data Analysis

Quantitative baseline data were collected using REDCap (Research Electronic Data Capture) [17] and analyzed using descriptive statistics with Stata Statistical Software (version 17, StataCorp LLC) [18].

Qualitative data were audio recorded and transcribed verbatim. Transcripts from the semistructured interviews were analyzed using inductive and deductive thematic analyses, using the stepped approach described by Braun and Clarke [19]. All coding was undertaken by EH, a health services researcher, with a subsample coded by JDE, an academic general practitioner (GP); discrepancies were discussed and resolved as a team. The team also included a second academic GP and a dermatologist. All individuals in the team brought their perspectives to the analysis. Data saturation was reached when the team agreed that no new themes were arising from the transcripts. All analyses were performed using Dedoose (version 8.3.17) [20].

Results

Participant Demographics

A total of 54 participants (28/54, 52% female; mean age 57.3 years, SD 12.5 years) were recruited in the study between June and September 2018. A total of 20 participants were recruited from primary care and 34 from secondary care. Among the 54 participants who completed the baseline questionnaire, 34 (63%) were interviewed about their experiences (12 from primary care and 22 from secondary care). The demographic characteristics are presented in Table 1. The median interview time was 21 (range 5-39) minutes. Nine participants were lost to follow-up, and 11 participants withdrew during the study period. The main reasons for withdrawal were competing health issues (n=3), difficulty using the apps (n=3), and being too busy to participate (n=2). These participants were mostly older and from rural areas.

Table 2 presents data on patterns of use of apps by participants. Of the 34 participants interviewed, 88% (30) had downloaded an app in the last year and 73% (25) often use the apps on their phone more than once a day. More than half of the participants (20/34, 59%) had health-related apps on their phone.

Table 1. Demographic characteristics (N=54).

Variable	Total recruited, n (%)	Total interviewed (n=34), n (%)	Total not interviewed (n=20), n (%)
Gender			
Female	28 (52)	15 (44)	13 (65)
Male	26 (48)	19 (56)	7 (35)
Age (years)			
18-44	8 (15)	6 (18)	2 (10)
45-54	9 (16)	6 (18)	3 (15)
55-64	21 (39)	16 (47)	5 (25)
65-74+	16 (30)	6 (17)	10 (50)
Education			
Year 11 or below	15 (28)	8 (23)	7 (35)
Year 12 or equivalent	8 (15)	5 (15)	3 (15)
Trade or apprenticeship	10 (19)	7 (20)	3 (15)
Tertiary certificate or diploma	6 (11)	4 (12)	2 (10)
Undergraduate	4 (7)	2 (6)	2 (10)
Postgraduate	11 (20)	8 (24)	3 (15)
ARIA[a] postcode classification			
City	36 (67)	30 (88)	6 (30)
Rural	18 (33)	4 (12)	14 (70)
Phone operating system			
iOS	36 (67)	21 (62)	15 (75)
Android	18 (33)	13 (38)	5 (25)

[a]ARIA: Accessibility or Remoteness Index of Australia.

Table 2. Baseline survey responses (N=54).

Question	Total recruited, n (%)	Total interviewed (n=34), n (%)	Total not interviewed (n=20), n (%)
Number of apps downloaded in the last year			
0	7 (13)	4 (12)	3 (15)
1-4	16 (29)	9 (26)	7 (35)
5-10	21 (39)	14 (41)	7 (35)
11-20	8 (15)	6 (18)	2 (10)
≥20	2 (4)	1 (3)	1 (5)
What types of apps do you use on your phone?[a]			
Games	21 (39)	10 (29)	11 (55)
Social networking	37 (69)	23 (68)	14 (70)
Video or movies	2 (4)	2 (6)	0 (0)
News	22 (41)	15 (44)	7 (35)
Maps or navigation	45 (83)	28 (82)	7 (35)
Weather	43 (80)	25 (73)	18 (90)
Banking or finance	38 (70)	24 (71)	14 (70)
Shopping or retail	19 (35)	11 (32)	8 (40)
Health-related	20 (37)	13 (38)	7 (35)
How often do you typically use the apps on your smartphone?			
More than 10 times a day	15 (28)	8 (23)	7 (35)
2-10 times per day	24 (44)	17 (50)	7 (35)
Once a day	8 (15)	4 (12)	4 (20)
Less than once a day	7 (13)	5 (15)	2 (10)
How many health-related apps do you have on your phone?			
0	24 (44)	14 (41)	10 (50)
≥1	30 (56)	20 (59)	10 (50)

[a]More than 1 option could be chosen; on average, 4.5 were selected, with a median of 5.

Use of the Skin Self-monitoring Apps

Overall, although a minority of the participants who were interviewed thought the skin self-monitoring apps were helpful and used them for the entire duration of the study (n=8), most participants either did not use the apps at all (n=12) or tried them once and did not continue (n=14). Participants spoke about their preferences for the different apps, which mostly referred to their user experience of the apps. Of the 4 apps used in the study, no app was preferred over the other by a majority of users. There were no discernible differences in views about the skin self-monitoring apps between those with a previous melanoma and those recruited from primary care. We present the results of the qualitative data analysis in relation to the following core themes: perceived benefits of early detection and experiences of skin self-monitoring, the experience of using the apps to support skin self-monitoring, skin self-monitoring routines and the role of app reminders, and the apps and their positioning within existing relationships with health care providers (HCPs). Data saturation was reached by the last 3 interviews, where no new themes were arising for both primary and secondary care participants. All relevant quotes are provided in Multimedia Appendix 2.

Benefits of Early Detection

Many participants, regardless of their use, discussed the importance of early detection of melanoma and how these apps could support patients in identifying melanomas at an early stage. As a result, all participants who used the app throughout the study thought that using the app provided peace of mind and reduced some of the uncertainty about checking their skin for signs of melanoma. Despite recognizing the potential benefits of using apps for the early detection of melanoma, there were variable degrees of engagement with them. Some participants felt that they were more relevant to their needs, and this was driven, in part, by their perceived increased risk of melanoma.

Experience of Skin Self-monitoring

In the context of the perceived benefits of early detection of melanoma, all participants discussed skin self-monitoring and recognized the importance of checking their own skin regularly. Some participants discussed the importance of routine to engage in regular skin self-monitoring, for example, performing it while they were dressing for the day. However, some participants felt that skin self-monitoring was not appropriate for them, describing the challenges of skin self-monitoring on having large numbers of moles and the challenges of deciding which ones to monitor, especially when they had many to choose from.

Experience of Using Apps to Support Skin Self-monitoring

Although individual opinions on skin self-monitoring varied, most participants perceived skin self-monitoring positively and continued to perform it regardless of their engagement with the apps. Participants described several factors that influenced their perceptions of the quality of the apps, which affected their engagement with them. People were more likely to engage with an app that they felt was of high quality, although what exactly determined this perception differed among users. Primarily, users described the importance of intuitive design and the simplicity of use to foster engagement. This was key as the app was only recommended to be used once a month and not on a more frequent basis, as in most other apps.

When discussing their experience of the different apps, participants described the importance of simple navigation through the app and the ability to move through the app easily as they checked individual moles. Not surprisingly, key functions in the apps were considered better in some apps compared to others—a critical function related to the ability to capture good quality images of the mole to enable comparison over time.

Technical Challenges of Using the Apps

In addition to such key aspects of image capture, the participants discussed other important technical challenges they experienced. A particular one, relevant to skin self-monitoring more broadly, is viewing moles in less accessible parts of the body, including the back. For many, this required seeking assistance from a partner or carer but was a greater challenge for those who lived alone.

Although all participants were regular users of smartphones, there were varying levels of reported proficiency in their use. Some were, therefore, not confident enough to use the app in the way it was intended. There were concerns related to this issue about the amount of time needed to learn how to use the individual apps and maintain the photos.

Participants also experienced specific technical issues with the apps; some participants complained about the apparent impact on battery life, whereas others had difficulties reinstalling the app when purchasing a new phone.

App Reminders and Skin Self-monitoring Routines

All the apps had a reminder function to prompt users to examine their skin. There was mixed feedback on these reminders. Most participants thought they were helpful and used them to help keep on track with monitoring their skin. However, there were problems with the reminders not coinciding with individuals' skin self-monitoring routines. For younger participants who were less regular with conducting skin self-monitoring, the app reminders were insufficient to prompt them to check their skin.

The Apps and Their Positioning Within Existing Relationships With HCPs

Participants discussed the importance of the HCPs involved in managing their skin, and this often involved seeing multiple doctors, even for those participants recruited in primary care who had not been previously diagnosed with melanoma. Many participants spoke to their GPs regarding concerns about a specific mole, and some participants also attended primary care skin clinics; those with a previous melanoma also consulted their specialists for signs of recurrence and a whole-body examination. Participants also discussed how the app fit into these relationships with their HCP and how they could share and discuss the photographs they had been taking.

They felt that the ability to compare photographs over time within the app and have all their photographs stored in a single accessible place could help communicate with their doctors.

However, some participants felt that there was no place for the app because they were already being monitored closely by their doctors.

Related to this was the issue of greater trust in continuing to see their doctor than relying on an app. This model of care provided them with greater peace of mind and was more effective for the early detection of melanoma.

Others thought the apps were potentially more relevant to a rural audience, who did not have such good access to health care.

There was some support for the potential use of the apps to enable a telehealth model and change the way they interacted with their health professionals about their skin. They supported the idea of sending images directly to a specialist through an app for review, whereas others were more skeptical about this model of care. By assuming that even if they did send a photograph in for review, they would be asked to consult a doctor every time.

Discussion

Principal Findings

To our knowledge, this is one of the first studies to assess the experiences of people at higher risk of melanoma using mobile apps for skin self-monitoring. This qualitative study found that participants were receptive to the potential benefits of using mobile apps for skin self-monitoring. Not all participants engaged on a monthly basis with the use of apps, despite acknowledging their potential benefits. This is related to technical and practical barriers, including infrequent use limiting learning about app use. Additional barriers to adoption were the relationship of the apps to existing skin self-monitoring routines and skin checks provided by HCPs.

We found that perceptions of the quality of the apps were integral to its use and how it was experienced. Technology literacy was highly variable; although almost all participants used their smartphones regularly, they did not necessarily perceive the apps to be easy to use. Although some of these technical barriers could potentially be overcome by better app design, we must recognize the practical challenges related to the specific task; obtaining a high-quality image of a skin lesion, especially in certain parts of the body, is difficult, more so without assistance.

To our knowledge, this is the first qualitative study reporting the lack of actual use of skin self-monitoring apps in people at increased risk of melanoma. Only a quarter of the participants regularly used the app for the entire duration of the study. This was in an at-risk population who already had an increased personal incentive to use these melanoma skin self-monitoring apps. It is possible that even fewer people would actively engage with mobile app use among people at population-level risk. A recent randomized controlled trial of skin self-monitoring app use among a UK primary care population who were at increased risk of melanoma found no evidence of increased consulting about skin lesions over a 12-month period [21]. This study was unable to collect data on the actual use of the mobile app; however, according to our findings, the lack of effect in that trial may well have been due to limited engagement with the app.

Previous qualitative research has focused on patients' intentions and attitudes toward using skin self-monitoring apps [14,22]. Dieng et al [22] interviewed patients who had a previous diagnosis of melanoma and asked about the possible use of digital technology to assess changes in skin lesions over time. Similar to our findings, participants had positive attitudes toward this type of technology and thought it would prompt them to visit their HCP if a concern was found ahead of their regular appointments. Our study suggests a large gap between intentions and actual engagement with the currently available skin self-monitoring apps.

Our study has highlighted the many technical and practical factors at play when patients experience skin self-monitoring apps. It emphasizes the importance of participants' personal circumstances and their context as to whether they engage with these apps. It is important to understand patients' existing relationships with HCPs and their access to regular clinical skin examinations, their current skin self-monitoring routines, and the role of partners or carers for assistance using the app. Only a minority of people in our study were regular users of these apps after 3 months. We do not know if they continued to use them for longer-term skin self-monitoring, but we suggest that both personal and contextual issues as well as the app-related technical issues are likely to determine this. This is echoed in many studies on health apps more broadly, where uptake is low and dropout is high. This has been observed in mental health apps [23], asthma apps [24], and diabetes apps [25]. Using depression health apps as an example, the completion of apps within the real-world setting was as low as 1%-28% [23].

Strengths and Limitations

We conducted qualitative interviews in a relatively large sample, providing a rich, in-depth understanding of the factors influencing app use.

We recruited participants from two different populations: those at increased risk of melanoma in the general practice setting and those who have had a previous diagnosis of melanoma in the hospital setting. Both populations represent potential target users of these apps. We had initially expected app engagement to be higher in those with a previous melanoma but found that this may not hold true.

There were some limitations to this study. Although we recruited a large sample for a qualitative study, we experienced moderate attrition. A third of the participants withdrew or were lost to follow-up before completion, likely representing people who were even less inclined to engage with the apps. Nonetheless, it is clear that the sample we interviewed did not represent a self-selected group that was highly motivated to use these apps.

Considering the use of commercially available apps, we were unable to record the exact amount of time or the frequency of actual interactions with the apps used during the study and relied on self-reporting. We had no control over changes to app functions or updates. Therefore, we deliberately monitored use for a relatively short period of follow-up, which limits our understanding of or additional barriers to long-term adoption.

Finally, the participants themselves did not choose the apps but were only given 2 apps to try on the basis of their phone's operating system. We do not know how the public currently selects skin self-monitoring apps from app stores or how payment for an app might influence whether users persevere with them for longer.

Conclusions

This qualitative study provides important new findings about engagement with skin self-monitoring apps in people at increased risk of melanoma. The findings can make useful contributions to designing future apps or interventions for promoting skin self-monitoring. If such apps are to play a role in the early detection of melanoma, we must move beyond a focus on app design and diagnostic accuracy. This will require acknowledgment of the complex contextual factors affecting app use and incorporating app-based skin self-monitoring into existing models of care and skin assessments.

Acknowledgments

The authors would like to thank all the participants in this study and the general practice staff who supported the recruitment. This research arises from the CanTest Collaborative, which was funded by Cancer Research UK (C8640/A23385): FMW is the Director, JDE is the Associate Director, and EH's PhD was supported by CanTest. The researchers gratefully acknowledge the Primary Care Collaborative Cancer Clinical Trials Group for their support of this project. The UK MelaTools programme was supported by FMW's Clinician Scientist Award from the National Institute for Health Research (RG 68235). JDE was supported by the National Health and Medical Research Council Practitioner Fellowship. The views expressed in this publication are those of the authors and not necessarily those of the National Health Service, the National Institute for Health Research, or the Department of Health.

References

1. Melanoma of the skin statistics. Cancer Australia. 2020. URL: https://melanoma.canceraustralia.gov.au/statistics [accessed 2020-07-02]
2. Körner A, Coroiu A, Martins C, Wang B. Predictors of skin self-examination before and after a melanoma diagnosis: the role of medical advice and patient's level of education. Int Arch Med 2013 Feb 27;6(1):8 [FREE Full text] [doi: 10.1186/1755-7682-6-8] [Medline: 23446040]
3. Early detection of skin cancer. RACGP Redbook Clinical Guidelines. 2012. URL: https://www.racgp.org.au/clinical-resources/clinical-guidelines/key-racgp-guidelines/view-all-racgp-guidelines/guidelines-for-preventive-activities-in-general-pr/early-detection-of-cancers/skin-cancer [accessed 2020-07-02]
4. Clinical practice guidelines for the diagnosis and management of melanoma. Cancer Council Australia Clinical Guidelines. 2020. URL: https://wiki.cancer.org.au/australiawiki/index.php?oldid=212613, [accessed 2021-07-16]
5. Coups EJ, Manne SL, Stapleton JL, Tatum KL, Goydos JS. Skin self-examination behaviors among individuals diagnosed with melanoma. Melanoma Res 2016 Feb;26(1):71-76. [doi: 10.1097/CMR.0000000000000204] [Medline: 26426762]
6. Tellez W, Nieto-Gutierrez W, Taype-Rondan A. Sunscreen mobile apps: a content analysis. Eur Res Telemed / La Recherche Européenne en Télémédecine 2017 Nov;6(3-4):157-163. [doi: 10.1016/j.eurtel.2017.08.001]
7. Kassianos AP, Emery JD, Murchie P, Walter FM. Smartphone applications for melanoma detection by community, patient and generalist clinician users: a review. Br J Dermatol 2015 Jun;172(6):1507-1518. [doi: 10.1111/bjd.13665] [Medline: 25600815]
8. Yas QM, Zaidan AA, Zaidan BB, Hashim M, Lim CK. A systematic review on smartphone skin cancer apps: coherent taxonomy, motivations, open challenges and recommendations, and new research direction. J Circuit Syst Comp 2018 Feb 06;27(05):1830003. [doi: 10.1142/s0218126618300039]
9. Ersser SJ, Effah A, Dyson J, Kellar I, Thomas S, McNichol E, et al. Effectiveness of interventions to support the early detection of skin cancer through skin self-examination: a systematic review and meta-analysis. Br J Dermatol 2019 Jun;180(6):1339-1347. [doi: 10.1111/bjd.17529] [Medline: 30561006]
10. Freeman K, Dinnes J, Chuchu N, Takwoingi Y, Bayliss SE, Matin RN, et al. Algorithm based smartphone apps to assess risk of skin cancer in adults: systematic review of diagnostic accuracy studies. Br Med J 2020 Feb 10;368:m127 [FREE Full text] [doi: 10.1136/bmj.m127] [Medline: 32041693]
11. Chuchu N, Takwoingi Y, Dinnes J, Matin RN, Bassett O, Moreau JF, Cochrane Skin Cancer Diagnostic Test Accuracy Group. Smartphone applications for triaging adults with skin lesions that are suspicious for melanoma. Cochrane Database Syst Rev 2018 Dec 04;12(12):CD013192 [FREE Full text] [doi: 10.1002/14651858.CD013192] [Medline: 30521685]
12. Bradbury K, Watts S, Arden-Close E, Yardley L, Lewith G. Developing digital interventions: a methodological guide. Evid Based Complement Alternat Med 2014;2014:561320 [FREE Full text] [doi: 10.1155/2014/561320] [Medline: 24648848]
13. Yardley L, Morrison L, Bradbury K, Muller I. The person-based approach to intervention development: application to digital health-related behavior change interventions. J Med Internet Res 2015;17(1):e30 [FREE Full text] [doi: 10.2196/jmir.4055] [Medline: 25639757]
14. Koh U, Horsham C, Soyer HP, Loescher LJ, Gillespie N, Vagenas D, et al. Consumer acceptance and expectations of a mobile health application to photograph skin lesions for early detection of melanoma. Dermatology 2019;235(1):4-10 [FREE Full text] [doi: 10.1159/000493728] [Medline: 30404081]
15. Habgood E, Walter FM, O'Hare E, McIntosh J, McCormack C, Emery JD. Using an electronic self-completion tool to identify patients at increased risk of melanoma in Australian primary care. Australas J Dermatol 2020 Feb 12;61(3):231-236. [doi: 10.1111/ajd.13244] [Medline: 32050041]
16. Williams LH, Shors AR, Barlow WE, Solomon C, White E. Identifying persons at highest risk of melanoma using self-assessed risk factors. J Clin Exp Dermatol Res 2011;2(6):1000129 [FREE Full text] [doi: 10.4172/2155-9554.1000129] [Medline: 22229112]
17. Harris PA, Taylor R, Thielke R, Payne J, Gonzalez N, Conde JG. Research electronic data capture (REDCap) - a metadata-driven methodology and workflow process for providing translational research informatics support. J Biomed Inform 2009 Apr;42(2):377-381 [FREE Full text] [doi: 10.1016/j.jbi.2008.08.010] [Medline: 18929686]
18. Stata Statistical Software: Release 15. StataCorp LLC. URL: https://www.stata.com/stata-news/news32-2/ [accessed 2021-07-16]
19. Braun V, Clarke V. Using thematic analysis in psychology. Qual Res Psychol 2006 Jan;3(2):77-101. [doi: 10.1191/1478088706qp063oa]
20. Dedoose Version 8.0.35 - Web application for managing, analyzing, and presenting qualitative and mixed method research data. SocioCultural Research Consultants, LLC, Los Angeles, CA. 2018. URL: https://www.dedoose.com/ [accessed 2021-07-16]
21. Walter FM, Pannebakker MM, Barclay ME, Mills K, Saunders CL, Murchie P, et al. Effect of a skin self-monitoring smartphone application on time to physician consultation among patients with possible melanoma: a phase 2 randomized clinical trial. JAMA Netw Open 2020 Feb 05;3(2):e200001 [FREE Full text] [doi: 10.1001/jamanetworkopen.2020.0001] [Medline: 32101302]

22. Dieng M, Smit AK, Hersch J, Morton RL, Cust AE, Irwig L, et al. Patients' views about skin self-examination after treatment for localized melanoma. JAMA Dermatol 2019 May 15;155(8):914-921 [FREE Full text] [doi: 10.1001/jamadermatol.2019.0434] [Medline: 31090868]
23. Fleming T, Bavin L, Lucassen M, Stasiak K, Hopkins S, Merry S. Beyond the trial: systematic review of real-world uptake and engagement with digital self-help interventions for depression, low mood, or anxiety. J Med Internet Res 2018 Jun 06;20(6):e199 [FREE Full text] [doi: 10.2196/jmir.9275] [Medline: 29875089]
24. Chan YY, Wang P, Rogers L, Tignor N, Zweig M, Hershman SG, et al. The Asthma Mobile Health Study, a large-scale clinical observational study using ResearchKit. Nat Biotechnol 2017 Mar 13;35(4):354-362 [FREE Full text] [doi: 10.1038/nbt.3826] [Medline: 28288104]
25. Holtz B, Lauckner C. Diabetes management via mobile phones: a systematic review. Telemed J E Health 2012 Apr;18(3):175-184. [doi: 10.1089/tmj.2011.0119] [Medline: 22356525]

Abbreviations

GP: general practitioner
HCP: health care provider
REDCap: Research Electronic Data Capture

10

Does Wearing a Face Mask During the COVID-19 Pandemic Increase the Incidence of Dermatological Conditions in Health Care Workers?

Robyn-Jenia Wilcha

Faculty of Biology, Medicine and Health, University of Manchester, Manchester, United Kingdom

Corresponding Author:
Robyn-Jenia Wilcha
Faculty of Biology, Medicine and Health
University of Manchester
Oxford Road
Manchester, M13 9PL
United Kingdom

Email: robynwilcha05@gmail.com

Abstract

Background: COVID-19 is a health emergency. SARS-CoV-2 was discovered in Wuhan (Hubei Province, China) and has rapidly spread worldwide, leaving no country untouched. COVID-19 is a respiratory infection characterized by a pneumonia of unknown etiology. It is transmitted through respiratory droplets; for example: through breathing, talking, and coughing. Transmission of the virus is high. Health care workers play important roles in helping those affected by COVID-19; this could not be done without the use of personal protective equipment (PPE). PPE involves the use of goggles, masks, gloves, and gowns and is known to reduce COVID-19 transmission; however, multiple reports of skin disease and damage associated with occupational mask-wearing have emerged.

Objective: The objective of this study is to review the literature for newly emerging dermatological conditions as a result of occupational mask-wearing during the COVID-19 pandemic.

Methods: A narrative review of new reports of dermatological conditions associated with occupational mask-wearing was carried out in May 2020 by referencing keywords including: "covid mask dermatology," "covid dermatological damage," "covid mask skin," "covid N95 mask damage," and "covid mask skin damage" from PubMed, supplemented by searches on both Google Scholar and ResearchGate. A total of 287 articles were found, of which 40 were successfully included in this study, and an additional 7 were selected from the reference lists of these 40 articles. The findings were tabulated and analyzed under the following headings: dermatological diagnosis, causes, and management.

Results: Qualitative analysis of the reviewed data was carried out. A number of dermatological conditions were found to increasingly occur owing to prolonged and frequent use of face masks. Pressure-related injuries were often the most serious complaint; recommendations to reduce this type of injury include the use of hydrocolloid dressings, plastic handles, education, and regular moisturization. Innovation in PPE as well as services, such as virtual clinics, need to be advanced to protect the welfare of health care staff.

Conclusions: In these unprecedented times, PPE has been an effective barrier to the transmission of COVID-19 among health care workers. This has allowed health care workers to provide care to patients, with minimal risk. However, our findings suggest that despite the obvious benefits of using face masks to protect the respiratory system, there are also considerable health consequences to the skin. Future research studies are required to focus on improving face masks to ensure both the protection of the respiratory system as well as skin care, which, according to our study, has been overlooked.

KEYWORDS

COVID-19; dermatology; face masks; health care worker; incidence; literature; mask; N95 mask; review; skin

Introduction

COVID-19, formerly known as the novel coronavirus infection, is a global public health emergency [1]. The causative virus was initially detected in Wuhan (Hubei Province, China) in December 2019; bats have subsequently been linked to the spread of the disease [1]. Typical symptoms of COVID-19 prominently include fever, cough, sore throat, breathlessness, fatigue, headache, and changes to cognition, although some infected individuals may be asymptomatic [1]. Human-to-human transmission of the virus occurs at high rates, and the virus can be spread through direct contact and respiratory particles [2]. Respiratory particles may be transmitted through breathing, talking, coughing, and sneezing [2].

As of May 2020, no drug nor antiviral vaccine has been officially approved for the treatment of COVID-19 [2]. The current state of emergency due to the COVID-19 pandemic has led to rapid acceleration of vaccine development. According to the World Health Organization, 10 vaccine candidates are currently in different clinical phases, and 123 vaccines are being evaluated in preclinical models [3]. Current management of COVID-19 includes infection prevention and supportive care, such as oxygen supplementation and maintenance of a continuous positive airway pressure [4]. Preventative strategies, such as face mask–wearing, help reduce respiratory transmission of COVID-19. The World Health Organization recommends the use of face masks among those who provide care to a person with suspected COVID-19 [5].

Protection against COVID-19 among health care workers is key to providing effective care; however, latest studies from China have reported a high number of adverse reactions caused by personal protective equipment (PPE), specifically surgical and N95 face masks. In a sample of 542 health care workers, 97% were found to have facial or hand dermatoses [6-10]. Despite published guidelines recommending to limit the time of wearing N95 masks to 2 hours, health care workers often wear masks for much longer periods [6]. The consequences of prolonged mask-wearing include the following: pressure-related injuries, various dermatoses, skin dryness, skin erythema, acne, eczema, urticaria, rosacea, secondary infections, nasal bridge ulceration, and exacerbation of known skin disorders [11,12]. The objective of this study is to review the emerging literature on newly emerging dermatological conditions as a result of occupational mask-wearing.

Methods

A narrative literature review was performed between May 1 and 29, 2020, in order to identify studies that evaluated the relationship between mask-wearing during the COVID-19 pandemic and the increase in the prevalence of certain dermatological conditions. Key search terms used herein included "covid mask dermatology," "covid dermatological damage," "covid mask skin," "covid N95 mask damage," and "covid mask skin damage." The term "covid" was also replaced by "coronavirus," "nCoV," and "SARSCoV2" to increase the number of studies churned by the search. PubMed was the main electronic database that was searched, with search supplementation from Google Scholar and ResearchGate to identify missing articles. On eliminating duplicated searches, we found that the majority of studies found on Google Scholar and ResearchGate were duplicates of those found on PubMed. Qualitative results were obtained by comparing and summarizing results from all relevant and emerging studies by an independent researcher.

The inclusion criteria set for this study were vast owing to the limited literature sources and the novel exploratory design of the literature review. All articles included within the review explored new cases of dermatological damage caused by occupational use of PPE, focusing specifically on the damage caused by surgical and N95 masks, during the COVID-19 pandemic. Articles were sought from multiple institutions worldwide. Moreover, all articles focused on the effects of skin damage among health care workers; by definition, health care workers include physicians, nurses, health care assistants, pharmacists, students, therapists, and laboratory staff. Study designs included within the literature review were randomized controlled trials, cohort studies, and case studies. To further expand the breadth of the literature assessed, the review also accepted letters to the editors, commentaries, editorials, and perspectives. Articles that were case reports of individual patients' dermatological findings in relation to COVID-19 were excluded from the study. Additionally, dermatological findings from previous pandemics including severe acute respiratory syndrome, Middle East respiratory syndrome, and Ebola were excluded.

On searching the aforementioned electronic databases, a total of 287 articles were found (PubMed: n=185, Google Scholar: n=67, and ResearchGate: n=35). After eliminating duplicate searches, 203 articles were screened by title and abstract, and a total of 120 articles were analyzed in full text. After full-text analysis, 40 articles, which satisfied the inclusion criteria, were included in the study. Through manual searches of the included articles' reference lists, an additional 7 articles were identified. Prominent findings from the literature review are presented in a table under the following headings: dermatological diagnosis, causes, and management.

Results

A total of 287 articles were found from various searches. After the elimination of duplicated articles, the title and abstract of 203 articles were screened. Of these, 120 articles were deemed appropriate for full-text screening, of which 40 articles met the inclusion criteria. Manual review of their reference lists yielded an additional 7 articles.

The findings of these 47 papers reviewed in this study are summarized in Table 1. The table documents reported dermatological diagnoses resulting from prolonged mask-wearing with their relevant causes and the management of conditions. Qualitative analysis of the included articles was conducted.

Table 1. A table summarizing the causes and management of dermatological conditions resulting from occupational mask-wearing.

Dermatological diagnosis	Causes	Management
Pressure-related injuries	• Facial protective equipment, such as masks, place a significant amount of pressure on different facial areas, most notably the nasal bridge [13]. This can often cause numerous injuries at different facial points [14]. Pressure, friction and the hyperhydration effect caused by masks and goggles often result in skin indentation, mechanical skin damage, and epidermal barrier breakdown [12,15]. N95 masks specifically have increased air impermeability and a higher local pressure, increasing the risk of dermatological symptoms [7]. • Risk factors for pressure damage are the following: prolonged wearing of personal protective equipment (PPE) [14-17], repeated wearing of PPE [15], use of grade 3 PPE [14], joint use of masks and goggles [7], high humidity [15], and heavy sweating [14]. Conflicting findings based on the relevance of gender and pressure-related injuries were reported in several studies [7,14,17].	• Measures to reduce pressure-related injuries include the following: education of health care workers [7,17], wearing a properly fitted mask to minimize friction at specific points [7,11], regular moisturizing before and after the use of facial protective equipment for skin barrier repair [6,7,11,16], and limiting the time spent using a mask; published guidelines suggest limiting mask-wearing to 2 hours [6,11,13,16]. • Pressure-related injuries that are progressive or cause discomfort to the user may be relieved by the use of a hydrocolloid dressing [6,16-18]. Hydrocolloid dressings are composed of water, sodium polyacrylate, cellulose gum, and sodium hyaluronate; these components serve as a cushion for soft tissue, thus reducing pressure and retaining skin moisture [18]. Dong et al [18] conducted a study to observe if hydrogel patches relieve skin damage in 19 health care workers; they reported that using hydrogel patches resulted in a lower mean score for skin reactions (3.47, SD 1.39, compared to nonuse scores of 13.32, SD 2.06), demonstrating that hydrogel patches are able to reduce the emergence and severity of skin damage [18]. Furthermore, they reported that the use of hydrogel patches reduced skin indentation as well as pain [18]. • Conflicting evidence was reported on whether hydrocolloid dressings impacted the seal of facial masks [6,16,19]. • High levels of humidity are reportedly a predisposing factor to skin barrier damage [15]; to reduce humidity levels, it is recommended to line masks with a paper towel or gauze [15].
Irritant contact dermatitis (ICD)	• ICD is a common problem reported by health care workers [7,17,20]; symptoms include burning, itching, and stinging [11]. Formaldehyde, a material used in both surgical and N95 masks, has been recognized to be a frequent contact sensitizer for many people [7,16]. Acute and chronic dermatitis may be a result of skin and mucus membrane damage [11]. Facial protective equipment may induce ICD through occlusion and friction from the mask and the hyper-hydration effect of PPE; in turn, this breaks down the epidermal barrier of the skin [20]. Factors that predispose individuals to ICD include the following: increased moisture, warm environments, occlusion due to local pressure, and friction [7,21].	• Protective measures include the following: ensuring the proper fit of the mask, labeling of contact sensitizers on face masks [17], cooling the skin by ensuring adequate air conditioning at the site, and wiping skin to remove sweat at appropriate times [20]. Staff should limit the duration of mask-wearing by having rotating shifts and regular mask-free breaks [20]. Furthermore, staying hydrated may also reduce symptoms of dermatitis [20]. • Treatment of ICD includes the use of emollients before wearing masks [11,20,22]; emollients should be applied at least 30 minutes before wearing the mask to prevent damage to the mask [20]. Staff may also choose to line the mask with gauze to reduce the humidity [11]. For moderate to severe ICD, topical glucocorticoids may be recommended [11,20,22].
Allergic contact dermatitis (ACD)	• Occupational ACD was also a common problem reported among health care workers [17]. ACD has a similar set of symptoms to ICD, which includes the following: pruritus, burning sensations, facial and periocular erythema, and subtle eczematous lesions [12,17]. Aggravating factors that may induce ACD include the following: prolonged use of PPE [7], increased moisture from perspiration, occlusion effects from the mask [7,23], friction [7,23], atopic predisposition [7], and contact sensitizers including formaldehyde [17,23]. Maliyar et al [23] reported that 22.8% of the population is sensitive to formaldehyde.	• The gold standard for the diagnosis of ACD is patch testing [7]. • The treatment for ACD is similar to that recommended for ICD. It is important to ensure correct fitting of PPE [23], the use of facial moisturizers before and after using PPE [11,23], the avoidance of facial cleansing with overheated water, 75% ethanol, or a facial cleanser [11], and the use of hydrogel dressings on damaged skin [23]. Layers of gauze inside the mask may be used to reduce moisture effects within the mask [11]. For mild dermatitis, the use of emollients is adequate; if the dermatitis progresses, topical glucocorticoid ointments may be used [11].

Dermatological diagnosis	Causes	Management
Retroauricular dermatitis	• Retroauricular dermatitis is characterized by itching, redness, and scaling within the auricular region [24]. Ear pressure through the use of ear-hook masks is a reported cause of this type of dermatitis [15].	• Recommendations to reduce dermatitis and ear pain include the following: the use of strings or hairpins to lengthen the ear-hook string [15] help reduce the tightness of masks [25]. Jiang et al [26] explored the use of a plastic handle to reduce ear pressure exerted by N95 masks; the advantage of this method was the simplicity of the idea and the increase in comfort on using the masks.
Skin lesions	• Pei et al [27] reported that 73.1% of participants developed skin lesions due to PPE in a cohort of 484 health care workers. Skin lesions included the following: erythema, prurigo, blisters, rhagades, papule, oedema, exudation, crusting, and lichenification [12,27]. The most common sites were the nasal bridge as well as the cheeks and forehead [12]. Factors attributed to skin lesions included the following: higher grades of PPE, higher working frequency within PPE, and prolonged use of PPE [9,25,27].	• Measures to reduce the incidence of skin lesions include the following: wearing the mask correctly, taking mask-free breaks, and frequently replacing of protective gear [25].
Skin dryness	• In a sample of 542 participants in China, skin dryness was the most commonly reported symptom (70.3%) [9]. Closed humid environments, such as those resulting from breathing in masks and the use of PPE [9], result in skin barrier dysfunction [11,28]. Skin barrier dysfunction may consequently lead to skin dryness and scaling [11].	• Management of skin dryness involves the use of high-potency moisturizers before and after PPE use [11].
Skin erythema	• Hua et al [29] reported increased erythema following PPE use; erythema results from cutaneous blood vessel dilation and increased blood supply to the skin [29]. Although this may be a normal reaction to heat and pressure, long-lasting erythema may be a sign of inflammation [29]. Significant differences between the use of N95 masks and surgical masks have been reported; N95 masks reportedly increase the facial temperature of the user and are perceived to be more uncomfortable [30]. Factors potentially causing skin erythema include long hours and prolonged mask-wearing [20]. Campbell et al [31] reported that skin erythema may progress to miliaria owing to the associations of immobility and humidity through prolonged mask-wearing.	• Measures to reduce skin erythema include the following: limiting shift length [20], having mask-free breaks [20], and using a surgical mask rather than an N95 mask when appropriate [30].
Skin injury due to the use of disinfectants	• Skin injury due to the use of disinfectants may result in ICD [32] and ACD [13]. Excessive stress among health care workers because of working with patients with COVID-19 may increase the frequency and duration of skin cleansing, which disrupts the skin barrier and inevitably leads to skin damage [13].	• Although it is important to clean the face using soap-based cleansers after contact with patients with COVID-19 owing to the high risk of disease transmission, health care workers should be wary of excessive washing and the repeated application of disinfectants to the skin [13].
Secondary infections	• Skin and mucous membrane injury, through the disruption of the epidermal barrier, may lead to secondary infections [11]. Factors aggravating membrane injury include the following: prolonged mask-wearing resulting in a closed environment, compression, friction, and humidity [33].	• Avoidance of PPE and the use of antihistamines and antibiotics are recommended for the treatment of secondary infections [13,33]. To prevent secondary infections, it is important to stop water from entering damaged skin; this can be done using waterproof plasters [33].
Acne vulgaris		• The management of acne vulgaris includes the following: liberal use of moisturizers before and after using facial protective equipment, topical antibiotic creams for mild papules and pustules, as well as topical retinoid creams for blackheads and whiteheads [11]. Cases of severe acne vulgaris should be referred to a dermatologist [11].

Dermatological diagnosis	Causes	Management
	• Flares of acne have been reported to result from the use of facial protective equipment; this is thought to be due to increased temperature and humidity caused by the mask [34]. High temperatures as well as high humidity facilitate the progression of acne due to bacterial proliferation and the portal occlusive effect of skin hydration and irritation to the upper parts of the pilosebaceous duct; in turn, this causes swelling of the epidermal keratinocytes, leading to acute blockage of the skin barrier [11,34]. Other underlying mechanisms potentially include pressure and friction [11]. Interestingly, Han et al [34] observed no correlation between acne severity and prolonged mask-wearing. Signs of acne include comedones, papules on the cheeks and nose, as well as nodules or cysts on the forehead, submaxillary, and neck region [34].	
Eczema	• Navarro - Triviño et al [35] found eczema to be one of the most frequently reported skin diseases associated with PPE use. The risk of eczema increased with continuous use of masks and protective glasses [32,35] as a result of increased heat owing to the closed environment, and increased stress [28].	• Use of topical glucocorticoid creams or ointments is suggested for eczematous skin changes [13].
Rosacea	• Rosacea has been frequently reported in association with PPE use [35]. Increased heat and stress is linked to the exacerbation of rosacea [28]. Prolonged PPE use is a risk factor for developing rosacea [32].	N/A[a]
Urticaria	• Urticaria of the face has been linked to the resulting vertical pressure of facial protective equipment [11]. Risk factors include the following: prolonged wearing of protective equipment and excessive personal hygiene [12].	• Preventative measures include the use of correctly fitted protective equipment and antihistamines [11].
Impetigo	• Yu et al [36] documented a case of impetigo due to occupational goggle-mask–wearing during the pandemic [36]. Increased humidity, skin trauma, and malnutrition can increase the skin's vulnerability to infection and create a moist occlusive environment, allowing *Staphylococcus aureus* to grow and infect the damaged skin [36].	• Management of this condition included rest away from PPE and the application of topical 2% fusidic acid cream twice daily [36].
Nasal bridge ulceration	• Owing to occupational use of PPE, the nasal bridge was reported to be damaged in 83.1% of health care workers [37]. Pressure, friction, and the hyperhydration effect are known risk factors for ulceration [12,15.]	• Hydrocolloid dressings may be of use to successfully treat nasal bridge ulceration [37].
Exacerbations of known skin disease	• Flares of pre-existing dermatoses have been reported to result from PPE use [17,28,32]. Stress, due to the pandemic, has been linked to the aggravation of skin conditions such as psoriasis, eczema, atopy, and neurodermatitis [28,32].	• Zheng et al [32] questioned the use of psychological counseling to reduce the stress experienced by health care workers in order to reduce exacerbations of skin diseases.

[a]N/A: not applicable.

Discussion

Principal Findings

This preliminary and exploratory review documents the different dermatological conditions associated with occupational mask-wearing, by causes and management, among health care workers during the COVID-19 pandemic from the existing literature (in May 2020) (Table 1).

Personal Perspectives of Health Care Workers in Relation to Dermatological Problems

The literature reveals a high number of health care workers who are affected by skin damage; in a sample of 546 individuals, 526 (97%) staff members reported negative skin consequences as a result of PPE use [6-10]. Symptoms of skin barrier damage, as reported by health care professionals, include burning, itching, and stinging [11]. The most common site of skin damage was the nasal bridge, and this occurred in 83.1% of health care workers [6-8,13].

Pei et al [27] conducted a study involving 484 health care workers and reported that 73.1% experienced various skin lesions including the following: erythema (38.8%), prurigo (22.9%), blisters (13.8%), rhagades (13.6%), papules (12.8%), exudation (6.8%), and lichenification.

Facial erythema was reported at varying rates; Pei et al [27] reported that 38.8% of health care workers experienced erythema, whereas Balato et al [38] found erythema rates to be higher at 60.4%. Singh et al [20] categorized two varying forms of erythema: whole face erythema (linked to prolonged hours) and lip lick erythema (linked to constant licking of lips from excessive thirst and fluid restriction). Scarano et al [30] investigated facial skin temperature in relation to occupational mask-wearing and reported a significant difference between surgical and N95 masks with regard to humidity, heat, breathing difficulty, and discomfort. Erythema, as a result of increased warmth, may cause health care workers to alter the position of their mask using contaminated hands, which may increase the risk of self-infection with COVID-19 [30].

Furthermore, skin papules have been reported to result from mask-wearing; papules are often a common sign of acne, alongside other symptoms such as comedones, nodules, and cysts [34]. Gheisari et al [21] reported that 35.5% of health care workers experienced acne as a consequence of occupational mask-wearing. Skin damage, such as an irritating pimples in the case of acne, may cause health care workers to repeatedly touch their face, thus increasing the risk of infection [34,39].

Iatrogenic skin damage, resulting from allergic and irritant contact dermatitis, is associated with occupational mask-wearing. In a sample of 14 health care workers, 35.7% of participants developed irritant contact dermatitis, and 28.6% of participants developed allergic contact dermatitis, which was associated with facial masks [24].

Another common complaint among health care workers concerned pressure-related injuries. Jiang et al [14] conducted a cross-sectional study, incorporating the views of 4308 health care workers and reported that 42.8% of respondents had skin injuries resulting from pressure (95% CI 41.30-44.30). Moreover, health care workers develop multiple skin lesions across different areas of the face; the disruption of the epidermal skin barrier across multiple sites may increase the risk of contracting COVID-19 among health care workers [14].

Lastly, Szepietowski et al [40] investigated the prevalence of pruritus among health care workers as a result of mask-wearing. From among 1393 participants, 273 (19.6%) reported an itching sensation. Higher incidences of pruritus have been reported in studies from Singapore and China; in Singapore, 51.4% of health care workers developed a facial itch [24], as opposed to 61.8% in China [27]. The risk of pruritus was further increased among those with an atopic predisposition, facial dermatoses, and prolonged PPE use [40]. Moreover, it was found that the sensation of pruritus caused health care workers to itch and touch their mask, reducing its protectiveness against COVID-19 [40].

Recommendations to Reduce the Adverse Effects Associated With Facial Masks

Despite evidence regarding the vast number of dermatological conditions resulting from mask-wearing, limited evidence is available on the occupational management of these problems. One study advocated the use of virtual occupational health checks to prevent serious skin damage among health care workers [41]. The virtual clinic was led by nurses who advised health care workers on protective self-care and skin care measures and triaged moderate and severe skin disorders to dermatologists if needed [42].

Pressure-related injuries associated with occupational mask-wearing has been common. Letters to the editor, written by multiple working health care professionals throughout the current pandemic, have highlighted the immense discomfort and pressure damage faced by staff on a regular basis [13,16,41]. Surprisingly, despite reports of discomfort and pressure damage, Jiang et al [14] reported that only 17.7% of health care professionals used prophylactic dressings and lotions. Hydrocolloid dressings have been suggested to reduce skin damage and improve comfort among health care workers who use facial masks [16]. A study by Dong et al [18] found that the use of hydrogel patches resulted in lower skin reaction mean scores (3.47, SD 1.39) compared to their nonuse (13.32, SD 2.06), demonstrating their ability to reduce the severity and incidence of skin damage. Furthermore, Payne [16] argued that a strip of hydrocolloid dressing over the area of pressure damage should not impair the mask seal and should be used by health care workers with pre-existing skin disease or those who wear masks for over 2 hours. Buckley et al [6] agreed with the use of hydrocolloid dressings; however, they recommended refit testing for staff members to ensure the seal was intact to prevent infection. In stark contrast, Yin et al [41] reported that hydrocolloid dressings may be harmful to the skin owing to the extreme stickiness of the dressing and the potential to rip away skin on removal. A recent study by Jiang et al [26] documented the use of a plastic handle on the N95 respirator to reduce pressure injuries to the ear and reduce mask adjustments made by health care workers. The advantages of using a plastic handle included improved comfort, intact mask seal, reduced risk of infection through a lower rate of mask adjustments, and easy disinfection of the handles [27]. Other methods to reduce pressure-related injuries include the following: education of health care professionals [7,38], use of a correctly fitted mask to minimize friction [7,11], regular moisturizing [6,7,11,16], and frequent mask-free breaks [6,11,13,16].

The alleviation of mental health conditions, such as stress and anxiety, within these unprecedented times also plays a key role in preventing skin damage. Li et al [33] reported that high mental stress may precipitate endocrine disorders such as acne through excessive secretion of androgens, which in turn stimulate excess sebum secretion from the sebaceous glands. This, along with mask-wearing, reduces local blood circulation and oxygen levels and causes occlusion of the sebaceous ducts in hair follicles [33]. Additional factors that exacerbate skin stress include high-intensity work, irregular eating habits, and poor rest [32]. Other studies further corroborated the findings of Li et al, linking stress to acne [28], dermatitis [28], and pre-existing skin disorders [28,32].

In addition, anxiety has proved to be a problem among health care workers. A study conducted in Malaysia [41] reported that several pressure-related injuries were self-inflicted by health care professionals owing to overtightening of their N95 masks. Although overtightening of the masks provided the staff with mental relief of improved protection, it consequently increased the risk of skin damage and inadvertently increased the risk of COVID-19 infection through disrupted skin [41]. Staff members responsible for providing care to patients with COVID-19 should be educated on the efficacy of masks to reduce overtightening as well as anxiety [41].

Furthermore, nonmodifiable risk factors, such as gender, influenced the progression of skin damage. One study [25] reported that rashes were more likely to affect women. Zuo et al [39] found that women had a lower threshold for reporting symptoms of skin damage. However, Gefen et al [43] surveyed 4308 health care workers and found that the male prevalence of pressure injuries was significant and 1.6-fold that among women. Possible theories for this finding include differences in the facial architecture between men and women [41]. Moreover, this result may demonstrate the need for gender-specific PPE to prevent skin damage among men [41].

Limitations

Notable limitations of our study include the exploratory direction of the literature review; the available literature was restricted owing to the emerging nature of COVID-19 and lack of studies during the search period (May 1-29, 2020). Moreover, the data included within the review may be constrained by PubMed being the only legitimate scientific database being used herein; this may raise concerns that other important studies may have been missed. As a result of limitations arising from the aforementioned reasons, our literature review accepted all types of articles, which may have limited the applicability of the results to the broader population. Furthermore, numerous studies included within our literature review reported their findings on the basis of a small cohort, which may have decreased the reliability of the results. Furthermore, articles included in this literature review were from multiple institutions worldwide, most notably the United Kingdom and Asia. Difficulties, such as finding reliable translations of articles as well as a lack of literature from other countries, may also skew the results of this literature review.

Conclusions

PPE has been invaluable throughout the COVID-19 pandemic; it has allowed health care workers to safely provide care to the most vulnerable individuals, with minimal risk. Masks have provided the main form of essential protection to the respiratory system against COVID-19; however, owing to the rapid global threat COVID-19 presents, it is clear that the risk of skin damage resulting from mask-wearing has not been considered. The effects of skin damage can be dangerous among health care workers; the risk of infection may be increased through disruptions in the skin barrier as well as self-contamination through mask adjustments. The highly contagious nature of SARS-CoV-2 increases the likelihood that protective measures may stay in place from this day forward; innovation and advancements in PPE need to be sought to protect the skin and to reduce the currently increasing incidence of dermatological conditions among health care workers.

References

1. Singhal T. A Review of Coronavirus Disease-2019 (COVID-19). Indian J Pediatr 2020 Apr 13;87(4):281-286 [FREE Full text] [doi: 10.1007/s12098-020-03263-6] [Medline: 32166607]
2. Zhang L, Wang M, Wang Y, Zhu J, Zhang N. Focus on the 2019 novel coronavirus (SARS-CoV-2). Future Microbiol 2020 Jul;15:905-918 [FREE Full text] [doi: 10.2217/fmb-2020-0063] [Medline: 32524843]
3. Al-Kassmy J, Pedersen J, Kobinger G. Vaccine Candidates against Coronavirus Infections. Where Does COVID-19 Stand? Viruses 2020 Aug 07;12(8):861 [FREE Full text] [doi: 10.3390/v12080861] [Medline: 32784685]
4. Abd El-Aziz TM, Stockand JD. Recent progress and challenges in drug development against COVID-19 coronavirus (SARS-CoV-2) - an update on the status. Infect Genet Evol 2020 Sep;83:104327 [FREE Full text] [doi: 10.1016/j.meegid.2020.104327] [Medline: 32320825]
5. Feng S, Shen C, Xia N, Song W, Fan M, Cowling BJ. Rational use of face masks in the COVID-19 pandemic. Lancet Respir Med 2020 May;8(5):434-436 [FREE Full text] [doi: 10.1016/S2213-2600(20)30134-X] [Medline: 32203710]
6. Buckley D, Stone N, British Society for Cutaneous Allergy Committee. British Society for Cutaneous Allergy advice on skin damage from FFP3 masks. BMJ 2020 Jun 09;369:m2268. [doi: 10.1136/bmj.m2268] [Medline: 32518080]
7. Bhatia R, Sindhuja T, Bhatia S, Dev T, Gupta A, Bajpai M, et al. Iatrogenic dermatitis in times of COVID-19: a pandemic within a pandemic. J Eur Acad Dermatol Venereol 2020 Oct;34(10):e563-e566 [FREE Full text] [doi: 10.1111/jdv.16710] [Medline: 32495393]
8. Fahmy D, El-Amawy HS, El-Samongy MA, Fouda A, Soliman S, El-Kady A, et al. COVID-19 and dermatology: a comprehensive guide for dermatologists. J Eur Acad Dermatol Venereol 2020 Jul;34(7):1388-1394 [FREE Full text] [doi: 10.1111/jdv.16545] [Medline: 32428303]

9. Lan J, Song Z, Miao X, Li H, Li Y, Dong L, et al. Skin damage among health care workers managing coronavirus disease-2019. J Am Acad Dermatol 2020 May;82(5):1215-1216 [FREE Full text] [doi: 10.1016/j.jaad.2020.03.014] [Medline: 32171808]
10. Elston DM. Occupational skin disease among health care workers during the coronavirus (COVID-19) epidemic. J Am Acad Dermatol 2020 May;82(5):1085-1086 [FREE Full text] [doi: 10.1016/j.jaad.2020.03.012] [Medline: 32171807]
11. Yan Y, Chen H, Chen L, Cheng B, Diao P, Dong L, et al. Consensus of Chinese experts on protection of skin and mucous membrane barrier for health-care workers fighting against coronavirus disease 2019. Dermatol Ther 2020 Jul;33(4):e13310 [FREE Full text] [doi: 10.1111/dth.13310] [Medline: 32170800]
12. Darlenski R, Tsankov N. COVID-19 pandemic and the skin: what should dermatologists know? Clin Dermatol 2020;38(6):785-787 [FREE Full text] [doi: 10.1016/j.clindermatol.2020.03.012] [Medline: 33341217]
13. Zhang B, Zhai R, Ma L. 2019 novel coronavirus disease epidemic: skin protection for healthcare workers must not be ignored. J Eur Acad Dermatol Venereol 2020 Sep;34(9):e434-e435 [FREE Full text] [doi: 10.1111/jdv.16573] [Medline: 32358808]
14. Jiang Q, Song S, Zhou J, Liu Y, Chen A, Bai Y, et al. The Prevalence, Characteristics, and Prevention Status of Skin Injury Caused by Personal Protective Equipment Among Medical Staff in Fighting COVID-19: A Multicenter, Cross-Sectional Study. Adv Wound Care (New Rochelle) 2020 Jul;9(7):357-364. [doi: 10.1089/wound.2020.1212] [Medline: 32320359]
15. Yu N, Xiao Y, Su J, Huang K, Zhao S. Practical tips for using masks in the COVID-19 pandemic. Dermatol Ther 2020 Jul;33(4):e13555 [FREE Full text] [doi: 10.1111/dth.13555] [Medline: 32390307]
16. Payne A. Covid-19: skin damage with prolonged wear of FFP3 masks. BMJ 2020 May 04;369:m1743. [doi: 10.1136/bmj.m1743] [Medline: 32366499]
17. Aerts O, Dendooven E, Foubert K, Stappers S, Ulicki M, Lambert J. Surgical mask dermatitis caused by formaldehyde (releasers) during the COVID-19 pandemic. Contact Dermatitis 2020 Aug;83(2):172-173. [doi: 10.1111/cod.13626] [Medline: 32468589]
18. Dong L, Yang L, Li Y, Yang J, An X, Yang L, et al. Efficacy of hydrogel patches in preventing facial skin damage caused by mask compression in fighting against coronavirus disease 2019: a short-term, self-controlled study. J Eur Acad Dermatol Venereol 2020 Sep;34(9):e441-e443 [FREE Full text] [doi: 10.1111/jdv.16638] [Medline: 32421878]
19. Smart H, Opinion FB, Darwich I, Elnawasany MA, Kodange C. Preventing Facial Pressure Injury for Health Care Providers Adhering to COVID-19 Personal Protective Equipment Requirements. Adv Skin Wound Care 2020 Aug;33(8):418-427 [FREE Full text] [doi: 10.1097/01.ASW.0000669920.94084.c1] [Medline: 32530822]
20. Singh M, Pawar M, Bothra A, Maheshwari A, Dubey V, Tiwari A, et al. Personal protective equipment induced facial dermatoses in healthcare workers managing Coronavirus disease 2019. J Eur Acad Dermatol Venereol 2020 Aug;34(8):e378-e380 [FREE Full text] [doi: 10.1111/jdv.16628] [Medline: 32396675]
21. Gheisari M, Araghi F, Moravvej H, Tabary M, Dadkhahfar S. Skin reactions to non-glove personal protective equipment: an emerging issue in the COVID-19 pandemic. J Eur Acad Dermatol Venereol 2020 Jul;34(7):e297-e298 [FREE Full text] [doi: 10.1111/jdv.16492] [Medline: 32302444]
22. Preventing and Treating Occupationally Induced Dermatologic Conditions During COVID-19. American Academy of Dermatology Association. URL: https://www.aad.org/public/diseases/coronavirus/occ-induced [accessed 2020-06-02]
23. Maliyar K, Sachdeva M, Mufti A, Yeung J. Reply to: "Skin damage among health care workers managing coronavirus disease 2019". J Am Acad Dermatol 2020 Aug;83(2):e169-e170 [FREE Full text] [doi: 10.1016/j.jaad.2020.05.037] [Medline: 32417418]
24. Bothra A, Das S, Singh M, Pawar M, Maheswari A. Retroauricular dermatitis with vehement use of ear loop face masks during COVID-19 pandemic. J Eur Acad Dermatol Venereol 2020 Oct;34(10):e549-e552 [FREE Full text] [doi: 10.1111/jdv.16692] [Medline: 32491204]
25. Hu K, Fan J, Li X, Gou X, Li X, Zhou X. The adverse skin reactions of health care workers using personal protective equipment for COVID-19. Medicine (Baltimore) 2020 Jun 12;99(24):e20603 [FREE Full text] [doi: 10.1097/MD.0000000000020603] [Medline: 32541493]
26. Jiang W, Cao W, Liu Q. Wearing the N95 mask with a plastic handle reduces pressure injury. J Am Acad Dermatol 2020 Jun;82(6):e191-e192 [FREE Full text] [doi: 10.1016/j.jaad.2020.04.001] [Medline: 32283239]
27. Pei S, Xue Y, Zhao S, Alexander N, Mohamad G, Chen X, et al. Occupational skin conditions on the front line: a survey among 484 Chinese healthcare professionals caring for Covid-19 patients. J Eur Acad Dermatol Venereol 2020 Aug;34(8):e354-e357 [FREE Full text] [doi: 10.1111/jdv.16570] [Medline: 32362062]
28. Goldust M, Shivakumar S, Kroumpouzos G, Murrell DF, Mueller SM, Navarini AA. Where do we stand as dermatologists in combat with COVID-19. Dermatol Ther 2020 Jul;33(4):e13638 [FREE Full text] [doi: 10.1111/dth.13638] [Medline: 32441435]
29. Hua W, Zuo Y, Wan R, Xiong L, Tang J, Zou L, et al. Short-term skin reactions following use of N95 respirators and medical masks. Contact Dermatitis 2020 Aug;83(2):115-121 [FREE Full text] [doi: 10.1111/cod.13601] [Medline: 32406064]
30. Scarano A, Inchingolo F, Lorusso F. Facial Skin Temperature and Discomfort When Wearing Protective Face Masks: Thermal Infrared Imaging Evaluation and Hands Moving the Mask. Int J Environ Res Public Health 2020 Jun 27;17(13):4624 [FREE Full text] [doi: 10.3390/ijerph17134624] [Medline: 32605056]

31. Campbell V, Middleton D, Donnelly J, Hunter H. Localized mid-face miliaria as a consequence of filtering face piece respirator use during the COVID-19 pandemic. J Eur Acad Dermatol Venereol 2020 Aug;34(8):e375-e376 [FREE Full text] [doi: 10.1111/jdv.16624] [Medline: 32386442]
32. Zheng Y, Lai W. Dermatology staff participate in fight against Covid-19 in China. J Eur Acad Dermatol Venereol 2020 May;34(5):e210-e211. [doi: 10.1111/jdv.16390] [Medline: 32201983]
33. Li C, Shen J, Ju Y, Huang X, Huang L, Zeng K. [Management and prevention of common skin problems during epidemic prevention and control of COVID-19]. Nan Fang Yi Ke Da Xue Xue Bao 2020 Mar 29;40(2):168-170 [FREE Full text] [doi: 10.12122/j.issn.1673-4254.2020.02.05] [Medline: 32376531]
34. Han C, Shi J, Chen Y, Zhang Z. Increased flare of acne caused by long-time mask wearing during COVID-19 pandemic among general population. Dermatol Ther 2020 Jul;33(4):e13704 [FREE Full text] [doi: 10.1111/dth.13704] [Medline: 32472634]
35. Navarro-Triviño FJ, Ruiz-Villaverde R. Therapeutic approach to skin reactions caused by personal protective equipment (PPE) during COVID-19 pandemic: An experience from a tertiary hospital in Granada, Spain. Dermatol Ther 2020 Nov;33(6):e13838 [FREE Full text] [doi: 10.1111/dth.13838] [Medline: 32543015]
36. Yu Q, Li W, Yang L. A case of goggle-mask-related impetigo at the time of the COVID-19 pandemic. Dermatol Ther 2020 Jul;33(4):e13636 [FREE Full text] [doi: 10.1111/dth.13636] [Medline: 32436604]
37. Sernicola A, Chello C, Cerbelli E, Adebanjo GAR, Parisella FR, Pezzuto A, et al. Treatment of nasal bridge ulceration related to protective measures for the COVID-19 epidemic. Int Wound J 2020 Oct;17(5):1520-1522 [FREE Full text] [doi: 10.1111/iwj.13397] [Medline: 32379379]
38. Balato A, Ayala F, Bruze M, Crepy M, Gonçalo M, Johansen J, et al. European Task Force on Contact Dermatitis statement on coronavirus disease-19 (COVID-19) outbreak and the risk of adverse cutaneous reactions. J Eur Acad Dermatol Venereol 2020 Aug;34(8):e353-e354. [doi: 10.1111/jdv.16557] [Medline: 32356382]
39. Zuo Y, Hua W, Luo Y, Li L. Skin reactions of N95 masks and medial masks among health-care personnel: A self-report questionnaire survey in China. Contact Dermatitis 2020 Aug;83(2):145-147 [FREE Full text] [doi: 10.1111/cod.13555] [Medline: 32297349]
40. Szepietowski J, Matusiak L, Szepietowska M, Krajewski P, Białynicki-Birula R. Face Mask-induced Itch: A Self-questionnaire Study of 2,315 Responders During the COVID-19 Pandemic. Acta Derm Venereol 2020 May 28;100(10):adv00152 [FREE Full text] [doi: 10.2340/00015555-3536] [Medline: 32449781]
41. Yin Z. Covid-19: countermeasure for N95 mask-induced pressure sore. J Eur Acad Dermatol Venereol 2020 Jul;34(7):e294-e295 [FREE Full text] [doi: 10.1111/jdv.16490] [Medline: 32302449]
42. Chowdhury MM, Bevan N, Ryan K. Covid-19: virtual occupational skin health clinics for healthcare workers. BMJ 2020 Jun 18;369:m2281. [doi: 10.1136/bmj.m2281] [Medline: 32554389]
43. Gefen A, Ousey K. Prevention of skin damage caused by the protective equipment used to mitigate COVID-19. J Wound Care 2020 Jun 02;29(6):311 [FREE Full text] [doi: 10.12968/jowc.2020.29.6.311] [Medline: 32530779]

Abbreviations

ACD: allergic contact dermatitis
ICD: irritant contact dermatitis
PPE: personal protective equipment

11

Global Burden of Skin Disease Representation in the Literature: Bibliometric Analysis

Kayd J Pulsipher[1], BS; Mindy D Szeto[2], MS; Chandler W Rundle[3], MD; Colby L Presley[4], BA, BS; Melissa R Laughter[2], PhD; Robert P Dellavalle[2,5,6], MSPH, MD, PhD

[1]College of Osteopathic Medicine, Rocky Vista University, Parker, CO, United States
[2]Department of Dermatology, University of Colorado Anschutz Medical Campus, Aurora, CO, United States
[3]Department of Medicine, St. Joseph's Hospital, Denver, CO, United States
[4]Division of Dermatology, Lehigh Valley Health Network, Allentown, PA, United States
[5]Department of Epidemiology, Colorado School of Public Health, University of Colorado Anschutz Medical Campus, Aurora, CO, United States
[6]Dermatology Service, Rocky Mountain Regional Medical Center, US Department of Veteran Affairs, Aurora, CO, United States

Corresponding Author:
Robert P Dellavalle, MSPH, MD, PhD
Dermatology Service
Rocky Mountain Regional Medical Center
US Department of Veteran Affairs
1700 N Wheeling St
Rm E1-342
Aurora, CO, 80045
United States

Email: robert.dellavalle@cuanschutz.edu

Abstract

Background: The global burden of skin disease may be reduced through research efforts focused on skin diseases with the highest reported disability-adjusted life years.

Objective: This study evaluates the representation of dermatologic conditions comprising the highest disability-adjusted life years in dermatology literature to identify areas that could benefit from greater research focus.

Methods: The top 10 skin disorders according to their respective disability-adjusted life years as per the 2013 Global Burden of Disease were identified using previous studies. The top 5 dermatology journals ranked by the 2019 h-index were also identified. A PubMed search of each journal was performed using individual skin disease terms. From 2015 to 2020, all indexed publications pertaining to each disease were recorded and compared to the total number of publications for each journal surveyed.

Results: A total of 19,727 papers were published in the 5 journals over the span of 2015-2020. Although melanoma ranked as the eighth highest in disability-adjusted life years, it had the highest representation in the literature (1995/19,727, 10.11%). Melanoma was followed in representation by psoriasis (1936/19,727, 9.81%) and dermatitis (1927/19,727, 9.77%). These 3 conditions comprised a total of 29.69% (5858/19,727) of the total publications, while the remaining 7 skin conditions were represented by a combined 6.79% (1341/19,727) of the total publications.

Conclusions: This research identifies gaps in the literature related to the top skin diseases contributing to the global burden of disease. Our study provides insight into future opportunities of focused research on less-studied skin diseases to potentially aid in reducing the global burden of skin disease.

KEYWORDS

global burden of disease; global health; global dermatology; disability-adjusted life years; GBD; DALYs; journalology; dermatology; skin disorders

Introduction

The 2013 Global Burden of Disease (GBD) Morbidity and Mortality report identified skin diseases as the fourth leading cause of global disability-adjusted life years (DALYs) [1]. One DALY is the sum of years of life lost to a disease plus years lived with disability, with 1 DALY equating to 1 year of healthy life lost [1]. Research pertaining to skin disorders with higher reported DALYs has potential to reduce the global burden of skin disease through improvements in management guidelines, public health initiatives, policy changes, and increased awareness within the scientific and greater community [2]. This study evaluates the representation of dermatologic conditions comprising the highest DALYs in dermatology literature to identify areas that could benefit from increased research focus.

Methods

A comprehensive search was performed using PubMed to identify peer-reviewed papers. A previous GBD study has identified and ranked individual skin disorders according to their respective DALYs [1]. This GBD study was used to select our specific search terms such as dermatitis, acne vulgaris, psoriasis, urticaria, viral skin diseases, fungal skin diseases, scabies, melanoma, pyoderma, and cellulitis. The h-index is a noted metric used to measure individual author and journal research influence and impact [3]. The top 5 dermatology journals ranked by the 2019 h-index were identified using the Scimago Journal and Country Rank [4]. PubMed searching was performed by pairing individual skin disease terms with each journal title (eg, "dermatitis" AND "Journal of the American Academy of Dermatology"). From 2015 to 2020, all indexed publications pertaining to each disease were recorded and compared to the total number of publications for each journal surveyed. All article types were included to obtain a complete picture of relevant skin disease research. Duplicate papers were excluded.

Results

Over the span of 2015-2020, 19,727 publications were recorded from the previously mentioned journals. Melanoma (eighth in DALYs) had the highest representation in the literature at 10.11% (1995/19,727) of the total publications, followed by psoriasis (1936/19,727, 9.81%) and dermatitis (1927/19,727, 9.77%) (Table 1). Melanoma, psoriasis, and dermatitis comprised a total of 29.69% (5858/19,727) of all the publications from 2015 to 2020. The remaining 7 skin diseases comprised only 6.79% (1341/19,727) of the total publications. Acne vulgaris, the second highest contributor to skin GBD, followed dermatitis with a much lower representation in the literature (477/19,727, 2.42%). Scabies accumulated the lowest percentage of the total publications (54/19,727, 0.27%). The proportions of publications by year for each disease are shown in Figure 1.

Table 1. Top 10 skin conditions contributing to the global burden of disease [1] and their representation in the dermatology literature.[a]

Skin disease search term	Global burden of skin disease rank	Rank by percentage of total publications	Percentage of global burden of disease (measured in disability-adjusted life years)[b]	Proportion of global burden of skin disease measured in disability-adjusted life years, fraction (%)[c]	Publications in 2015-2020 (N=19,727), n (%)	Percentage of total publications/Percentage of global burden of skin disease
Dermatitis	1	3	0.38	0.38/1.70 (22.35)	1927 (9.77)	0.44
Acne	2	4	0.29	0.29/1.70 (17.06)	477 (2.42)	0.14
Psoriasis	3	2	0.19	0.19/1.70 (11.18)	1936 (9.81)	0.88
Urticaria[d]	3	7	0.19	0.19/1.70 (11.18)	139 (0.70)	0.06
Viral skin disease	5	5	0.16	0.16/1.70 (9.41)	283 (1.38)	0.15
Fungal skin disease	6	6	0.15	0.15/1.70 (8.82)	193 (0.98)	0.11
Scabies	7	10	0.07	0.07/1.70 (4.12)	54 (0.27)	0.07
Melanoma	8	1	0.06	0.06/1.70 (3.53)	1995 (10.11)	2.86
Pyoderma	9	8	0.05	0.05/1.70 (2.94)	124 (0.63)	0.21
Cellulitis	10	9	0.04	0.04/1.70 (2.35)	81 (0.41)	0.17
All other skin and subcutaneous diseases	N/A[e]	N/A	0.12	0.12/1.70 (7.00)	N/A	N/A

[a]The following journals ranked by the 2019 h-index were searched: rank 1, Journal of the American Academy of Dermatology; rank 2, Journal of Investigative Dermatology; rank 3, British Journal of Dermatology; rank 4, Journal of the American Medical Association Dermatology; and rank 5, Dermatologic Surgery.

[b]The percentage values in this column have been directly taken from the global burden of disease paper [1]. Total skin-related percentage of global burden of disease=1.70%.

[c]This column shows the fractions of the total skin-related global burden of disease over the total percentage of global burden of disease (1.70%) calculated for the 10 skin diseases.

[d]Urticaria has the same ranking as psoriasis in the calculation of the global burden of skin disease rankings [1].

[e]N/A: not applicable.

Figure 1. Proportion of publications by year for each global burden of skin disease condition.

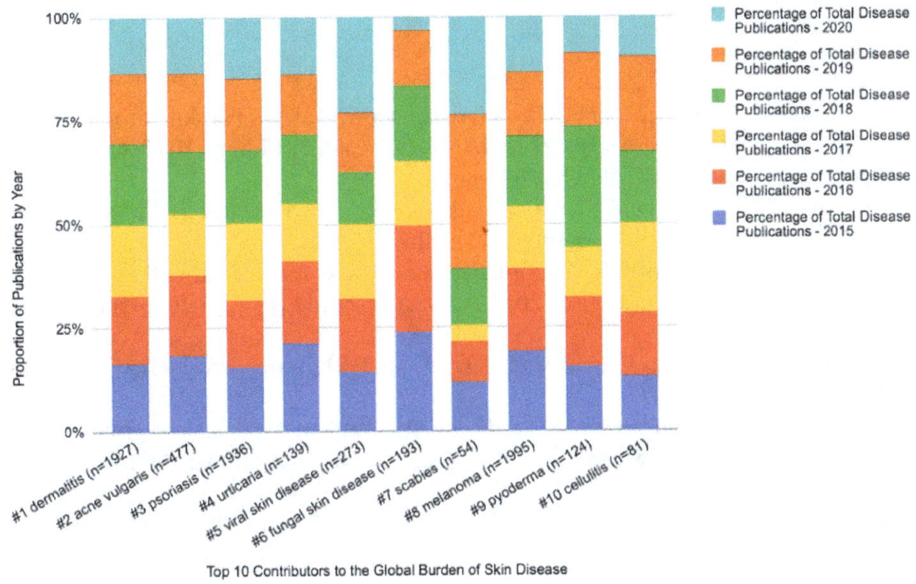

Discussion

The disproportionate representation of melanoma in the literature compared to overall GBD is likely explained by the increased mortality risk of melanoma relative to other skin diseases [5,6]. Additionally, a large portion of the examined publications originated from North American– and European-based journals, which are regions with high melanoma incidence reported globally [5]. Notably, these regions have minimal incidence of scabies [1], which had the lowest representation in the literature. However, literature representation is likely multifactorial, with epidemiologic factors and research funding contributing to literature representation [7].

Although this study utilizes 2013 GBD data to guide our literature search, it does not implicate the literature gaps identified in this study. Our study was limited by the use of 1 specific search term pertaining to the individual skin diseases. We recognize that performing our search across 5 journals with a single term per skin disease could have led to possible omissions. Although a variety of terms could be searched for some skin diseases within our study, such as fungal skin diseases, we elected to use a single term for consistency across all the skin diseases studied and recognize that certain publications discussing multiple skin diseases may have been listed under more than one search term. Lastly, we acknowledge that many of the mentioned skin diseases may be represented outside of dermatology-specific journals, which our study did not examine. Nonetheless, we offer a valuable initial survey of these skin diseases in highly read and influential dermatology literature and hope that our study will prompt future necessary work to identify potential avenues for refinement of current research efforts.

Indeed, a primary purpose of the GBD collaboration is to aid clinical researchers in determining priority of research at local, national, and global levels [1]. Herein, our study provides insight into possible future investigative pathways for dermatologic research. For example, urticaria accounts for 11.18% (0.19/1.70) of skin-related DALYs (equal to psoriasis), yet these rank sixth and second in the percentage of the total publications, respectively [8]. Thus, researchers have opportunities to further elucidate causal mechanisms and the clinical impact of less-studied dermatologic conditions as a means to guide clinical decision-making, public health initiatives, policy changes, and education for dermatologists.

Dermatologic disease is a significant source of global DALYs. Although there has been significant research focus on dermatologic malignancies, dermatitis, and psoriasis in the last 5 years, this study highlights significant gaps and opportunities that remain in skin disease literature.

Authors' Contributions

KJP contributed to the project conceptualization, methodology, data collection, writing of manuscript, review, and editing. MDS contributed to the methodology, statistical analysis, review, and editing. CWR contributed to the writing of manuscript, review, and editing. CLP contributed to project conceptualization, writing of manuscript, review, and editing. MRL contributed to the methodology, statistical analysis, review, and editing. RPD contributed to the review and editing, project supervision, and project administration.

References

1. Karimkhani C, Dellavalle RP, Coffeng LE, Flohr C, Hay RJ, Langan SM, et al. Global skin disease morbidity and mortality: an update from the Global Burden of Disease study 2013. JAMA Dermatol 2017 May 01;153(5):406-412 [FREE Full text] [doi: 10.1001/jamadermatol.2016.5538] [Medline: 28249066]
2. Pagoto S, Waring ME, Xu R. A call for a public health agenda for social media research. J Med Internet Res 2019 Dec 19;21(12):e16661 [FREE Full text] [doi: 10.2196/16661] [Medline: 31855185]
3. El Emam K, Arbuckle L, Jonker E, Anderson K. Two h-index benchmarks for evaluating the publication performance of medical informatics researchers. J Med Internet Res 2012 Oct 18;14(5):e144 [FREE Full text] [doi: 10.2196/jmir.2177] [Medline: 23079075]
4. Journal rankings on dermatology. Scimago Journal & Country Rank. URL: https://www.scimagojr.com/journalrank.php?category=2708 [accessed 2020-09-27]
5. Karimkhani C, Green AC, Nijsten T, Weinstock MA, Dellavalle RP, Naghavi M, et al. The global burden of melanoma: results from the Global Burden of Disease Study 2015. Br J Dermatol 2017 Jul;177(1):134-140 [FREE Full text] [doi: 10.1111/bjd.15510] [Medline: 28369739]
6. Boyers LN, Karimkhani C, Naghavi M, Sherwood D, Margolis DJ, Hay RJ, et al. Global mortality from conditions with skin manifestations. J Am Acad Dermatol 2014 Dec;71(6):1137-1143.e17. [doi: 10.1016/j.jaad.2014.08.022] [Medline: 25282129]
7. Hagstrom EL, Patel S, Karimkhani C, Boyers LN, Williams HC, Hay RJ, et al. Comparing cutaneous research funded by the US National Institutes of Health (NIH) with the US skin disease burden. J Am Acad Dermatol 2015 Sep;73(3):383-91.e1. [doi: 10.1016/j.jaad.2015.04.039] [Medline: 26051697]

8. Maxim E, Aksut C, Tsoi D, Dellavalle RP. Global burden of urticaria: Insights from the 2016 Global Burden of Disease Study. J Am Acad Dermatol 2018 Sep;79(3):567-569 [FREE Full text] [doi: 10.1016/j.jaad.2018.02.026] [Medline: 29438758]

Abbreviations

DALY: disability-adjusted life year
GBD: Global Burden of Disease

12

Effects of Pain from Atopic Dermatitis: Interview and Focus Group Study with Patients and their Families

Ashley M Snyder[1,2], MPH; Vanina L Taliercio[1], MS, MD; Adelheid U Brandenberger[3], MD; Bianca E Rich[3], MD; Lisa B Webber[1], BS; Abram P Beshay[1], MD; Joshua E Biber[2], MBA, MS; Rachel Hess[2,4], MS, MD; Jamie L W Rhoads[1], MS, MD; Aaron M Secrest[1,2], MD, PhD

[1]Department of Dermatology, University of Utah, Salt Lake City, UT, United States

[2]Department of Population Health Sciences, University of Utah, Salt Lake City, UT, United States

[3]School of Medicine, University of Utah, Salt Lake City, UT, United States

[4]Department of Internal Medicine, University of Utah, Salt Lake City, UT, United States

Corresponding Author:
Aaron M Secrest, MD, PhD
Department of Dermatology
University of Utah
30 North 1900 East, 4A330
Salt Lake City, UT, 84132
United States

Email: Aaron.Secrest@hsc.utah.edu

Abstract

Background: Pain is an underappreciated symptom of atopic dermatitis that can affect the health-related quality of life (HRQL) of patients.

Objective: The aim of this study is to understand the effect of pain on patients with atopic dermatitis and their family members and to recognize how this symptom affects HRQL.

Methods: We conducted focus groups and interviews with patients with atopic dermatitis and their family members. Researchers independently coded the transcripts and reached a consensus on the major themes.

Results: A total of 33 adult participants, consisting of 21 patients with atopic dermatitis (median age 47 years, range 22-77) and 12 family members (median age 50, range 22-72), attended either focus groups (23/33, 70%) or interviews (10/33, 30%), where we assessed their experiences of pain. Four themes emerged in our study. Itchiness and pain can be intertwined: pain was often caused by or otherwise associated with itchiness and could result from open sores and excoriated skin. Characteristics of pain: pain was most often described as burning. Other descriptors included mild, persistent discomfort; stinging; and stabbing. Effects of pain: pain negatively affected various aspects of daily life, including choice of clothing, sleep, social activities, and relationships. The location of painful areas could also limit physical activity, including sex. Pain management: pain from atopic dermatitis could be managed to varying degrees with different over-the-counter and prescription treatments. Systemic agents that cleared the skin also resolved the pain associated with atopic dermatitis.

Conclusions: Pain can be a significant factor in the HRQL of patients with atopic dermatitis and should be considered by clinicians when caring for patients with atopic dermatitis.

KEYWORDS

atopic dermatitis; eczema; pain; qualitative research; quality of life

Introduction

Background

Atopic dermatitis is a chronic inflammatory skin disease with a highly symptomatic clinical course [1]. The hallmark symptom of atopic dermatitis is itch, or pruritus [1]. However, pain has also been recognized as an important and highly prevalent symptom in patients with atopic dermatitis [2]. An international web-based survey of 1111 patients with atopic dermatitis from 34 countries showed that pain was the second most common symptom of atopic dermatitis after itchiness [3]. A prospective practice-based study found that over 40% of patients with atopic dermatitis experienced some level of pain [4], and a more recent cross-sectional study found that 61% of participants reported experiencing pain from atopic dermatitis [2].

Several studies have analyzed the effect of chronic pain on the lives of patients, highlighting the strong correlation between pain and the deterioration of health-related quality of life (HRQL) [5-8], and atopic dermatitis is no exception. Some patients with atopic dermatitis find that their pain is related to scratching, fissures on the skin, inflamed red skin, or burning from creams or ointments [2]. Pain from atopic dermatitis can have a negative impact on the ability of patients to shop, make clothing decisions, and maintain relationships, among other aspects of daily life [4]. Moreover, although pain is not universally experienced, one study found that the proportion of patients with moderate or severe atopic dermatitis who reported pain as the most burdensome symptom was more than six times the proportion of patients with mild atopic dermatitis who reported the same [9].

Objective

Due to the time constraints of clinical practice, dermatologists are often unable to gain an in-depth understanding of all symptoms that the patient has and how they affect the HRQL of a patient. Dermatologists' assessment of the frequency of primary symptoms of a patient (often itchiness with atopic dermatitis) may not accurately reflect the perspectives of the patient. For diseases in which symptoms become debilitating, the primary goal of treatment is symptom control. Failure to understand how debilitating symptoms are for patients may leave them undertreated. We aimed to document the qualitative experience of atopic dermatitis from the perspectives of patients and their families, specifically focusing on the understudied symptoms of pain with atopic dermatitis.

Methods

Study Design

We conducted a qualitative study using focus groups and interviews to understand the effect of pain on HRQL in patients with atopic dermatitis and their family members. Our study was approved by the University of Utah institutional review board (#98441).

Participants and Setting

Participants were recruited either by recommendation from their dermatologist or by identifying patients with a diagnosis of atopic dermatitis in the electronic medical record with an upcoming appointment and having the study coordinator ask them about participating in the study at the time of the appointment. To be included, patients had to be aged ≥18 years, speak English, and have atopic dermatitis diagnosed by a University of Utah dermatologist. Family members had to be a partner or first-degree relative of a patient with atopic dermatitis, be aged ≥18 years, and speak English.

We attempted to recruit a sufficiently large sample to achieve thematic saturation. In total, 21 patients and 12 family members participated in the focus groups or interviews. Each participant provided demographic data via a written survey and written informed consent before the focus group or interview. One family member also had atopic dermatitis, so they contributed data from both family member and patient perspectives.

Data Collection and Analysis

Semistructured interview guides with open-ended questions were developed regarding experiences with itchiness, pain, sleep quality, and personal relationships because of atopic dermatitis (Textbox 1). The principle of theory-driven qualitative research was used, including basing themes and interview questions on theoretical considerations, expert discussions, and an extensive literature review. Investigators used an integrative model of patient-centeredness to guide the development of guidelines [10,11]. Interviews lasted about 15-35 minutes, and focus groups lasted about 60-70 minutes. Meetings were audiorecorded and transcribed verbatim, though some utterances were left out if not considered important for meaning, for example, "mm-hmm."

Textbox 1. Interview guide questions about pain from atopic dermatitis (eczema).

Interview guide questions

Please tell me more about the pain associated with the eczema.

- What words would you use to describe the pain of the eczema?
    - Prompts: burning, stinging, pins and needles, aching, stabbing, tingling.
- What time of day is the eczema most painful?
- What are things that cause pain with eczema?
    - Prompts: scratching too much, putting creams/lotions on your eczema
- What helps when the pain is worst, what provides relief?
- How does eczema's pain affect your sleep? The sleep of your significant other?
    - How often is pain affecting sleep? How does it affect your bedroom relationship?
- How does eczema's pain affect your mood? The mood of your loved ones?
- How does pain from eczema affect relationships?
- What other areas of your life are affected by the pain of eczema?

A thematic analysis approach was used to assess transcripts [12,13]. Two investigators (AM Snyder and VLT) with previous training in qualitative methods assessed several transcripts for themes and ideas for an initial codebook, and themes evolved as they continued to code all the transcripts and analyzed the final set of codes. The two investigators reached a consensus on the major themes. Although no changes were made to the meaning of the quotes, it should be noted that minor aspects of some quotes (eg, punctuation and grammatical errors) were changed to account for errors during transcription. For the presentation of quotes, words inserted into quotes or replacing specific words to help convey meaning are shown in brackets; descriptions of actions during the interview or focus group are italicized and shown in brackets; and any text left out of a quote, whether to shorten the quote or replace the text where there was uncertainty about the transcription, was replaced by bracketed ellipses. NVivo version 12 (QSR International) was used in assessing the codes. STATA version 16 (StataCorp) was used to calculate the demographic statistics.

Results

Demographic Characteristics

Participants attended either focus groups (23/33, 70%) or interviews (10/33, 30%), where we assessed the experiences of 21 patients with atopic dermatitis and 12 family members. Most participants identified as female and non-Hispanic White (Table 1). Four themes emerged that indicated that pain had a significant effect on HRQL (Figure 1). Not all participants reported pain, but for those who did, pain created many different sensations and a variety of effects on daily life.

Table 1. Demographic characteristics of patients and family members (N=33).

Characteristics	Patients (n=21)	Family members (n=12)
Age (years), median (range)	47 (22-77)	50 (22-72)
Gender, n (%)		
Female	16 (76)	8 (67)
Male	5 (24)	4 (33)
Race and ethnicity, n (%)		
Non-Hispanic White	20 (95)	10 (83)
Other	1 (5)	2 (17)
Education, n (%)		
High school	3 (14)	2 (17)
College degree	7 (33)	6 (50)
Bachelor's degree	7 (33)	3 (25)
Master's degree or higher	3 (14)	1 (8)
Not reported	1 (5)	0 (0)
Marital status, n (%)		
Married or domestic partner	16 (76)	11 (92)
Single, widowed, or divorced	5 (24)	1 (8)
Employment status, n (%)		
Employed	11 (52)	10 (83)
Retired	4 (19)	2 (17)
Unable to work	1 (5)	0 (0)
Unemployed	4 (19)	0 (0)
Not reported	1 (5)	0 (0)

Figure 1. Four main themes regarding pain were elucidated from the transcripts of focus groups and interviews with patients with atopic dermatitis and their family members.

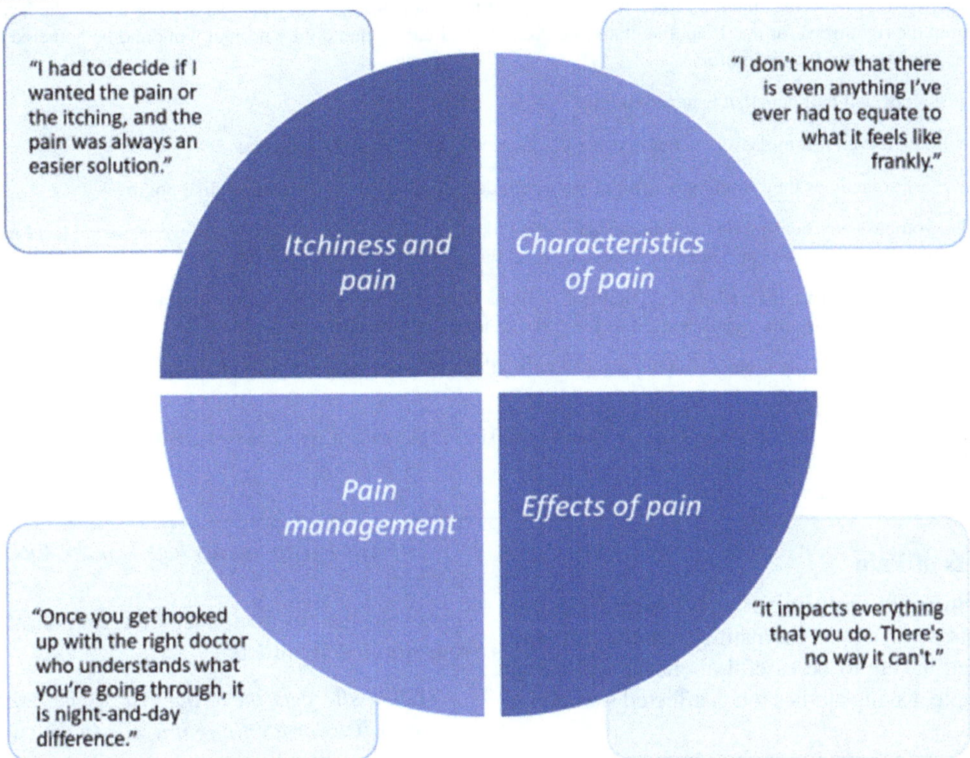

Theme 1: Itchiness and Pain

Scratching was a necessity for some patients with atopic dermatitis, and pain was sometimes an unfortunate consequence of scratching to try to relieve itchiness. The urge to provide relief from itchiness could be more powerful than the desire to avoid further consequences. This behavior of *inducing pain* led to physical consequences for some, such as open sores and denuded skin:

> *[That] is probably where the pain is coming from [...] he's scratched it raw and then it, especially on the inner crooks of his elbows and stuff like where he's bending them a lot, it just kind of opens those wounds back up.*

Conversely, scratching was not always viewed as a negative as scratching could provide relief from the pain:

> *[Sometimes] you get the pain, but sometimes if you scratch it, now you have the sensation of scratching and now it's not hurting like it did in that moment before the scratch. You jarred it up a little bit so your body can get a break from the pain, some relief.*

Itchiness and pain were sometimes difficult to distinguish from each other. This *painful itch* phenomenon experienced by some patients appeared to be a significant component of the effects of the condition. One patient explained:

> *[It] doesn't feel like it's just itching on top of the skin; it itches down in the skin [...] if you rub it and scratch it, feels almost like a thrill going through your body but it's a hurting thrill or [...] it's like you're having sex or something and you get that climax. It is like that but the only thing is it's pain.*

This pain, described as *coming from deep within*, might not be stopped simply by scratching an itch. Patients in our study generally struggled with itchiness, but coexistent pain worsened daily struggles with atopic dermatitis.

Theme 2: Characteristics of Pain

Itchiness was not always a part of the pain sensation for patients; instead, some patients felt a burning sensation that could be just as irritating. A *burning pain* was a somewhat common description of the pain experienced:

> *[It's] amazing how there aren't any scars from it, because it's like a fire. I mean it's like you got burnt.*

One patient explained:

> *There are times that my skin just feels like it's on fire and there is nothing [that] will put it out.*

Additional descriptors of pain included: *hot and burning, stabbing, dull, sharp, sunburn, sting,* needle-like, or even a persistent *discomfort* (Textbox 2). Some participants had difficulty describing their experience, and one patient expressed having trouble even talking about it:

> *Pain [...] is hard to talk to people about, because people don't view [atopic dermatitis] in terms of pain.*

Textbox 2. Example descriptions of pain from atopic dermatitis.

Descriptions of pain

- Burning: "It is hot and burning. It's true. And it's like you just feel so helpless and nothing makes it feel better."
- Discomfort: "I think...it's not so much like the little bit of itchiness bothers me. It's not so much that a little bit of pain that bothers me. It is more of the persistence of the two. You know what I mean? If I had it for a day and it went away, I'd be like, 'Alright, that wasn't so bad.' Once it gets [to be], like, two to three weeks, then it's like, 'Alright, I've got to do something.' They always ask me what's the level of pain. I always felt that pain is not the right word for me. I feel like it's more discomfort. I can sit and do my normal work and be bothered by it but not like in pain [...] just the persistence of the discomfort."
- Dull: "there is just an overall dull pain that is never-ending."
- Itching: "You will itch it even if it hurts to itch, because the itch feels way better than the pain does."
- Needle-like: "because sometimes they would get infected, he would describe it as like, like needles, like poking."
- Sharp: "I am glad you guys are focusing on the pain, because I feel like that is one aspect that is not even considered [...] I mean, it is just never stopping. It [is] like dull pain, sharp pain. Like you were saying, all the time."
- Stabbing: "it is like a stabbing pain that radiates. If you think of like a reverse lightning bolt, there is one spot that hurts more than others, but it is also radiating to different areas—like a jab or a jolt. It feels like an itch, like a painful itch."
- Sting: "When mine breaks out, I say it burns, but it's not heat burn. It's more probably a sting. But I always say burn, but when I think about it, it's probably more like a sting."
- Sunburn: "it rubbed and I couldn't hardly walk. I couldn't hardly stand it, and [...] I was achy. [...] You know how you feel when you get sunburnt? Your skin just burns. [...] It doesn't go away."

Theme 3: Effects of Pain

When present, pain could result in various consequences for daily life. Patients with atopic dermatitis and their family members expressed having to be careful about their clothing choices. For example, having clothes touch affected skin could lead to pain:

> *[It] was mostly on his legs [...] the socks will really hurt.*

This could lead to avoidance of certain clothes to avoid pain from atopic dermatitis:

> *When she gets these open sores [...] she could not wear bras or anything if it was in the sweat line.*

Conversely, as one patient expressed, clothes that cover more skin could be a necessity:

> *[When] it's so hot, I watch everyone else and they've got short-sleeved shirts. I'm all covered up, because the sun is so hard on my skin then. [...] I cannot wear sleeveless or short-sleeve clothes at all.*

The pain of an atopic dermatitis flare-up can also affect daily activities. Pain was not always limited to one time of day: "my pain goes all day long." However, the time of day was reported to make a difference for some and could particularly affect sleep:

> *It does hurt more when you lay down to go to sleep because I think you are starting to think about it more when you're just lying there.*

Sleep was also affected for some family members. One family member expressed concern over the consequences of their loved one's pain during the night:

> *...when I know it's flaring up, I might sleep a little bit lighter just because I don't want him to wake up super, you know, bloody and in a ton a pain, and so I have a tendency to wake up a couple times a night and be like, "Hey, let's put some lotion [on it]." But that's really only when it's flaring up really bad.*

However, if the patient cannot control their reactions, family member comments are not helpful:

> *He will say, "Do not itch it. It is going to hurt." But I can't control it; it's really itchy.*

Daytime activities are also affected by atopic dermatitis–related pain. A hobby such as gardening became too painful to continue for a patient with atopic dermatitis:

> *My mom used to like gardening, but she doesn't anymore because her hands are so affected by it. But she tries to wear gloves, but it still just, like, kills her.*

However, as one patient expressed, other hobbies may then become favorable for their lack of resulting pain:

> *I read, because that's one thing I can do in spite of the pain.*

Showering can also be painful:

> *If he just gets out of the shower, he'll say it feels like it burns.*

The skin care regimen of a patient can be tedious and limited:

> *I use surgical soap as a body soap at this point. I miss pretty smells, just smelling pretty, smelling like a girl.*

Warm environments can be problematic:

> *In the summertime just, the sweat. [...] She spent a lot of time indoors with the air condition on, but if we have to go out, or we go to the store and she starts sweating, you know, I can tell that she will get uncomfortable.*

Furthermore, going out can be painful both physically and emotionally:

> *[It's] depressing to go out. I'll put on makeup. [...] I haven't been able to wear eyeshadows or anything because my eyes are so sensitive [and they] swell up, and it's caused me to have a depression, just the itching and burning.*

Activities influenced specifically by pain were mentioned less often than those influenced by itchiness, but the range of effects was broad.

Similarly, social experiences can be affected by pain, and relationships can be strained by trying to care for pain in the affected patients. Physical relationships with a partner can be limited by pain from atopic dermatitis, and the location of the painful areas can limit sexual intimacy, as one patient explained:

> *It affected [...] our sex life, because I have sores all over my chest [...] It is painful [...] I am so self-conscious of it. [...] now this has been going on for eight years, so there's been nothing in this area going on intimately, you know, with my husband.*

For family members, the pain of atopic dermatitis can be difficult simply because they see the burden of the disease:

> *Every time she scratches, she's talking about it hurting and wishes she could get something to stop it from scratching.*

However, for family members, the effects of pain can be difficult to understand without knowing what the pain is like: "I can't feel the pain." However, the understanding of the family members of the effects may still be better than the understanding of others outside the family:

> *You pick up on it a lot faster if you're living with them. We go over to friends' houses, and they don't understand it.*

This lack of understanding, both from family members and others, can be frustrating for the patient:

> *The explaining to everyone what it is. You're at the grocery store and you have a big cut on your hand, and people are like, "Did you get in a fight?" and you are like, "No!" Yeah, it's just a crazy situation that is hard to explain. I wish they had groups for it because it is nice to talk to you [others in the focus group] because it is this connection that nobody else can understand, because even your partner doesn't understand the exact level to which it affects you on a daily basis.*

Theme 4: Pain Management

Another important component was the use of over-the-counter and prescription treatments to control the symptoms. Prescription treatments could be very helpful in improving the HRQL of the patient:

> *I started the Dupixent and, oh my gosh, what a life-saver. [...] I can't believe the difference.*

One patient found cannabidiol helpful:

> *[She] has been using CBD oil and [...] that really has helped the pain and helped her sleep.*

Steroids, such as triamcinolone, as well as over-the-counter treatments, such as acetaminophen and ibuprofen, were mentioned as ways to relieve pain. However, not all treatments work:

> *[Betamethasone] really doesn't help. But I will put it on as soon as they pop out.*

Some medications, such as pregabalin, were mentioned as being ineffective for atopic dermatitis–associated pain:

> *It kind of helps with these things [patient pointing to atopic dermatitis on hand]. But it wasn't necessarily nerve pain.*

One patient explained that it could also take time for a medication to start working:

> *It takes some time; I mean like when I was taking cyclosporine and it didn't happen, like, overnight where it just stopped.*

In addition to pain directly associated with atopic dermatitis flares, open wounds can become infected, requiring special treatment:

> *I think he scratches them to the point where they are open wounds and then they get a little infected, and so a lot of times we use a lot of Neosporin and stuff like that on his arms just, like, to keep the pain and everything at bay.*

One patient expressed difficulty in discerning between atopic dermatitis–related pain and treatment-related pain:

> *I think certain ones are painful. [...] I'm trying to think if the creams cause the pain, and I don't think creams cause the pain.*

The pain for some patients was a direct result of medication use:

> *[He's] been on steroids; it's made his skin super thin [...], so he gets cuts all the time [...] he can't even go get stitches anymore 'cause his skin's so thin it just tears it. [...] it makes him not want to do stuff, which is hard for me 'cause I like to go out and do stuff and try new things and be active and he's a little more hesitant because he's just prone to getting hurt and sores and they take months to heal.*

Finding clinicians who could significantly help was difficult for some participants. Patients with atopic dermatitis and their family members had a variety of experiences with clinicians when figuring out treatments for symptoms of atopic dermatitis—some positive and some negative.

Discussion

Principal Findings

Atopic dermatitis is known for its itchiness; however, our study found that focusing only on itchiness does not capture the full range of experiences of patients with atopic dermatitis and their family members. This study found that pain could coincide with itchiness, be difficult to describe, and influence all aspects of daily life for patients (and their family members). In addition, systemic agents could clear atopic dermatitis while also resolving the pain associated with this condition. The effects of pain from atopic dermatitis are relatively understudied but deserve further attention, both to identify the effects of pain on HRQL and to determine how to appropriately measure and potentially manage this symptom [14].

Increased frequency and intensity of pain from atopic dermatitis leads to worse HRQL, and for some, pain can affect relationships and numerous daily activities [2]. A study assessing the effects of pain from atopic dermatitis on patients and their caretakers found that 80% of participants had experienced effects on sleep, nearly as many (78%) experienced effects on leisure activities, and most (63%) experienced effects on other activities of daily living [15]. Although most comments in our study related to effects on HRQL were made about itchiness or atopic dermatitis more generally, we found that some patients experienced pain that affected the activities of daily living (eg, clothing choices, exercise, environmental exposures, and sexual relations) and could further affect overall HRQL. However, not all participants shared the same level of impact, likely due to differences in disease severity.

Some expressed having regained control over symptoms through medications. The use of systemic treatments, such as dupilumab, greatly improved both symptoms and HRQL outcomes for some participants, an observation supported by the literature [16]. However, not all systemic treatments share the same level of success [16], and prescribing systemic treatments must be carefully considered based on side effects, as was expressed by some participants in our study.

One of the most challenging aspects of pain is defining it. The root cause of pain from atopic dermatitis can be difficult to identify; one study found that about 17% of patients with atopic dermatitis thought pain was part of itchiness, whereas 72% thought it was part of both scratching and itchiness [4]. This is consistent with our results, as itchiness and pain overlapped for several patients. The two symptoms could be almost indistinguishable, and for some, scratching due to itchiness led to pain, although this trade-off was worth it when the pain felt better than an itch. The sensation of pain could be difficult to describe, underlining the problem that pain is a poorly understood and ill-defined symptom of atopic dermatitis.

Helping patients express concerns and how symptoms affect their daily lives is a necessity when addressing HRQL, and we believe that appropriate methods of identifying and defining pain are needed to further address this concern with patients. One approach to measuring pain is through pain-specific patient-reported outcome (PRO) measures [17]. PROs capture information of interest from the patient perspective and have demonstrated utility in identifying concerns otherwise left unexpressed in a dermatology visit [18]. These measures track patient progress and problems over time when administered regularly at visits [19], and numerous PROs currently exist for a wide range of concerns, giving clinicians many options to choose from when deciding the best measures to use with their patients. However, further studies are needed to determine which methods work best for identifying pain specific to atopic dermatitis.

Limitations of the Study

Our study is limited in generalizability because it took place at a single academic medical center in a high-altitude, low-humidity environment conducive to increased atopic dermatitis severity. Expanding to other institutions and other geographic locations outside Utah may produce different results. Furthermore, our study only included adults, and thus our results might not be generalizable to the experiences of children and adolescents with atopic dermatitis. Although investigators used open-ended questions to capture the participants' voices, it is possible that the way the questions were worded influenced participant responses. In using prompts to aid discussion, the interviewers may have directed a conversation toward those specifics, and some aspects were talked about more than others due to how questions were worded. This study is also limited in its interpretability because of its qualitative nature. Qualitative research provides an opportunity to learn about patient experiences and produce ideas for future research [20]. However, a small, nonrandom, single-institution cohort makes the findings from this study difficult to generalize if the data were quantified. The thematic analysis for this study does not involve quantification of themes or individual components of these themes but does provide information to help generate ideas for future studies that can appropriately quantify the phenomena presented here.

This study presents the experiences of patients and their family members in dealing with the effects of pain caused by atopic dermatitis. We found that many aspects of daily life can be affected by this symptom, and although pain can be very bothersome and significantly impact HRQL, it can be difficult for some patients to explain what they are experiencing. Clinicians must be aware that atopic dermatitis can cause pain and should ask patients about the presence and effects of pain when treating patients with atopic dermatitis.

Acknowledgments

This research project was funded by a grant from the National Eczema Association awarded to AM Secrest. AM Secrest is also supported by the Public Health Career Development Award from the Dermatology Foundation.

Authors' Contributions

All authors were involved in the conceptualization of this paper, although AM Secrest led conceptualization and acquired funding.

References

1. Boguniewicz M, Leung DY. Atopic dermatitis: a disease of altered skin barrier and immune dysregulation. Immunol Rev 2011 Jul;242(1):233-246 [FREE Full text] [doi: 10.1111/j.1600-065X.2011.01027.x] [Medline: 21682749]
2. Silverberg JI, Gelfand JM, Margolis DJ, Boguniewicz M, Fonacier L, Grayson MH, et al. Pain is a common and burdensome symptom of atopic dermatitis in United States adults. J Allergy Clin Immunol Pract 2019;7(8):2699-2706. [doi: 10.1016/j.jaip.2019.05.055] [Medline: 31228619]
3. von Kobyletzki LB, Thomas KS, Schmitt J, Chalmers JR, Deckert S, Aoki V, et al. What factors are important to patients when assessing treatment response: an international cross-sectional survey. Acta Derm Venereol 2017 Jan 04;97(1):86-90 [FREE Full text] [doi: 10.2340/00015555-2480] [Medline: 27305646]
4. Vakharia PP, Chopra R, Sacotte R, Patel KR, Singam V, Patel N, et al. Burden of skin pain in atopic dermatitis. Ann Allergy Asthma Immunol 2017 Dec;119(6):548-552 [FREE Full text] [doi: 10.1016/j.anai.2017.09.076] [Medline: 29223299]
5. Lerman SF, Rudich Z, Brill S, Shalev H, Shahar G. Longitudinal associations between depression, anxiety, pain, and pain-related disability in chronic pain patients. Psychosom Med 2015 Apr;77(3):333-341. [doi: 10.1097/PSY.0000000000000158] [Medline: 25849129]
6. VanDenKerkhof EG, Hopman WM, Towheed T, Wilson R, Murdoch J, Rimmer M, et al. Pain, health-related quality of life and health care utilization after inpatient surgery: a pilot study. Pain Res Manag 2006;11(1):41-47. [doi: 10.1155/2006/320461] [Medline: 16511613]
7. Tüzün EH. Quality of life in chronic musculoskeletal pain. Best Pract Res Clin Rheumatol 2007 Jun;21(3):567-579. [doi: 10.1016/j.berh.2007.03.001] [Medline: 17603000]
8. Blyth FM, March LM, Nicholas MK, Cousins MJ. Chronic pain, work performance and litigation. Pain 2003 May;103(1-2):41-47. [doi: 10.1016/s0304-3959(02)00380-9] [Medline: 12749957]
9. Silverberg JI, Gelfand JM, Margolis DJ, Boguniewicz M, Fonacier L, Grayson MH, et al. Patient burden and quality of life in atopic dermatitis in US adults: A population-based cross-sectional study. Ann Allergy Asthma Immunol 2018 Sep;121(3):340-347 [FREE Full text] [doi: 10.1016/j.anai.2018.07.006] [Medline: 30025911]
10. Scholl I, Zill JM, Härter M, Dirmaier J. An integrative model of patient-centeredness - a systematic review and concept analysis. PLoS One 2014 Sep 17;9(9):e107828 [FREE Full text] [doi: 10.1371/journal.pone.0107828] [Medline: 25229640]
11. Rogers CR. Client-Centered Therapy: Its Current Practice, Implications and Theory. Boston: Houghton Mifflin; 1951.
12. Bengtsson M. How to plan and perform a qualitative study using content analysis. NursingPlus Open 2016;2:8-14 [FREE Full text] [doi: 10.1016/j.npls.2016.01.001]

13. Vaismoradi M, Turunen H, Bondas T. Content analysis and thematic analysis: Implications for conducting a qualitative descriptive study. Nurs Health Sci 2013 Sep 11;15(3):398-405 [FREE Full text] [doi: 10.1111/nhs.12048] [Medline: 23480423]
14. Drucker AM, Wang AR, Qureshi AA. Research gaps in quality of life and economic burden of atopic dermatitis: The National Eczema Association Burden of Disease Audit. JAMA Dermatol 2016 Aug 01;152(8):873-874. [doi: 10.1001/jamadermatol.2016.1978] [Medline: 27305113]
15. Maarouf M, Kromenacker B, Capozza KL, Kempton D, Hendricks A, Tran K, et al. Pain and itch are dual burdens in atopic dermatitis. Dermatitis 2018;29(5):278-281. [doi: 10.1097/DER.0000000000000406] [Medline: 30179978]
16. Drucker AM, Ellis AG, Bohdanowicz M, Mashayekhi S, Yiu ZZ, Rochwerg B, et al. Systemic immunomodulatory treatments for patients with atopic dermatitis: a systematic review and network meta-analysis. JAMA Dermatol 2020 Jun 01;156(6):659-667. [doi: 10.1001/jamadermatol.2020.0796] [Medline: 32320001]
17. Intro to PROMIS. HealthMeasures. URL: https://www.healthmeasures.net/explore-measurement-systems/promis/intro-to-promis [accessed 2020-09-11]
18. Secrest AM, Chren MM, Hopkins ZH, Chen SC, Ferris LK, Hess R. Benefits to patient care of electronically capturing patient-reported outcomes in dermatology. Br J Dermatol 2019 Oct;181(4):826-827. [doi: 10.1111/bjd.18027] [Medline: 31017651]
19. Secrest AM, Hopkins ZH, Frost ZE, Taliercio VL, Edwards LD, Biber JE, Dermatology PRO Consortium. Quality of life assessed using skindex-16 scores among patients with acne receiving isotretinoin treatment. JAMA Dermatol 2020 Jul 08:1098-1106. [doi: 10.1001/jamadermatol.2020.2330] [Medline: 32639529]
20. Creswell JW, Creswell JD. Research Design: Qualitative, Quantitative, and Mixed Methods Approaches, 5th Ed. Kindle e-Book. Thousand Oaks, CA: SAGE Publications; 2018.

Abbreviations

HRQL: health-related quality of life
PRO: patient-reported outcome

13

Evaluation of Spin in the Abstracts of Systematic Reviews and Meta-Analyses Focused on the Treatment of Acne Vulgaris

Ryan Ottwell, BS; Taylor C Rogers, BS; J Michael Anderson, BS; Austin Johnson, BS; Matt Vassar, PhD

Oklahoma State University Center for Health Sciences, Tulsa, OK, United States

Corresponding Author:
Ryan Ottwell, BS
Oklahoma State University Center for Health Sciences
1111 W 17th St
Tulsa, OK, 74107
United States

Email: ryan.ottwell@okstate.edu

Abstract

Background: Spin is the misrepresentation of study findings, which may positively or negatively influence the reader's interpretation of the results. Little is known regarding the prevalence of spin in abstracts of systematic reviews, specifically systematic reviews pertaining to the management and treatment of acne vulgaris.

Objective: The primary objective of this study was to characterize and determine the frequency of the most severe forms of spin in systematic review abstracts and to evaluate whether various study characteristics were associated with spin.

Methods: Using a cross-sectional study design, we searched PubMed and EMBASE for systematic reviews focusing on the management and treatment of acne vulgaris. Our search returned 316 studies, of which 36 were included in our final sample. To be included, each systematic review must have addressed either pharmacologic or nonpharmacologic treatment of acne vulgaris. These studies were screened, and data were extracted in duplicate by two blinded investigators. We analyzed systematic review abstracts for the nine most severe types of spin.

Results: Spin was present in 31% (11/36) of abstracts. A total of 12 examples of spin were identified in the 11 abstracts containing spin, with one abstract containing two instances of spin. The most common type of spin, *selective reporting of or overemphasis on efficacy outcomes or analysis favoring the beneficial effect of the experimental intervention,* was identified five times (5/12, 42%). A total of 44% (16/36) of studies did not report a risk of bias assessment. Of the 11 abstracts containing spin, six abstracts (55%) had not reported a risk of bias assessment or performed a risk of bias assessment but did not discuss it. Spin in abstracts was not significantly associated with a specific intervention type, funding source, or journal impact factor.

Conclusions: Spin is present in the abstracts of systematic reviews and meta-analyses covering the treatment of acne vulgaris. This paper raises awareness of spin in abstracts and emphasizes the importance of its recognition, which may lead to fewer incidences of spin in future studies.

KEYWORDS
acne vulgaris; systematic review; abstracts; dermatology

Introduction

Background

Acne vulgaris is one of the most common medical diagnoses made by dermatologists each year, with over 50 million Americans affected by this condition [1]. In 2013 alone, more than 5 million people with acne vulgaris sought medical treatment, resulting in over US $1.2 billion spent annually on the disease [1]. This condition can cause physical and emotional discomfort for those affected and can lead to long-term scarring [2]. Owing to the prevalence of acne vulgaris, it is important for the providers to be well informed about the current treatment options that are supported with the highest level of evidence.

Systematic reviews offer valuable insights to clinicians about current treatments [3]. Clinicians will often look specifically at the abstract of systematic reviews—which may be all that is accessible to them—as a succinct summary of results to guide treatment decisions. Barry et al [4] found that abstracts influenced the treatment decisions of nearly three-quarters of family physicians. Similarly, Marcelo et al [5] reported that nearly two-thirds of the residents used the abstracts of papers alone to guide them in their clinical decision making. Johnson et al [6] reported that the majority of nurse practitioner students found abstracts useful in guiding their clinical decision making. Haynes et al [7], investigating the usefulness of Medical Literature Analysis and Retrieval System Online (MEDLINE) in the clinical setting, showed that almost half of the searches performed influenced clinical decision making. They also found that, more often than not, decisions were made from limited information such as the abstract, article title, subject heading, or a combination of these. Therefore, it is imperative that the information provided in the abstracts of publications be representative of the study findings and devoid of spin. Boutron et al [8] defined spin as "a specific way of reporting, intentional or not, to highlight that the beneficial effect of the experimental treatment in terms of efficacy or safety is greater than that shown by the results." Spin, specifically in abstracts, can influence the interpretation of data, which can lead to misinformation and, ultimately, misguided decisions about treatment.

Objectives

Spin has been demonstrated to be prevalent in the abstracts of randomized controlled trials [9-14]. Similar lines of inquiry have noted poor reporting quality in systematic reviews [15-18]. On the basis of these two complementary lines of work, we hypothesized that spin would also be present in the abstracts of systematic reviews on the topic of treatment of acne vulgaris. This study aimed to characterize and determine the frequency of each type of spin in systematic review abstracts. More specifically, this study evaluated the top nine most severe types of spin, as previously outlined by Yavchitz et al [8]. The secondary objective was to evaluate whether various study characteristics corresponded with the presence of spin in systematic review abstracts focusing on acne vulgaris.

Methods

Publication Search

This study was performed in accordance with a previously written protocol available publicly on Open Science Framework (OSF) [19]. A search of PubMed and EMBASE, which incorporates MEDLINE, was performed on September 2, 2019. The search string for PubMed was as follows: "acne vulgaris"[MeSH Terms] OR acne vulgaris[Text Word] AND (systematic[sb] OR Meta-Analysis[ptyp]). The search string for EMBASE was as follows: 'acne vulgaris'/exp AND ('meta analysis'/de OR 'systematic review'/de). These searches were modeled from the search strategies provided by a number of Cochrane systematic reviews on acne vulgaris [20,21]. Search results were then added to Rayyan [22], a screening platform.

Training

Before screening, training was conducted, which included face-to-face training sessions for the authors RO and CR. Author MV led the training sessions as his studies regarding the presence of spin in randomized controlled trials have previously been published. During these training sessions, the authors (RO and CR) received instruction and education using example abstracts and full studies from different areas of medicine. During this training, the most severe types of spin described by Yavchitz et al [8] were discussed, and agreement was reached on the definition of each item. A Google form containing the nine most severe types of spin was developed and pilot tested for ease of use and to ensure that all the necessary data elements were included. The Google form was pilot tested by the authors (RO and CR) on numerous papers known to contain spin to ensure the form contained all the items needed for data extraction and that the Google form worked correctly. Studies were then screened independently by title and abstract by RO and CR. To be included in this study, a published article had to be a systematic review or meta-analysis designed to address either the pharmacological or nonpharmacological treatment of acne vulgaris.

Data Extraction

Data extraction was performed in duplicate fashion using the Google form, and the investigators were blinded during the extraction process. After data extraction was completed, the investigators were unblinded and met to discuss any inconsistency until agreement was reached. On items for which agreement could not be reached, a third investigator was available for adjudication. The process of dual extraction of data was used to substantiate the work of each individual investigator. The items extracted on the Google form included the study title, journal title, number of studies included, number of subjects included, types of studies included, types of interventions, when the review was performed, databases searched, funding source, and if the review/primary outcome was significant. Furthermore, we evaluated whether the article contained any of the nine most severe examples of spin in abstracts [8].

To characterize and determine the frequency of spin in the abstracts of systematic reviews on the topic of the treatment of acne vulgaris, we employed the classification system previously developed by Yavchitz et al [8], specifically evaluating the top nine most severe examples of spin found in the abstracts of systematic reviews. These nine types of spin are outlined in Table 1.

Table 1. Frequency of each type of spin (N=12).

Type of spin	Value, n (%)[a]
Conclusion contains recommendations for clinical practice not supported by the findings.	0 (0)
Title claims or suggests a beneficial effect of the experimental intervention not supported by the findings.	0 (0)
Selective reporting of or overemphasis on efficacy outcomes or analysis favoring the beneficial effect of the experimental intervention.	5 (42)
Conclusion claims safety based on nonstatistically significant results with a wide confidence interval.	0 (0)
Conclusion claims the beneficial effect of the experimental treatment despite a high risk of bias in primary studies.	4 (33)
Selective reporting of or overemphasis on harm outcomes or analysis favoring the safety of the experimental intervention.	1 (83)
Conclusion extrapolates the review's findings to a different intervention (ie, claiming efficacy of a specific intervention although the review covers a class of several interventions).	2 (17)
Conclusion extrapolates the review's findings from a surrogate marker or a specific outcome to the global improvement of the disease.	0 (0)
Conclusion claims the beneficial effect of the experimental treatment despite reporting bias.	0 (0)

[a]More than one type of spin may have been present in the same systematic review.

Data Synthesis

To evaluate the most common forms of spin within systematic review abstracts, we calculated frequencies and percentages. To evaluate particular study characteristics associated with spin in systematic review abstracts, we planned in our protocol, *a priori*, to conduct a logistic regression in which the presence or absence of spin would be coded as a dichotomous criterion variable (0=presence of spin and 1=no spin), and intervention type, journal impact factor, funding source, whether there was medical writer assistance, and whether the journal requires adherence to Preferred Reporting Items for Systematic Reviews and Meta-Analyses (PRISMA) or PRISMA for Abstracts (PRISMA-A) [23,24] would be included in the predictor set. However, the final sample size of 36 systematic reviews suggested that examining the associations between categorical variables using the Chi-square test and point biserial correlations between categorical and continuous variables would be more appropriate, and it was thus decided upon before data analysis was conducted. Only two systematic reviews were written by medical writers; thus, we did not include this variable. Furthermore, none of the systematic reviews reported the use of PRISMA-A, so this variable was also eliminated from the analysis. Interrater reliability was estimated using Gwet's AC1. All statistical analyses were performed using Stata 15.1. [25].

Results

Simple Characteristics

Our search string retrieved 316 studies, of which 58 studies were deleted as duplicates and 204 studies were excluded by the title and abstract. The studies excluded from this study are mentioned in Figure 1. We further excluded 20 studies after screening the full text. This screening process left 36 studies that met the inclusion criteria (Figure 1). Among the 36 systematic reviews included, pharmacological intervention for acne vulgaris treatment was the most common intervention type (23/36, 64%), and 31% (11/36) of studies focused on nonpharmacological interventions. The most common source of funding was through public mechanisms (12/36, 33%); however, equally as many studies made no mention of funding (12/36, 33%). The median impact factor was 3.092 for the journals with the systematic reviews included in this study's sample. Detailed characteristics of the included studies can be found in Table 2.

Figure 1. Flow diagram of study selection.

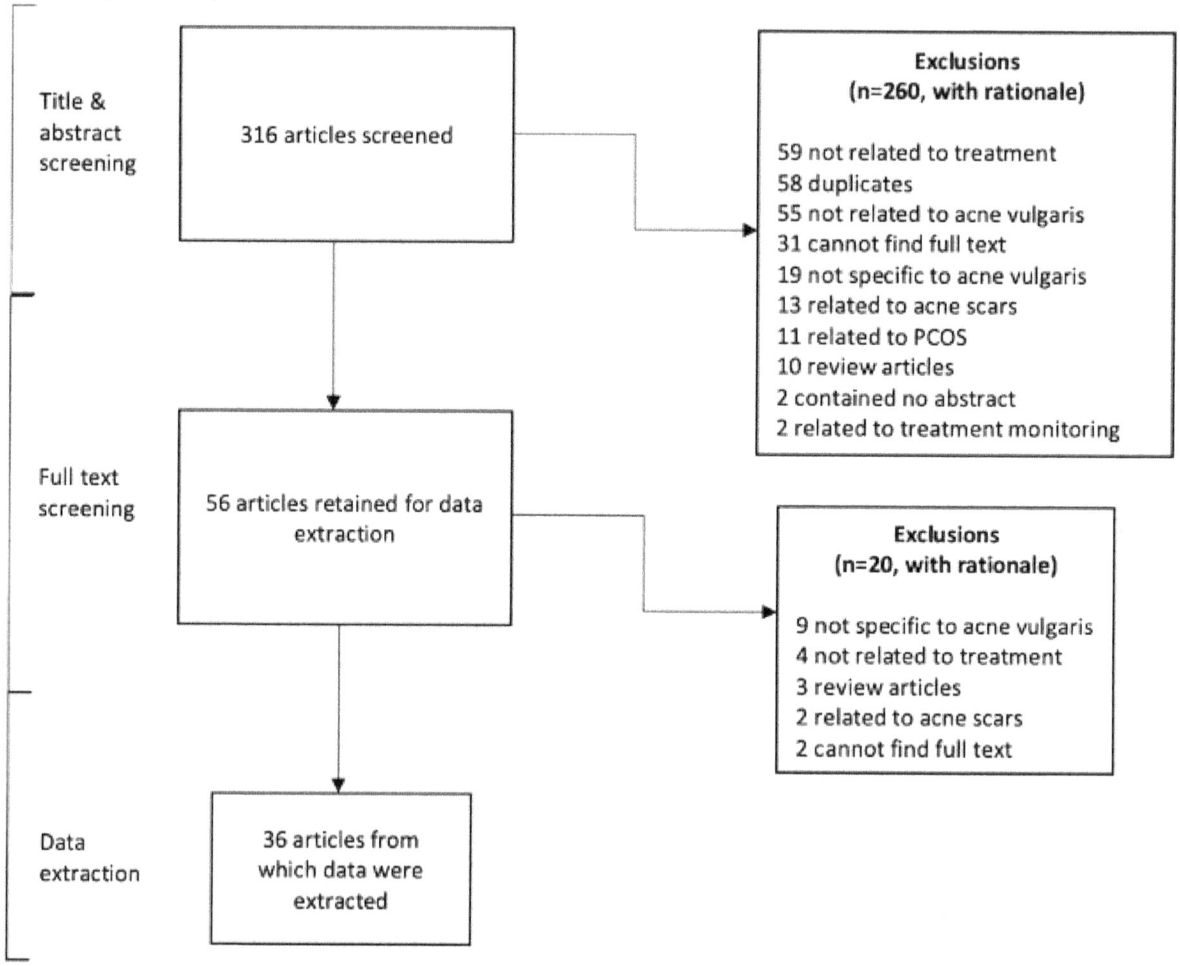

Table 2. Characteristics of included studies (N=36).

Characteristics	Total (N=36), n (%)	With spin (n=11), n (%)
Source of funding		
Public	12 (33)	3 (27)
Industry	6 (17)	2 (18)
Not funded	6 (17)	3 (27)
Funding not mentioned	12 (33)	3 (27)
Intervention type		
Pharmacologic	23 (64)	8 (73)
Nonpharmacologic	11 (31)	3 (27)
Combined	2 (6)	0 (0)
Journal requirement for Preferred Reporting Items for Systematic Reviews and Meta-Analyses		
Yes	21 (58)	7 (64)
No	15 (42)	4 (36)
Journal requirement for Preferred Reporting Items for Systematic Reviews and Meta-Analyses for Abstracts		
Yes	0 (0)	0 (0)
No	0 (0)	0 (0)
Use of a medical writer		
Yes	2 (6)	1 (9)
No	34 (94)	0 (0)

Primary Outcome

For the primary outcome, interrater reliability was assessed using Gwet's AC1, which was 0.68 (95% CI 0.44-0.92). Each discrepancy was subsequently resolved by group discussion, achieving an agreement of 100%. Spin was determined to be present in 31% (11/36) of abstracts in this study's sample. A total of 12 separate instances of spin were identified in the 11 abstracts containing spin, with one of the abstracts containing two examples of spin. The most common type of spin identified was type 3, *selective reporting of or overemphasis on efficacy outcomes or analysis favoring the beneficial effect of the experimental intervention* (5/12, 42%); followed by type 5, *conclusion claims the beneficial effect of the experimental treatment despite a high risk of bias in primary studies* (4/12, 33%); type 6, *conclusion extrapolates the review's findings to a different intervention (ie, claiming efficacy of one specific intervention although the review covers a class of several interventions*; 2/12, 17%); and type 7, *selective reporting of or overemphasis on harm outcomes or analysis favoring the safety of the experimental intervention* (1/12, 8%). Table 1 summarizes this study's findings for the top nine most severe types of spin in the abstracts of systematic reviews.

Although we found no instances of spin type number 4 regarding safety (Table 1), safety was not mentioned in 61% (22/36) of abstracts. For the purpose of this study, we also considered the discussion of adverse events or treatment side effects as the author inferring safety. A total of 16 studies did not provide a risk of bias assessment (16/36, 44%), and four studies assessed the risk of bias but did not discuss it (4/36, 11%). Of the 11 abstracts that did contain a form of spin, six (55%) did not report a risk of bias assessment or performed a risk of bias assessment but did not discuss it. If an article mentioned a risk of bias assessment but did not provide explanation of risk assessment or data concerning the risk of bias, then we considered this as assessed but not discussed. Spin in the abstracts was not significantly associated with a specific intervention type, funding source, or journal impact factor.

Discussion

Principal Findings

Spin is prevalent in the abstracts of systematic reviews and meta-analyses focused on the treatment of acne vulgaris. We identified spin in nearly one-third of the included studies in this study's sample. The most common type of spin found was type 3, *selective reporting of or overemphasis on efficacy outcomes or analysis favoring the beneficial effect of the experimental intervention*. For example, Koo et al [26] performed a meta-analysis comparing the efficacy of oral antibiotics with that of oral contraceptives for the treatment of acne vulgaris at 3 and 6 months. The oral contraceptive pills were shown to be less effective than oral antibiotics at 3 months but were equivalent to oral antibiotics at 6 months. However, the author suggests in the abstract that oral contraceptive pills may be a better alternative to oral antibiotics while providing no data to support that oral contraceptive pills would be more effective.

We were limited in our assessment of spin type 5, *conclusion claims the beneficial effect of the experimental treatment despite a high risk of bias in primary studies,* as bias was not assessed or was assessed and not discussed, in many of the included studies. This issue is of concern as we noticed six of our 11 studies, which contained spin, either did not assess for the risk of bias or assessed for bias but did not discuss it or further account for it. Providing a risk of bias assessment in systematic reviews is important as it guides the reader in determining the extent to which the included study results should be trusted [27]. Another reason it is essential to perform a risk of bias assessment is that a study may have an important risk of bias, even though the study was performed to the highest possible standards. A few of the reviews included stated that their studies had methodological limitations but did not provide a proper risk of bias assessment. Without a risk of bias assessment, the reader does not have a promising tool to assess the validity of the study. Therefore, it is imperative that systematic reviews perform and discuss a risk of bias assessment of their primary studies.

Recommendations

To our knowledge, we are the first to investigate the presence of spin in the abstracts of systematic reviews and meta-analyses focused on acne vulgaris treatment options. In the field of dermatology, Motosko et al [28] found that 100% (20/20) of the randomized controlled trials on topical treatments for photoaged skin contained some form of spin, most broadly classified as either inappropriate statistical analyses or inappropriate interpretation of results. Other studies in various fields have previously demonstrated the presence of spin in the abstracts of randomized controlled trials. For example, Boutron et al [29], in the field of oncology, showed that spin in the abstract of a randomized controlled trial can influence clinicians' understanding of the study's results, to the degree that they are more likely to rate a treatment as beneficial, even though the primary outcome is statistically nonsignificant. This finding could have significant clinical implications across all fields of medicine and research in general. A total of four studies conducted by the members of our research team identified spin within abstracts of randomized controlled trials. Austin et al [9] identified spin in the abstracts of nearly half of randomized obesity trials. Cooper et al [10] demonstrated the presence of spin in 70% of the trials published in highly ranked otolaryngology journals. Checketts et al [14] identified spin in 58% of the lower extremity joint trials. Kinder et al [11] reported spin being present in 23% abstracts of the randomized control trials in the field of anesthesiology. Outside of our team's research, others have found similar results. Khan et al [30] reported spin in the abstracts of 53% of the cardiovascular randomized clinical trials. The prevalence of spin in these previously mentioned studies and others led us to ask the question whether spin was also prevalent in the abstracts of systematic reviews. Considering previous studies have shown that abstracts may influence clinical decision making [4-7], the presence of spin in the abstracts of systematic reviews may lead to the dissemination of misinformation and, ultimately, misguided decisions in clinical practice. The steps to minimize spin rest on the shoulders of all research stakeholders, including peer reviewers. Previous studies have demonstrated that reviewers often fail to recognize the misrepresentation of results in study abstracts. For example, Lazarus et al [31] demonstrated that peer reviewers failed to identify spin in abstract conclusions in 76% of the reports reviewed, and 15% of the reviewers actually requested the authors to add some type of spin. Therefore, the task of reducing spin includes the ability to recognize it. Increasing the knowledge of spin could be implemented through education and training so that reviewers, editors, and authors are better equipped to identify and eliminate spin. Guidelines have been developed and published, which will assist reviewers in the detection and interpretation of misleading claims [32,33]. Making use of these guidelines a common practice may help in identifying and eliminating spin.

The PRISMA Statement [34] is an evidence-based minimum set of items for reporting in systematic reviews and meta-analyses, which is widely used by authors, peer reviewers, and editors for reporting and critical appraisal of published systematic reviews [24]. PRISMA-A is an extension to the PRISMA Statement, which provides guidelines for reporting in the abstracts of systematic reviews. Beyond authors and reviewers, we advocate that clinicians, who ultimately make treatment decisions, should be trained to evaluate for the presence of spin in abstracts. Methodologists have performed interesting work to aid in establishing the confidence of the results and conclusions of systematic reviews; however, more work is needed regarding systematic review abstracts. A study performed by Gómez-García et al [35] found that, on average, only 57% of the PRISMA-A items were included in the abstracts of systematic reviews and meta-analyses covering psoriasis treatments. They reported that studies with low-risk bias and high methodological quality had significantly more PRISMA-A items reported compared with studies with high-risk bias and low methodological quality. On the basis of these findings, examining a study's adherence to PRISMA-A may be a useful screening tool for journal editors, reviewers, and clinicians to assess a study's methodological quality and risk of bias. Currently, the PRISMA-A guideline does not specifically address spin; therefore, we recommend mandatory adherence to PRISMA and a revision to the PRISMA extension, PRISMA-A, which focuses on the minimization of spin.

Strengths and Limitations

This study has several strengths and limitations. Regarding strengths, investigators underwent extensive training to ensure the understanding of the concept of spin in publications. A group consensus was reached on the definition of each of the nine types of spin in an effort to ensure standardized responses. We fostered an atmosphere of reproducibility by posting the full study protocol on OSF before extraction. Each data extractor was blinded during the screening and data extraction process. Data were then extracted in duplicate fashion in accordance with the recommendations of the Cochrane Handbook for Systematic Reviews of Interventions [27]. Despite these efforts, this study is not without limitations. The identification of spin is inherently subjective in nature. To reduce some of this subjectivity, data extractors underwent rigorous training before data extraction and then met to discuss and resolve any discrepancies between extraction responses. A third-party arbitrator was consulted where agreement could not be reached. Another limitation of this study was the low availability of studies that met our inclusion criteria, which limited our sample size. The results of this study are applicable to the field of dermatology with regard to the treatment of acne vulgaris alone. Further studies are needed to investigate the presence of spin in publications regarding other areas of dermatology. Finally, the results of this study should not be generalized across other timelines or publication types other than systematic reviews regarding acne vulgaris treatment options.

Conclusions

In conclusion, a sizable amount of spin was found in the abstracts of systematic reviews focused on the treatment of acne vulgaris. Moving forward, we recommend that peer reviewers and editors should be educated about the identification of spin. We also recommend the development of strict reporting guidelines for abstracts. Further research is needed to evaluate the types of spin that most significantly affect clinical decision making, which was outside of the purview of this study. We recommend future studies to assess the frequency of spin in other specialties.

Acknowledgments

All authors of this study had access to all data. This study was not funded by any institution or sponsor.

Authors' Contributions

RO and TR contributed equally to this paper. RO contributed to data extraction, manuscript writing, manuscript editing, and project design. TR contributed to data extraction, manuscript writing, manuscript editing, and project design. MA contributed to manuscript editing, data collection, analysis, and project design. AJ contributed to data analysis, manuscript editing, and approval. CC contributed to project design, training, and project oversight. MV contributed to project design, manuscript editing, project oversight, and training.

References

1. American Academy of Dermatology. Skin Conditions by the Numbers URL: https://www.aad.org/media/stats/conditions/skin-conditions-by-the-numbers [accessed 2019-09-09]
2. Hosthota A, Bondade S, Basavaraja V. Impact of acne vulgaris on quality of life and self-esteem. Cutis 2016 Aug;98(2):121-124. [Medline: 27622255]
3. Gopalakrishnan S, Ganeshkumar P. Systematic reviews and meta-analysis: understanding the best evidence in primary healthcare. J Family Med Prim Care 2013 Jan;2(1):9-14 [FREE Full text] [doi: 10.4103/2249-4863.109934] [Medline: 24479036]
4. Barry HC, Ebell MH, Shaughnessy AF, Slawson DC, Nietzke F. Family physicians' use of medical abstracts to guide decision making: style or substance? J Am Board Fam Pract 2001;14(6):437-442 [FREE Full text] [Medline: 11757886]
5. Marcelo A, Gavino A, Isip-Tan IT, Apostol-Nicodemus L, Mesa-Gaerlan FJ, Firaza PN, et al. A comparison of the accuracy of clinical decisions based on full-text articles and on journal abstracts alone: a study among residents in a tertiary care hospital. Evid Based Med 2013 Apr;18(2):48-53 [FREE Full text] [doi: 10.1136/eb-2012-100537] [Medline: 22782923]
6. Johnson HL, Fontelo P, Olsen CH, Jones MK, Gimbel RW. Family nurse practitioner student perception of journal abstract usefulness in clinical decision making: a randomized controlled trial. J Am Assoc Nurse Pract 2013 Nov;25(11):597-603. [doi: 10.1111/1745-7599.12013] [Medline: 24170534]
7. Haynes RB, McKibbon KA, Walker CJ, Ryan N, Fitzgerald D, Ramsden MF. Online access to MEDLINE in clinical settings. A study of use and usefulness. Ann Intern Med 1990 Jan 1;112(1):78-84. [doi: 10.7326/0003-4819-112-1-78] [Medline: 2403476]
8. Yavchitz A, Ravaud P, Altman DG, Moher D, Hrobjartsson A, Lasserson T, et al. A new classification of spin in systematic reviews and meta-analyses was developed and ranked according to the severity. J Clin Epidemiol 2016 Jul;75:56-65. [doi: 10.1016/j.jclinepi.2016.01.020] [Medline: 26845744]
9. Austin J, Smith C, Natarajan K, Som M, Wayant C, Vassar M. Evaluation of spin within abstracts in obesity randomized clinical trials: a cross-sectional review. Clin Obes 2019 Apr;9(2):e12292. [doi: 10.1111/cob.12292] [Medline: 30576083]
10. Cooper CM, Gray HM, Ross AE, Hamilton TA, Downs JB, Wayant C, et al. Evaluation of spin in the abstracts of otolaryngology randomized controlled trials. Laryngoscope 2018 Dec 21:2036-2040. [doi: 10.1002/lary.27750] [Medline: 30578543]
11. Kinder NC, Weaver MD, Wayant C, Vassar M. Presence of 'spin' in the abstracts and titles of anaesthesiology randomised controlled trials. Br J Anaesth 2019 Jan;122(1):e13-e14 [FREE Full text] [doi: 10.1016/j.bja.2018.10.023] [Medline: 30579417]
12. Reynolds-Vaughn V, Riddle J, Brown J, Schiesel M, Wayant C, Vassar M. Evaluation of spin in the abstracts of emergency medicine randomized controlled trials. Ann Emerg Med 2019 May 14:pii: S0196-0644(19)30230-6. [doi: 10.1016/j.annemergmed.2019.03.011] [Medline: 31101371]

13. Jellison S, Roberts W, Bowers A, Combs T, Beaman J, Wayant C, et al. Evaluation of spin in abstracts of papers in psychiatry and psychology journals. BMJ Evid Based Med 2019 Aug 5:pii: bmjebm-2019-111176. [doi: 10.1136/bmjebm-2019-111176] [Medline: 31383725]
14. Checketts JX, Riddle J, Zaaza Z, Boose MA, Whitener JH, Vassar MB. An evaluation of spin in lower extremity joint trials. J Arthroplasty 2019 May;34(5):1008-1012. [doi: 10.1016/j.arth.2019.01.016] [Medline: 30733070]
15. O'Donohoe TJ, Dhillon R, Bridson TL, Tee J. Reporting quality of systematic review abstracts published in leading neurosurgical journals: a research on research study. Neurosurgery 2019 Jul 1;85(1):1-10. [doi: 10.1093/neuros/nyy615] [Medline: 30649511]
16. Nagendrababu V, Pulikkotil SJ, Sultan OS, Jayaraman J, Peters OA. Methodological and reporting quality of systematic reviews and meta-analyses in Endodontics. J Endod 2018 Jun;44(6):903-913. [doi: 10.1016/j.joen.2018.02.013] [Medline: 29602531]
17. Maticic K, Martinic MK, Puljak L. Assessment of reporting quality of abstracts of systematic reviews with meta-analysis using PRISMA-A and discordance in assessments between raters without prior experience. BMC Med Res Methodol 2019 Feb 14;19(1):32 [FREE Full text] [doi: 10.1186/s12874-019-0675-2] [Medline: 30764774]
18. Tan WK, Wigley J, Shantikumar S. The reporting quality of systematic reviews and meta-analyses in vascular surgery needs improvement: a systematic review. Int J Surg 2014 Dec;12(12):1262-1265 [FREE Full text] [doi: 10.1016/j.ijsu.2014.10.015] [Medline: 25448643]
19. Ottwell RL. OSF. 2019. Evaluation of Spin in the Abstracts of Systematic Reviews Regarding the Treatment of Acne Vulgaris URL: https://osf.io/z59bq/ [accessed 2019-09-18]
20. Cao H, Yang G, Wang Y, Liu JP, Smith CA, Luo H, et al. Complementary therapies for acne vulgaris. Cochrane Database Syst Rev 2015 Jan 19;1:CD009436 [FREE Full text] [doi: 10.1002/14651858.CD009436.pub2] [Medline: 25597924]
21. Barbaric J, Abbott R, Posadzki P, Car M, Gunn L, Layton A, et al. Cochrane systematic review: light therapies for acne. J Am Acad Dermatol 2017;76(6 Suppl 1):AB75 [FREE Full text] [doi: 10.1016/j.jaad.2017.04.307]
22. Rayyan QCRI. URL: https://rayyan.qcri.org/reviews/81224 [accessed 2019-09-10]
23. PRISMA Statement. The PRISMA for Abstracts Checklist URL: http://www.prisma-statement.org/documents/PRISMA%20Abstracts%20Checklist.pdf [accessed 2019-10-09]
24. Moher D, Liberati A, Tetzlaff J, Altman DG, PRISMA Group. Preferred reporting items for systematic reviews and meta-analyses: the PRISMA statement. PLoS Med 2009 Jul 21;6(7):e1000097 [FREE Full text] [doi: 10.1371/journal.pmed.1000097] [Medline: 19621072]
25. Stata: Software for Statistics and Data Science. Version 15. College Station, TX, USA: StataCorp; 2017. URL: https://www.stata.com/ [accessed 2020-02-05]
26. Koo EB, Petersen TD, Kimball AB. Meta-analysis comparing efficacy of antibiotics versus oral contraceptives in acne vulgaris. J Am Acad Dermatol 2014 Sep;71(3):450-459. [doi: 10.1016/j.jaad.2014.03.051] [Medline: 24880665]
27. Higgins J, Green S. Cochrane Handbook For Systematic Reviews Of Interventions. England: Wiley; 2008.
28. Motosko CC, Ault AK, Kimberly LL, Zakhem GA, Gothard MD, Ho RS, et al. Analysis of spin in the reporting of studies of topical treatments of photoaged skin. J Am Acad Dermatol 2019 Feb;80(2):516-22.e12. [doi: 10.1016/j.jaad.2018.04.034] [Medline: 29689326]
29. Boutron I, Altman DG, Hopewell S, Vera-Badillo F, Tannock I, Ravaud P. Impact of spin in the abstracts of articles reporting results of randomized controlled trials in the field of cancer: the SPIIN randomized controlled trial. J Clin Oncol 2014 Dec 20;32(36):4120-4126. [doi: 10.1200/JCO.2014.56.7503] [Medline: 25403215]
30. Khan MS, Lateef N, Siddiqi TJ, Rehman KA, Alnaimat S, Khan SU, et al. Level and prevalence of spin in published cardiovascular randomized clinical trial reports with statistically nonsignificant primary outcomes: a systematic review. JAMA Netw Open 2019 May 3;2(5):e192622 [FREE Full text] [doi: 10.1001/jamanetworkopen.2019.2622] [Medline: 31050775]
31. Lazarus C, Haneef R, Ravaud P, Hopewell S, Altman DG, Boutron I. Peer reviewers identified spin in manuscripts of nonrandomized studies assessing therapeutic interventions, but their impact on spin in abstract conclusions was limited. J Clin Epidemiol 2016 Sep;77:44-51. [doi: 10.1016/j.jclinepi.2016.04.012] [Medline: 27164274]
32. Montori VM, Jaeschke R, Schünemann HJ, Bhandari M, Brozek JL, Devereaux PJ, et al. Users' guide to detecting misleading claims in clinical research reports. Br Med J 2004 Nov 6;329(7474):1093-1096 [FREE Full text] [doi: 10.1136/bmj.329.7474.1093] [Medline: 15528623]
33. Sutherland WJ, Spiegelhalter D, Burgman M. Policy: twenty tips for interpreting scientific claims. Nature 2013 Nov 21;503(7476):335-337. [doi: 10.1038/503335a] [Medline: 24273799]
34. PRISMA Statement. URL: http://www.prisma-statement.org [accessed 2019-05-29]
35. Gómez-García F, Ruano J, Aguilar-Luque M, Alcalde-Mellado P, Gay-Mimbrera J, Hernández-Romero JL, et al. Abstract analysis method facilitates filtering low-methodological quality and high-bias risk systematic reviews on psoriasis interventions. BMC Med Res Methodol 2017 Dec 29;17(1):180 [FREE Full text] [doi: 10.1186/s12874-017-0460-z] [Medline: 29284417]

Abbreviations

MEDLINE: Medical Literature Analysis and Retrieval System Online
PRISMA: Preferred Reporting Items for Systematic Reviews and Meta-Analyses
PRISMA-A: Preferred Reporting Items for Systematic Reviews and Meta-Analyses for Abstracts
OSF: Open Science Framework

14

Consumer Preference of Products for the Prevention and Treatment of Stretch Marks: Systematic Product Search

Pengyi Zhu*, BS; Andrew Fung*, BSN, RN; Benjamin K P Woo*, MD

Olive View–University of California Los Angeles Medical Center, Sylmar, CA, United States

*all authors contributed equally

Corresponding Author:
Pengyi Zhu, BS
Olive View–University of California Los Angeles Medical Center
14445 Olive View Drive, Cottage H1
Sylmar, CA, 91342
United States

Email: sharonpzhu2@gmail.com

Abstract

Background: Striae distensae, or stretch marks, are a common and distressing condition affecting females two-and-a-half times more frequently than males. Despite the numerous products available for stretch mark prevention and treatment, there have been few studies that consider consumer product preference.

Objective: The aim of this study was to determine which products were preferred by consumers for the prevention and treatment of stretch marks based on product vehicle and product ingredients.

Methods: In January 2020, a search was conducted on internet retailer Amazon for products related to stretch marks. The top products were identified as those with 100 reviews or greater and a rating of 4 or higher. The products were classified as either stretch mark–specific or non stretch mark–specific. Price, rating, type of vehicle, and specific ingredients of both product groups were compared. Vehicle-type and ingredients in both product groups were compared with two-tailed two-sample proportion tests to determine if certain vehicles or ingredients were more likely to be found in stretch mark–specific products. $P<.05$ indicated statistical significance.

Results: Out of over 10,000 products, 184 were selected as the top products according to the review and rating criteria of which 117 (63.6%) were stretch mark–specific and 67 (36.4%) were non stretch mark–specific. Oil was the most common vehicle (131/184, 71.2%) while vitamin E was the most common ingredient (58/184, 31.5%). Oil, as a vehicle, was more likely to be found in stretch mark–specific products than in non stretch mark–specific products (P=.001). Olive oil (P=.02) and cocoa butter (P=.08), *Centella asiatica* (P=.01), and shea butter (P=.003) were the ingredients more likely to be found in stretch mark–specific products than in non stretch mark–specific products.

Conclusions: This study demonstrated that there are many products available for the prevention and treatment of stretch marks and identified specific ingredients in the products preferred by customers. There are few studies investigating the effectiveness of the major ingredients in the stretch mark products that are preferred by consumers. Future studies can focus on the effectiveness of the ingredients found in the products that are preferred by consumers.

KEYWORDS

Amazon; consumer preference; stretch mark; striae distensae; striae gravidarum

Introduction

Striae distensae, more commonly known as stretch marks, are a common and disfiguring dermatological condition in which the layer of dermis becomes scarred. Striae distensae occur two-and-a-half times more frequently in females than in males [1]. Striae distensae are more likely to develop during pregnancy (striae gravidarum), with obesity, with Cushing syndrome, during adolescence, with steroidal drug use, and after surgery [2].

The pathogenesis of striae distensae is multifactorial. Striae distensae are typically associated with rapid weight gain (such as in pregnancy) and rapid growth (such as in adolescence) as a result of tissue stretching [3]. Striae distensae are more common on the abdomen, breast, thigh, and buttocks [1,4]. Striae distensae caused by mechanical stress have been found to exhibit altered extracellular matrix components, primarily fibronectin, fibrillin, elastin, and collagen [5], through potential mechanisms such as low expression of genes for collagen and fibronectin, reduced fibroblast function, and disorganized fibrils or elastic fiber networks [3-5]. Studies of hormonal changes occurring in pregnancy, during steroid use, and in Cushing syndrome contribute to the understanding of the development of striae distensae; increased steroid levels cause increased protein catabolism and decreased production of collagen by fibroblasts resulting in less elastic fibers in the matrix of the dermis [1,6].

Because of the distress caused by the disfiguring nature of stretch marks, studies have attempted to find methods to prevent and treat stretch marks [7]. Different topical agents have been used to target processes that lead to the development of stretch marks. Trofolastin, a product which contains *Centella asiatica* was found to stimulate fibroblasts and counteract the glucocorticoid effect [8]. Oils and cocoa butter assist with maintaining skin hydration, which influences the expression of cytokines and growth factors via occlusive mechanisms [5,9]. Tretinoin (a derivative of vitamin A) has been found to stimulate fibroblasts to increase collagen I production in tissue while ascorbic acid (vitamin C) has also been found to increases collagen production [5]. Despite the numerous topical therapies available, therapy efficacy has not been well studied.

Because of the lack of evidence regarding the effectiveness of prevention or treatment of stretch marks, individuals look to other sources when determining which products to purchase. In this study, we assess which products are available to consumers, which are popular among consumers, and factors determining which products are used for stretch marks.

Methods

A search was performed in January 2020 on United States internet retailer Amazon to identify the top products used for stretch marks. The searches performed were (1)"stretch mark" in All Departments: Beauty & Personal Care, (2)"stretch mark cream" in All Departments, and (3) "stretch mark" in Beauty & Personal Care: Skin Care: Maternity. Products were included based on average customer rating (4 stars and higher out of a possible 5 stars) and number of customer reviews (100 reviews and greater). Product titles, product descriptions, customer question and answer sections, and customer review sections were reviewed for the phrase "stretch mark." Products were excluded if they were nontopical products such as masks, massage balls, massage cups, or socks; product sets with more than one type of item; or if there was no mention of "stretch mark" in the title, product description, customer question and answer section, or customer review section. The product listing with the highest number of reviews was included if the product had multiple listings for different quantities and sizes. Median rating, average rating, average number of reviews, vehicle-type, ingredient list, and median price per ounce or fluid ounce were determined for the overall sample of products. Because of the large variety of ingredients, only ingredients that had been investigated in previous studies for effectiveness in treating stretch marks were included in the analysis [3,5,10,11].

Products were divided into two groups—stretch mark–specific products were those that included "stretch mark" in the product title, product description, or both and non stretch mark–specific products were those that included "stretch mark" in the customer question and answer section or the customer review section. To determine if a specific vehicle-type or specific ingredient was more likely to be found in a stretch mark–specific product, two-tailed two-sample proportion tests were used. $P<.05$ indicated statistical significance.

Results

Out of over 10,000 products on the United States internet retailer Amazon, 184 products met the required criteria. This group of products had a median consumer rating of 4.5 and a median of 409 reviews per product (range 103-10,573; total 183,366). The median price per ounce or per fluid ounce was $3.19 (range $0.17- $48; products that did not provide volume or weight information were not included: silicone sheet products, Crocodile acne scar removal cream, and Aliver TCM scar and acne mark removal gel ointment).

Products were categorized by vehicle-type. Out of 184 products, 131 (71.2%) were oils, 21 (11.4%) were creams, 9 (4.9%) were butters, 9 (4.9%) were gels, 5 (2.7%) were silicone sheets, 3 (1.6%) were lotions, 2 (1.1%) were scrubs, and the remaining 4 (2.2%) were categorized as other (balm, salve, ointment, and stick).

Of all 184 products, there were 117 (63.6%) stretch mark–specific and 67 (36.4%) non stretch mark–specific. Of the stretch mark-specific products, "stretch mark" was mentioned in the product title (6/117, 5.1%), product description (75/117, 64.1%), or both (36/117, 30.8%). "Stretch mark" was mentioned in the customer question and answer section (84/184, 45.7%) and customer review section (138/184, 75.0%). Customers mentioned "stretch mark" in relation to pregnancy or postpartum use in 70.1% of products (129/184). The top 10 most reviewed products are listed in Table 1. The top 10 most reviewed stretch mark–specific products are listed in Table 2.

Of the 117 stretch mark–specific products, 76 (65.0%) were oils, 17 (14.5%) were creams, 8 (6.8%) were butters, 6 (5.1%) were gels, 3 (2.6%) were silicone sheets, 3 (2.6%) were lotions, 2 (1.7%) were scrubs, 1 (0.9%) was a balm, and 1(0.9%) was a salve. Of the 67 non stretch mark–specific products, 55 (82.0%) were oils, 4 (6%) were creams, 1 (1.5%) was a butter, 3 (4.5%) were gels, 2 (3%) were silicone sheets, 1 (1.5 %) was an ointment, and 1 (1.5%) was a stick. Oil as a vehicle was more likely to be found in the stretch mark–specific product group than in the non stretch mark–specific product group ($P=.001$).

Of all 184 products, 7 (3.8%) contained allantoin, 11 (6%) contained aloe, 10 (5.4%) contained *C. asiatica*, 20 (10.9%) contained cocoa butter, 9 (4.9%) contained collagen, 4 (2.2%) contained hyaluronic acid, 23 (12.5%) contained shea butter, 3 (1.6%) contained vitamin A, 7 (3.8%) contained vitamin C, and

58 (31.5%) contained vitamin E. Out of the 117 stretch mark–specific products, 5 contained allantoin (4.3%), 9 contained aloe (7.7%), 10 (8.5%) contained *C. asiatica*, 18 (15.4%) contained cocoa butter, 7 (6%) contained collagen, 4 (3.4%) contained hyaluronic acid, 21 (17.9%) contained shea butter, 2 (1.6%) contained vitamin A, 6 (5.1%) contained vitamin C, and 40 (34.2%) contained vitamin E. Out of the 67 non stretch mark–specific products, 2 (3%) contained allantoin, 2 (3%) contained aloe, 0 (0%) contained *C. asiatica*, 2 (3%) contained cocoa butter, 0 (0%) contained hyaluronic acid, 2 (3%) contained shea butter, 1 (1.5%) contained vitamin A, 1 (1.5%) contained vitamin C, and 18 (26.9%) contained vitamin E. Three ingredients were more likely to be found in stretch mark–specific products—cocoa butter (P=.08), *C. asiatica* (P=.01), and shea butter (P=.003).

Specific types of oil as ingredients were also investigated [5]. While there were a variety of oils present in the products, almond oil, coconut oil, and olive oil have been found to be present frequently in other literature and were the focus of this analysis. Of all 184 products, 40 (21.7%) contained almond oil, 33 (17.9%) contained coconut oil, and 18 (9.8%) contained olive oil with remaining products containing other oils or no oils. Of the 117 stretch mark–specific products, 22 (18.8%) contained almond oil, 22 (18.8%) contained coconut oil, and 16 (13.7%) contained olive oil. Of the 67 non stretch mark–specific products, 18 (26.9%) contained almond oil, 11 (16.4%) contained coconut oil, and 2 (3%) contained olive oil. Olive oil was more likely to be found in stretch mark–specific products (P=.02).

Table 1. Top 10 most reviewed products.

	Manufacturer name	Product name	Number of reviews	Mean rating (out of 5)
1	Pura D'or	Organic Jojoba Oil	10,573	4.5
2	Bio-Oil	Skincare Oil	9732	4.4
3	Sky Organics	Organic Castor Oil	7164	4.5
4	Now Solutions	Sweet Almond Oil	6861	4.7
5	M3 Naturals	Anti Cellulite Massage Oil	5048	4.6
6	First Botany Cosmeceuticals	Arabica Coffee Scrub	4839	4.0
7	Burt's Bees Mama Bee	Belly Butter	4660	4.4
8	Pura D'or	Organic Rosehip Seed Oil	4332	4.6
9	Ancient Greek Remedy	Ancient Greek Remedy Oil	4249	4.6
10	Honeyskin	Ultimate Face & Body Cream	3359	4.3

Table 2. Top 10 most reviewed stretch mark–specific products.

	Manufacturer name	Product name	Number of reviews	Mean rating (out of 5)
1	Bio-Oil	Skincare Oil	9732	4.4
2	Sky Organics	Organic Castor Oil	7164	4.5
3	M3 Naturals	Anti Cellulite Massage Oil	5048	4.6
4	First Botany Cosmeceuticals	Arabica Coffee Scrub	4839	4.0
5	Burt's Bees Mama Bee	Belly Butter	4660	4.4
6	Ancient Greek Remedy	Ancient Greek Remedy Oil	4249	4.6
7	Honeyskin	Ultimate Face & Body Cream	3359	4.3
8	Coco & Co.	The Purest Coconut Virgin Oil	2858	4.7
9	Palmer's Cocoa Butter Formula	Massage Lotion For Stretch Marks	2654	4.3
10	Majestic Pure Cosmeceuticals	Rosehip Oil	2647	4.4

Discussion

Principal Findings

Over 10,000 products for stretch marks were found on Amazon, indicating the broad and diverse array of products ranging from topical to physical products (such as masks and socks) that are available for consumers. In this study, only topical products were assessed to limit the discussion of effectiveness to certain ingredients (those previously studied), but even with past studies, there has been no consensus regarding the effectiveness of topical products. As such, consumers rely upon information and suggestions posted by consumers on internet retail websites such as Amazon.

There is a disparity between the characteristics of products that are intended for use on stretch marks and the characteristics of products that are used on stretch marks based on customer reviews. Out of all 184 products, 63.6% (117) were intended for use on stretch marks, while 36.4% (67) were not intended for stretch marks but were used nonetheless based on customer reviews or customer questions and answers. This indicated that customers may be purchasing ineffective products by relying upon the opinions of others; 45.7% (84/184) of products had a question regarding stretch marks in the question and answer section, 75% (138/184) of products mentioned "stretch marks" in the reviews, and 70.1% (129/184) of products mentioned "stretch marks" related to pregnancy. The number of products that had a combination of "stretch marks" being mentioned in either question and answer section, reviews, and in relation to pregnancy was not differentiated. Previous studies have also shown that patients seek advice from friends, product advertisements, and the internet, particularly in the early stages of pregnancy [12].

The majority of the top products that were found when searching "stretch mark" were oils—131 (71.2%) of the top 184 products. Stretch mark–specific products were more likely to be oils than non stretch mark–specific products as demonstrated by the two-sample proportion test. Oils help retain moisture in the skin, but oils rich in linoleic acid and polyunsaturated fatty acids, such as olive oil, have also been found to reduce the formation of scars by reducing pro-inflammatory mediators (tumor necrosis factor alpha and peroxisome proliferator-activated receptors) which assists with wound healing [13]. Other studies, however, have produced conflicting findings. Studies have found that olive oil does not significantly reduce the incidence of striae gravidarum [14,15], while a study on almond oil demonstrated its possible effectiveness through its role in decreasing the progression of striae gravidarum by preventing itchiness when massaged into the skin [16,17]. In our study, specific oils that were found to be ingredients in the top products included, but were not limited to, apricot oil, argan oil, avocado oil, canola oil, castor oil, emu oil, grapefruit oil, jojoba oil, safflower oil, and sunflower oil. Recent studies have focused on almond oil, coconut oil, and olive oil [5]. This raises the question if enough studies on oils have been conducted, particularly because there have been contradictory findings on the effectiveness reported by studies. The amount of available studies on oils does not reflect the popularity of oils among consumers for stretch mark prevention and treatment. Furthermore, several studies suggest the therapeutic effect of massage in relation with oil for the prevention of stretch marks [1,16]. This further indicates that there is not enough understanding concerning oils and their use for stretch marks.

Out of the major ingredients assessed in this study, vitamin E was the most commonly used ingredient in both stretch mark–specific (40/117, 34.2%) and non stretch mark–specific products (18/67, 26.9%). A prior study showed that olive oils were rich in vitamin E, yet the findings did not suggest that olive oils were effective in the prevention of striae gravidarum [14]. Almond oil is also rich in vitamin E and vitamin D, yet a previous study also did not demonstrate the effectiveness of almond oil on its own for striae gravidarum [16]. Thus, future studies may wish to continue to assess which ingredients are effective for stretch mark prevention.

Creams comprised 11.4% (21/184) of the top products; creams comprised 14.5% (17/117) of stretch mark–specific products and 6% (4/67) of non stretch mark–specific products. Creams have been found to be the type of product most used by pregnant patients for prevention of stretch marks [4]. Previous studies stated an incidence of 50% to 90% for the development of striae gravidarum [18], indicating a large population of individuals who may seek out striae gravidarum products. Another cross-sectional study demonstrated high use of Bio-Oil by patients for the prevention of striae gravidarum [12], which is consistent with our finding that Bio-Oil was the most reviewed stretch mark–specific product. Product effectiveness and safety are of concern, especially during pregnancy. Furthermore, cream treatments such as Alphastria (containing hyaluronic acid, allantoin, vitamin A, and vitamin E) and Verum (containing vitamin E and hyaluronic acid) were not found to be in the top 10 product list, nor were their ingredients found in the top 10 products, despite having been studied and shown to have possible benefits in stretch mark prevention [1,5]. This demonstrates a discrepancy between the products that are being studied and the products that consumers are actually using, suggesting the need for consumers to be educated.

We focused our study on ingredients that had been mentioned in previous studies [3,5,10,11]. Cocoa butter, *C. asiatica*, and shea butter were more likely to be found as ingredients in products intended for stretch marks. In a previous study, the findings regarding the efficacy of cocoa butter for striae gravidarum prevention did not support its use despite cocoa butter's moisturizing effects [6,19]. Trofolastin (containing *C. asiatica*, vitamin E, and collagen-elastin hydrolysates) was also studied for the prevention of striae gravidarum and demonstrated significant prevention of stretch marks during pregnancy likely due to fibroblast stimulation and glucocorticoid antagonism [1,5,8]. Though shea butter is known to reduce fibroblasts [3], and there have been studies on whether shea butter is or is not effective for stretch marks, it is more likely to be found in products intended for stretch marks. Other products may have studies indicating their efficacy but may not be specifically indicated for the prevention of stretch marks. Aloe vera has been studied for its effectiveness in decreasing itchiness, and thus, the progression of stretch marks [17]. Tretinoin (or other vitamin A derivatives) has demonstrated some efficacy in preventing stretch marks, but is not found primarily in stretch mark–specific products [6]. Furthermore, tretinoin as well as ascorbic acid and hyaluronic acid are ingredients known to promote production of collagen [5]. Hyaluronic acid increases the skin's ability to resist tension, likely due to a mechanism of increased collagen production, yet minimal evidence has been found for its effectiveness [5,6]. These discrepancies show the gaps between what is effective and what is communicated to consumers about a product's effectiveness. Further studies should focus the ingredients being used the most by consumers in order to understand the ingredient's mechanism and effectiveness in stretch mark prevention.

Limitations

One limitation was the size of the overall study. There were over 10,000 products listed for "stretch mark" when searching the online retailer Amazon; however, we only included the top products by screening ratings and number of reviews. As such, we did not assess products with lower ratings and less reviews which would have been able to give us a broader idea of which products were being used by consumers for stretch marks. We also excluded products that did not mention "stretch mark" in the title, description, question and answer section, or review section, thus we did not assess what other types of ingredients were potentially being used for stretch marks. Another limitation of our study was that while we considered products that mentioned "stretch mark" in the product review, we did not assess whether the review was positive or negative. Future studies could potentially compare positive and negative consumer product reviews to understand the subjective effectiveness of products.

Conclusions

As demonstrated from our search on the internet retailer Amazon for products related to stretch marks, there are a plethora of products and ingredients for stretch marks; however, with few studies on the effectiveness of ingredients and products, consumers may rely upon consumer reviews when selecting products. More studies are needed to determine effectiveness and safety of ingredients, particularly with respect to pregnant women.

References

1. Elsaie ML, Baumann LS, Elsaaiee LT. Striae distensae (stretch marks) and different modalities of therapy: an update. Dermatol Surg 2009 Apr;35(4):563-573. [doi: 10.1111/j.1524-4725.2009.01094.x] [Medline: 19400881]
2. Tsuji T, Sawabe M. Elastic fibers in striae distensae. J Cutan Pathol 1988 Aug;15(4):215-222. [doi: 10.1111/j.1600-0560.1988.tb00547.x] [Medline: 3183137]
3. Ud-Din S, McGeorge D, Bayat A. Topical management of striae distensae (stretch marks): prevention and therapy of striae rubrae and albae. J Eur Acad Dermatol Venereol 2016 Feb 20;30(2):211-222 [FREE Full text] [doi: 10.1111/jdv.13223] [Medline: 26486318]
4. Al-Himdani S, Ud-Din S, Gilmore S, Bayat A. Striae distensae: a comprehensive review and evidence-based evaluation of prophylaxis and treatment. Br J Dermatol 2014 Mar 12;170(3):527-547. [doi: 10.1111/bjd.12681] [Medline: 24125059]
5. Lokhande A, Mysore V. Striae distensae treatment review and update. Indian Dermatol Online J 2019;10(4):380. [doi: 10.4103/idoj.idoj_336_18]
6. Korgavkar K, Wang F. Stretch marks during pregnancy: a review of topical prevention. Br J Dermatol 2015 Mar 08;172(3):606-615. [doi: 10.1111/bjd.13426] [Medline: 25255817]
7. Yamaguchi K, Suganuma N, Ohashi K. Prevention of striae gravidarum and quality of life among pregnant Japanese women. Midwifery 2014 Jun;30(6):595-599. [doi: 10.1016/j.midw.2013.07.011] [Medline: 23962637]
8. Mallol J, Belda M, Costa D, Noval A, Sola M. Prophylaxis of striae gravidarum with a topical formulation. a double blind trial. Int J Cosmet Sci 1991 Feb;13(1):51-57. [doi: 10.1111/j.1467-2494.1991.tb00547.x]
9. Rawlings AV, Bielfeldt S, Lombard KJ. A review of the effects of moisturizers on the appearance of scars and striae. Int J Cosmet Sci 2012 Dec 21;34(6):519-524. [doi: 10.1111/j.1468-2494.2012.00751.x] [Medline: 22994859]
10. Ross NA, Ho D, Fisher J, Mamalis A, Heilman E, Saedi N, et al. Striae distensae: preventative and therapeutic modalities to improve aesthetic appearance. Dermatol Surg 2017 May;43(5):635-648. [doi: 10.1097/DSS.0000000000001079] [Medline: 28375972]
11. Hague A, Bayat A. Therapeutic targets in the management of striae distensae: A systematic review. J Am Acad Dermatol 2017 Sep;77(3):559-568.e18. [doi: 10.1016/j.jaad.2017.02.048] [Medline: 28551068]
12. Brennan M, Clarke M, Devane D. The use of anti stretch marks' products by women in pregnancy: a descriptive, cross-sectional survey. BMC Pregnancy Childbirth 2016 Sep 21;16(1):276 [FREE Full text] [doi: 10.1186/s12884-016-1075-9] [Medline: 27654661]
13. Bielfeldt S, Blaak J, Staib P, Simon I, Wohlfart R, Manger C, et al. Observer-blind randomized controlled study of a cosmetic blend of safflower, olive and other plant oils in the improvement of scar and striae appearance. Int J Cosmet Sci 2018 Feb 12;40(1):81-86. [doi: 10.1111/ics.12438] [Medline: 29094366]
14. Taavoni S, Soltanipour F, Haghani H, Ansarian H, Kheirkhah M. Effects of olive oil on striae gravidarum in the second trimester of pregnancy. Complement Ther Clin Pract 2011 Aug;17(3):167-169. [doi: 10.1016/j.ctcp.2010.10.003] [Medline: 21742284]
15. Soltanipoor F, Delaram M, Taavoni S, Haghani H. The effect of olive oil on prevention of striae gravidarum: a randomized controlled clinical trial. Complement Ther Med 2012 Oct;20(5):263-266. [doi: 10.1016/j.ctim.2012.05.001] [Medline: 22863639]
16. Timur Taşhan S, Kafkasli A. The effect of bitter almond oil and massaging on striae gravidarum in primiparaous women. J Clin Nurs 2012 Jun 22;21(11-12):1570-1576. [doi: 10.1111/j.1365-2702.2012.04087.x] [Medline: 22594386]
17. Hajhashemi M, Rafieian M, Rouhi Boroujeni HA, Miraj S, Memarian S, Keivani A, et al. The effect of Aloe vera gel and sweet almond oil on striae gravidarum in nulliparous women. J Matern Fetal Neonatal Med 2018 Jul 19;31(13):1703-1708. [doi: 10.1080/14767058.2017.1325865] [Medline: 28521546]

18. Chang ALS, Agredano YZ, Kimball AB. Risk factors associated with striae gravidarum. J Am Acad Dermatol 2004 Dec;51(6):881-885. [doi: 10.1016/j.jaad.2004.05.030] [Medline: 15583577]
19. Osman H, Usta IM, Rubeiz N, Abu-Rustum R, Charara I, Nassar AH. Cocoa butter lotion for prevention of striae gravidarum: a double-blind, randomised and placebo-controlled trial. BJOG 2008 Aug;115(9):1138-1142 [FREE Full text] [doi: 10.1111/j.1471-0528.2008.01796.x] [Medline: 18715434]

15

The Use of Person-Centered Language in Medical Research Journals Focusing on Psoriasis

Ryan Ottwell, DO; Benjamin Heigle, BS; Arjun K Reddy, BA; Nicholas Sajjadi, BS; Alexis Wirtz, BS; Courtney Cook, DO; Hannah Howard, MD; Micah Hartwell, PhD; Matt Vassar, PhD

Oklahoma State University Center for Health Sciences, Tulsa, OK, United States

Corresponding Author:
Ryan Ottwell, DO
Oklahoma State University Center for Health Sciences
1111 W 17th Street
Tulsa, OK, 74107-1898
United States

Email: ryan.ottwell@okstate.edu

Abstract

Background: Person-centered language places a person's identity before any disability or medical condition they may have. Using person-centered language reduces stigma and improves the patient-physician relationship, potentially optimizing health outcomes. Patients with psoriasis often feel stigmatized due to their chronic skin condition.

Objective: We seek to evaluate the use of person-centered language in psoriasis literature and to explore whether certain article characteristics were associated with non–person-centered language.

Methods: We performed a systematic search on PubMed for recently published articles in journals that regularly publish psoriasis studies. After article reduction procedures, randomization, and screening, we reached our target sample of 400 articles. The following non–person-centered language terms were extracted from each article: "Psoriasis Patient," "Psoriasis subject," "Affected with," "Sufferer," "Suffering from," "Burdened with," "Afflicted with," and "Problems with." Screening and data extraction occurred in a masked duplicate fashion.

Results: Of the 400 included articles, 272 (68%) were not adherent to person-centered language guidelines according to the American Medical Association Manual of Style. The most frequent non–person-centered language term was "Psoriasis Patient," found in 174 (43.5%) articles. The stigmatizing language was associated with the type of article and funding status, with original investigations and funded studies having higher rates of stigmatizing language.

Conclusions: Articles about psoriasis commonly use non–person-centered language terms. It is important to shift away from using stigmatizing language about patients with psoriasis to avoid potential untoward influences. We recommend using "patients with psoriasis" or "patient living with psoriasis" to emphasize the importance of person-centered care.

KEYWORDS

psoriasis; dermatology; person-centered language; stigma; inclusive language; language

Introduction

It is estimated that 125 million people worldwide have psoriasis [1]—a chronic skin condition associated with arthritic disease; cardiovascular disease; and, namely, psychiatric disorders like depression [2]. Indeed, depression occurs in 9% to 55% of patients with psoriasis, and the impact of having psoriasis on the overall quality of life is comparable to that of patients with cancer [2-5]. Additionally, psychiatric morbidity in patients with chronic skin diseases, like psoriasis, is significantly associated with poorer medical compliance [6], which may lead to poorer health outcomes. The psychiatric distress experienced by patients with psoriasis may be exacerbated by feelings of stigma associated with psoriasis [7]. In numerous studies, patients living with psoriasis have reported feeling stigmatized due to this chronic skin condition [3-5]. Thus, reducing stigma among patients with psoriasis may serve to minimize untoward psychosocial influences and to optimize health outcomes.

Stigma is defined as "a mark of disgrace associated with a particular circumstance, quality, or person" [8], and the application of a generalized stigma to medical conditions may lead to decreased patient self-esteem, support, and likelihood of seeking medical care. Oftentimes, stigmatizing language is perpetuated by its widespread use in medical literature, which flows into medical education and ultimately into patient interactions [7]. The use of stigmatizing language is known to occur in other medical fields and is associated with negative health outcomes [3,6]. To decrease stigma experienced by patients with psoriasis in the dermatologic community, it is imperative to limit the use of stereotyping labels and to instead place an emphasis on the use of person-first language or person-centered language.

Person-centered language is based on the notion that it is most appropriate to place individuals ahead of the disabilities or medical conditions they have [9]. To treat individuals with psoriasis appropriately, we must first recognize the proper way to refer to them [10]. In 2010, the American Psychological Association defined the use of person-centered language, stating that the goal is to "maintain integrity of the individuals as human beings and to avoid language that objectifies a person by his or her condition" [11]. Similarly, many scholarly journals have begun to require the use of person-centered language in manuscripts submitted for publication [12], and the American Medical Association Manual of Style (AMAMS) requires authors to follow guidelines that include the avoidance of labeling people with their disabilities or diseases [13]. The use of person-centered language regarding patients with psoriasis is essential in fostering an advantageous relationship between the practitioner and patient. Most importantly, using person-centered language can promote a favorable environment for improving the overall well-being and quality of life for patients treated for psoriasis.

Thus, the primary objective of our study is to explore the use of person-centered language in journals that have published the most articles on psoriasis over the past 2 years. Additionally, we examined whether associations between person-centered language and particular study characteristics exist. Identifying areas for improvement regarding the use of person-centered language in the dermatologic community is necessary to reduce stigma experienced by patients with psoriasis.

Methods

Using a cross-sectional design, one author (MH) conducted a systematic search via PubMed on May 7, 2020. To include a broad range in the initial query, we searched for the term "psoriasis" in the title or abstract of articles with filters to include studies of humans that were available in English from May 1, 2018, to April 30, 2020. For article reduction, we included journals with 20 or more search returns to capture studies from journals who regularly publish psoriasis-related articles. The remaining articles were then randomized and distributed to authors (AR and BH) separately for article screening and data extraction, which were conducted in a masked duplicative fashion. Articles were screened until a final sample size of 400 articles was achieved among both authors, who then met for reconciliation of responses. For an article to be included the following criteria must be met: the article pertains to the topic of psoriasis, the article involves human subjects, and the article is available in English. All peer-reviewed original research articles, including research letters, brief reports, case reports, published abstracts, and commentaries pertaining to psoriasis were included. Extracted information included the article type, study method, type of intervention, funding source, country of the first author, and whether the article mentioned adherence to reporting guidelines.

To analyze person-centered language among articles, we systematically searched each article for a list of non–person-centered language labels and stigmatizing and euphemistic language that were established a priori to the data process. Searched terms were "Psoriatic(s)," "Psoriasis Patient," "Psoriasis subject," "Affected," "Sufferer," "Suffering from," "Burdened with," "Afflicted with," and "Problems with." Regarding the search term "Psoriatic," this includes referring to patients as either "psoriatics" or as a "psoriatic patient." Following completion of data extraction, investigators were unmasked and data reconciliation occurred to resolve any disagreements between investigators. If an agreement could not be reached, a third-party arbitrator (author RO) was consulted for adjudication.

Following data extraction, we calculated the proportion of articles with and without deviation from the AMAMS [13] guidelines compared to the total number of articles in this sample. Additionally, we evaluated the most common forms of non–person-centered language terminology used among these articles. Next, we measured the associations between adherence to person-centered language guidelines and extracted study characteristics using chi-square tests. The journal reduction process, article randomization, and statistical analyses were performed using STATA 16.1 (StataCorp) on February 19, 2021.

Results

Our query resulted in 3148 search returns from 670 journals. After article reduction procedures, randomization, and screening, we reached our target sample of 400 articles, which spanned 34 journals (Figure 1). A majority of the articles were original research (n=270, 67.5%; Table 1).

Figure 1. Flowchart of systematic investigation and outcomes of PCL in publications focused on psoriasis according to the AMAMS. AMAMS: American Medical Association Manual of Style; PCL: person-centered language.

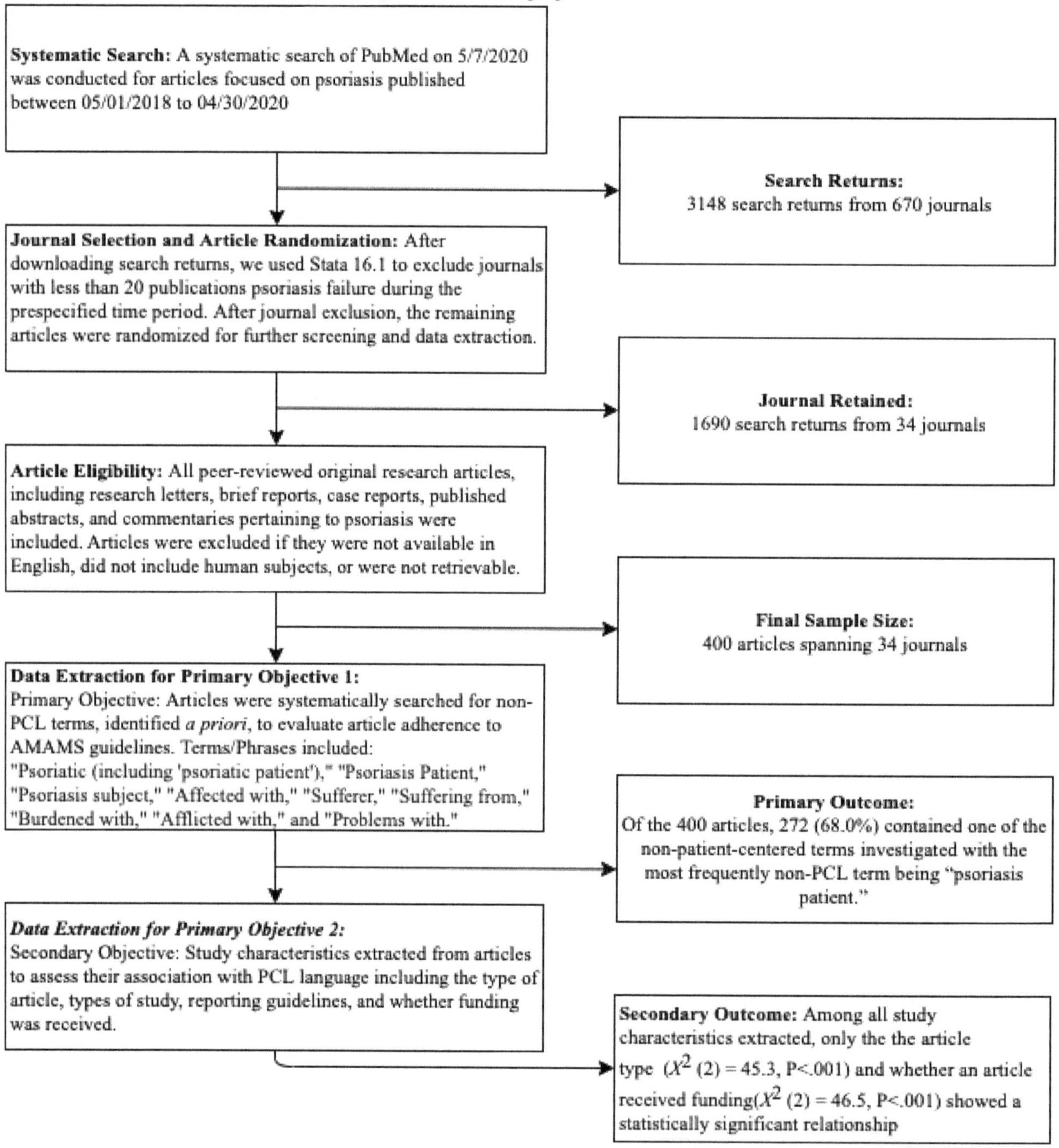

Table 1. Characteristics of studies and frequency of adherence to PCL.

Characteristics	Articles (N=400), n (%)	Articles with PCL[a] adherence, n (%)	Articles that were non-PCL adherent, n (%)	Chi-square (*df*)	*P* value
Type of article				45.3 (2)	<.001
Case report	40 (10.0)	22 (5.5)	18 (4.5)		
Editorial	90 (22.5)	49 (12.3)	41 (10.3)		
Original research	270 (67.5)	57 (14.3)	213 (53.3)		
Type of research				46.5 (4)	<.001
Clinical trial	49 (12.3)	12 (3)	37 (9.3)		
Literature review	36 (9)	6 (1.5)	30 (7.5)		
Editorials	131 (32.8)	71 (17.8)	60 (15)		
Observational	156 (39)	30 (7.5)	126 (31.5)		
Systematic review or meta-analysis	28 (7)	9 (2.3)	19 (4.8)		
Type of intervention				2.5 (3)	.48
Drug/pharmacologic	132 (33)	48 (12)	84 (21)		
Multiple therapies	7 (1.8)	2 (0.5)	5 (1.3)		
No treatment	250 (62.5)	76 (19)	174 (43.5)		
Nonpharmacologic	11 (2.9)	2 (0.6)	9 (2.3)		
Adherence to reporting guidelines				0.00 (1)	.95
Not mentioned	384 (96)	123 (30.8)	261 (65.3)		
Yes	16 (4)	5 (1.3)	11 (2.8)		
Study was funded				11.5 (1)	.001
No	239 (59.8)	92 (23)	147 (36.8)		
Yes	161 (40.3)	36 (9)	125 (31.3)		

[a]PCL: person-centered language.

The most prevalent type of research was cross-sectional or observational (n=156, 39%) followed by editorials (n=131, 32.8%). Of the 400 articles, 250 (62.5%) were not interventional studies, 384 (96%) did not mention adherence to any reporting guidelines, and 239 (59.8%) were not funded. According to the first author's affiliation, the majority of the articles were from the United States, Japan, and Italy (Table 2).

Table 2. Use of PCL by country.

Country[a]	Articles (N=400), n	Articles with PCL[b] adherence, n (%)	Articles that were non-PCL adherent, n (%)
Australia	5	3 (60)	2 (40)
Austria	3	2 (67)	1 (33)
Belgium	3	1 (33)	2 (67)
Brazil	5	0 (0)	5 (100)
Canada	22	8 (36)	14 (64)
Chile	1	0 (0)	1 (100)
China	23	6 (26)	17 (74)
Czech Republic	1	0 (0)	1 (100)
Denmark	22	5 (23)	17 (77)
Egypt	13	4 (31)	9 (69)
Estonia	1	0 (0)	1 (100)
France	12	4 (33)	8 (67)
Germany	23	4 (17)	19 (83)
Greece	3	2 (67)	1 (33)
Hungary	2	1 (50)	1 (50)
India	5	3 (60)	2 (40)
Ireland	11	7 (64)	4 (36)
Israel	2	0 (0)	2 (100)
Italy	28	9 (32)	19 (68)
Japan	31	12 (39)	19 (61)
Netherlands	3	1 (33)	2 (67)
New Zealand	2	0 (0)	2 (100)
Norway	6	1 (17)	5 (83)
Pakistan	1	0 (0)	1 (100)
Poland	7	0 (0)	7 (100)
Portugal	2	0 (0)	2 (100)
Scotland	1	0 (0)	1 (100)
Singapore	1	0 (0)	1 (100)
Slovenia	1	0 (0)	1 (100)
South Africa	1	0 (0)	1 (100)
South Korea	10	4 (40)	6 (60)
Spain	24	11 (46)	13 (54)
Sweden	4	0 (0)	4 (100)
Switzerland	7	1 (14)	6 (86)
Taiwan	9	1 (11)	8 (89)
Thailand	3	1 (33)	2 (67)
Turkey	7	1 (14)	6 (86)
UK	18	7 (39)	11 (61)
Ukraine	1	0 (0)	1 (100)
US	75	28 (37)	47 (63)
Venezuela	1	1 (100)	0 (0)
Total	400	128 (32)	272 (68)

[a]Country determined by first author's affiliation.

[b]PCL: person-centered language.

Of the 400 articles, 272 (68%) were not adherent to person-centered language guidelines according to AMAMS. Of these 272 articles with non–person-centered language, 129 (47.4%) included more than one non–person-centered language term. The most frequent non–person-centered language term identified was "Psoriasis Patient," found in 174 (43.5%) of the 400 articles, followed by "Psoriatic(s)," which was found in 103 (25.75%) articles (Table 3).

Table 3. Non-PCL terms and frequency within psoriasis articles.

Non-PCL[a] term searched	Articles in which non-PCL terms were present (N=400), n (%)
Psoriatic	103 (25.8)
Psoriasis patient	174 (43.5)
Psoriasis subject	2 (0.5)
Affected	63 (15.8)
Sufferer	2 (0.5)
Suffering from	39 (9.8)
Burden with	55 (13.8)
Afflicted with	2 (0.5)
Problem with	0 (0.0)

[a]PCL: person-centered language.

Significant associations were found between adherence to person-centered language guidelines and the type of article (χ^2_2=45.3; P<.001), as original research showed a higher proportion of studies with non–person-centered language terminology, and between person-centered language and type of research (χ^2_4=46.5; P<.001), where observational studies also contained a larger proportion of non–person-centered language studies. Additionally, there was a significant relationship between person-centered language and an article being funded (χ^2_1=11.5; P=.001) in which 38.5% (92/239) of the nonfunded articles were person-centered language adherent, compared to 22.4% (36/161) of the studies that were funded.

Discussion

We found that over two-thirds of the articles in our study contained non–person-centered language when referring to patients living with psoriasis. The most common non–person-centered language labels were "psoriasis patient" and "psoriatic"—to include "psoriatic patient" or "psoriatic subject." Efforts are needed to reduce the use of stigmatizing language in the medical community to prevent perpetuating non–person-centered language in medical literature and medical education. Clinicians and researchers may benefit from understanding that terms such as "psoriatic" or "psoriasis patient" are potentially stigmatizing to patients with psoriasis. Understanding that these terms are prevalent and undesirable may promote changing how we refer to patients with psoriasis. Additionally, the inappropriate use of stigmatizing language by medical professionals in medical records may elicit the clinician bias, leading to lower quality care for patients [14].

To our knowledge, no study has explored the use of stigmatizing and euphemistic language in medical literature about psoriasis or its influence on patients with psoriasis. Although the influence of non–person-centered language on patients with psoriasis is unknown, using stigmatizing language is known to have negative impacts on patients with other disorders. For example, patients with substance abuse disorders being referred to as "addicts" is associated with reduced medical compliance, lower quality care by clinicians secondary to bias, and poorer overall health outcomes [14-18]. In a specific case, the prevalence of stigmatizing language in recent publications regarding alcohol use disorder remains high [19]. The use of non–person-centered language in recent publications emphasizes the need to intentionally use inclusive language in scientific literature. Ensuring the proper use of person-centered language in scientific literature may require journals to update author guidelines. Additionally, reviewers may need to be more vigilant for non–person-centered language terms and labels when reviewing articles.

To increase the use of person-centered language in the field of dermatology, we recommend that the ubiquitous use of "patients with psoriasis" or "patients living with psoriasis" replace terms like "psoriatic patient" or "psoriatic subject" when publishing medical literature. Advocating for widespread implementation of person-centered language–specific reporting guidelines for dermatology research is necessary for creating a person-centered, patient-first approach to caring for patients with psoriasis. By incorporating inclusive language in professional dialogue, person-centered language will trickle down into patient interactions, potentially leading to reduced stigma and increased positive outcomes for patients living with psoriasis. We believe it is important to emphasize that the use of non–person-centered language by health care professionals is likely not malicious and is mostly a remnant of an uninformed, unchanged status quo. As the culture of medicine continues to shift toward inclusive, patient-centered dynamics, it is increasingly important that the field of dermatology maintain a high standard of care by normalizing the use of inclusive, person-centered language.

This study is not without limitations. For example, the AMAMS's definition of euphemistic language and emotional language is left to human interpretation and, therefore, subjective. Although we created a list of predefined non–person-centered language terms, other non–person-centered language terms may exist. An additional limitation lies within our study type; thus, our study's results should not be generalized beyond what our findings suggest. Regarding our results, due to the nature of editorials, and the fewer expectations and parameters of nonfunded research, we expected a greater number of articles with non–person-centered language among them; however, original and funded research included more stigmatizing language. Based on our results, future research may be needed to investigate this phenomenon. Lastly, we only searched PubMed for our literature search. PubMed was chosen as it is one of the largest online research databases and has been used in previous person-centered language research [19]; however, some studies focused on psoriasis may have been excluded. Future studies focused on person-centered language in other dermatologic conditions and other medical fields in which the condition is subject to labeling stigma is warranted.

Patients with psoriasis often feel stigmatized due to their chronic skin condition. We searched the psoriasis literature base for a representative sample of the most recent psoriasis studies to evaluate the prevalence of stigmatizing, non–person-centered language. We found that the majority of articles in our sample contained some form of stigmatizing language regarding patients with psoriasis. Efforts are needed to shift from using stigmatizing language to using inclusive, person-centered language regarding people with psoriasis. Our findings may be useful to clinicians and researchers striving to provide patients with high-quality person-centered care by using language that is more inclusive and empathetic toward patients living with psoriasis.

References

1. Psoriasis statistics. The National Psoriasis Foundation. URL: https://www.psoriasis.org/psoriasis-statistics/ [accessed 2021-02-23]
2. Rendon A, Schäkel K. Psoriasis pathogenesis and treatment. Int J Mol Sci 2019 Mar 23;20(6):1475 [FREE Full text] [doi: 10.3390/ijms20061475] [Medline: 30909615]
3. Hrehorów E, Salomon J, Matusiak L, Reich A, Szepietowski JC. Patients with psoriasis feel stigmatized. Acta Derm Venereol 2012 Jan;92(1):67-72 [FREE Full text] [doi: 10.2340/00015555-1193] [Medline: 21879243]
4. Ginsburg IH, Link BG. Psychosocial consequences of rejection and stigma feelings in psoriasis patients. Int J Dermatol 1993 Aug;32(8):587-591. [doi: 10.1111/j.1365-4362.1993.tb05031.x] [Medline: 8407075]
5. Ramsay B, O'Reagan M. A survey of the social and psychological effects of psoriasis. Br J Dermatol 1988 Feb;118(2):195-201. [doi: 10.1111/j.1365-2133.1988.tb01774.x] [Medline: 3348965]
6. Renzi C, Picardi A, Abeni D, Agostini E, Baliva G, Pasquini P, et al. Association of dissatisfaction with care and psychiatric morbidity with poor treatment compliance. Arch Dermatol 2002 Mar;138(3):337-342. [doi: 10.1001/archderm.138.3.337] [Medline: 11902984]
7. Bewley A, Burrage DM, Ersser SJ, Hansen M, Ward C. Identifying individual psychosocial and adherence support needs in patients with psoriasis: a multinational two-stage qualitative and quantitative study. J Eur Acad Dermatol Venereol 2014 Jun;28(6):763-770. [doi: 10.1111/jdv.12174] [Medline: 23663069]
8. Stigma. Merriam-Webster. URL: https://www.merriam-webster.com/dictionary/stigma [accessed 2020-05-12]
9. Wehmeyer M, Bersani H, Gagne R. Riding the third wave. Focus Autism Other Developmental Disabilities 2016 Sep 14;15(2):106-115. [doi: 10.1177/108835760001500206]
10. Crocker AF, Smith SN. Person-first language: are we practicing what we preach? J Multidiscip Healthc 2019;12:125-129. [doi: 10.2147/JMDH.S140067] [Medline: 30799931]
11. Granello DH, Gibbs TA. The power of language and labels: "The Mentally Ill" versus "People With Mental Illnesses". J Counseling Dev 2016 Jan 03;94(1):31-40. [doi: 10.1002/jcad.12059]
12. Jensen ME, Pease EA, Lambert K, Hickman DR, Robinson O, McCoy KT, et al. Championing person-first language: a call to psychiatric mental health nurses. J Am Psychiatr Nurses Assoc 2013;19(3):146-151. [doi: 10.1177/1078390313489729] [Medline: 23698977]
13. AMA Manual of Style Committee. Contents. AMA Manual of Style: A Guide for Authors and Editors (11th ed). 2020. URL: https://www.amamanualofstyle.com/view/10.1093/jama/9780190246556.001.0001/med-9780190246556 [accessed 2020-05-23]
14. P Goddu A, O'Conor KJ, Lanzkron S, Saheed MO, Saha S, Peek ME, et al. Do words matter? Stigmatizing language and the transmission of bias in the medical record. J Gen Intern Med 2018 May;33(5):685-691 [FREE Full text] [doi: 10.1007/s11606-017-4289-2] [Medline: 29374357]
15. Ashford RD, Brown AM, Curtis B. Substance use, recovery, and linguistics: the impact of word choice on explicit and implicit bias. Drug Alcohol Depend 2018 Aug 01;189:131-138 [FREE Full text] [doi: 10.1016/j.drugalcdep.2018.05.005] [Medline: 29913324]

16. Kelly JF, Westerhoff CM. Does it matter how we refer to individuals with substance-related conditions? A randomized study of two commonly used terms. Int J Drug Policy 2010 May;21(3):202-207. [doi: 10.1016/j.drugpo.2009.10.010] [Medline: 20005692]
17. Johnson ME, Dowling-Guyer S. Effects of inclusive vs. exclusive language on evaluations of the counselor. Sex Roles 1996 Mar;34(5-6):407-418. [doi: 10.1007/bf01547809]
18. Richter L, Vuolo L, Salmassi MS. Stigma and addiction treatment. In: Avery JD, Avery JJ, editors. The Stigma of Addiction: An Essential Guide. Cham: Springer; 2019:93-130.
19. Hartwell M, Naberhaus B, Arnhart C, Ottwell R, Dunn K, Rogers TC, et al. The use of person-centered language in scientific research articles focusing on alcohol use disorder. Drug Alcohol Depend 2020 Nov 01;216:108209. [doi: 10.1016/j.drugalcdep.2020.108209] [Medline: 32801060]

Abbreviations

AMAMS: American Medical Association Manual of Style

Assessing Sunscreen Protection Using UV Photography: Descriptive Study

Caitlin Horsham[1], MSc; Helen Ford[1], MSc; Jeremy Herbert[2], PhD; Alexander Wall[2], GradDip(IndDus); Sebastian Walpole[3], PhD; Elke Hacker[1], PhD

[1]School of Public Health and Social Work, Queensland University of Technology, Brisbane, Australia

[2]Designworks Group Pty Ltd, Brisbane, Australia

[3]Genetics & Population Health Division, QIMR Berghofer, Brisbane, Australia

Corresponding Author:
Elke Hacker, PhD
School of Public Health and Social Work
Queensland University of Technology
60 Musk Avenue
Kelvin Grove
Brisbane, 4059
Australia

Email: elke.hacker@qut.edu.au

Abstract

Background: Photography using a UV transmitting filter allows UV light to pass and can be used to illuminate UV blocking lotions such as sunscreens.

Objective: The aim of this study is to compare currently available UV photography cameras and assess whether these devices can be used as visualization tools for adequate coverage of sun protection lotions.

Methods: This study was conducted in 3 parts: in phase 1, 3 different UV cameras were tested; in phase 2, we explored whether UV photography could work on a range of sun protection products; and in phase 3, a UV webcam was developed and was field-tested in a beach setting. In phase 1, volunteers were recruited, and researchers applied 3 sun protection products (ranging from sun protection factor [SPF] 15 to 50+) to the participants' faces and arms. UV photography was performed using 3 UV cameras, and the subsequent images were compared. In phase 2, volunteers were recruited and asked to apply their own SPF products to their faces in their usual manner. UV photographs were collected in the morning and afternoon to assess whether the coverage remained over time. Qualitative interviews were conducted to assess the participants' level of satisfaction with the UV image. In phase 3, a small portable UV webcam was designed using a plug-and-play approach to enable the viewing of UV images on a larger screen. The developed webcam was deployed at a public beach setting for use by the public for 7 days.

Results: The 3 UV camera systems tested during phase 1 identified the application of a range of sun protection lotions of SPF 15 to 50+. The sensitivity of the UV camera devices was shown to be adequate, with SPF-containing products applied at concentrations of 2 and 1 mg/cm^2 clearly visible and SPF-containing products applied at a concentration of 0.4 mg/cm^2 having lower levels of coverage. Participants in phase 2 reported high satisfaction with the UV photography images, with 83% (29/35) of participants likely to use UV photography in the future. During phase 2, it was noted that many participants used tinted SPF-containing cosmetics, and several tinted products were further tested. However, it was observed that UV photography could not identify the areas missed for all tinted products. During phase 3, the electrical components of the UV webcam remained operational, and the camera was used 233 times by the public during field-testing.

Conclusions: In this study, we found that UV photography could identify the areas missed by sun protection lotions with chemical filters, and participants were engaged with personalized feedback.

KEYWORDS

skin neoplasms; melanoma; health promotion; public health; preventive medicine; sunburn; sunscreening agents; UV photography; mobile phone

Introduction

Background

Reflected UV photography provides a unique method of assessing sunscreen application. A camera using a UV transmitting filter allows UV radiation to pass but absorbs or blocks visible and infrared light. The subject is illuminated by either UV emitting lamps or sunlight, and a photo is taken, which then highlights the areas where sunscreens have been applied. Sunscreen application followed by UV photography is a potential method to objectively measure the visibility of sunscreen on the skin [1]. Pratt et al [2] have shown that UV photography can detect commonly missed areas during sunscreen application on the face, with participants missing the eyelids and the medial canthal area around the eyes. Molecular analysis of normal eyelids has also shown that over a quarter of cells carry mutations that exhibit characteristic signatures of UV light exposure [3]. The eyebrow and eyelid have also been reported as high-risk anatomical sites for locally destructive basal cell carcinoma skin cancers [4].

Skin cancer is estimated to account for more cases diagnosed than all other cancers combined in Australia, costing over Aus $800 million (US $622 million) to treat each year [5-7]. Sunlight or UV radiation is the main risk factor for skin cancers, and sunburn remains highly prevalent in the northern Australian state of Queensland, with 49% of adults and 45% of children sunburnt in the previous 12 months [8]. Of the children who were sunburnt in the past 12 months, 69% were most recently sunburnt during a water-based activity [8]. These findings are concerning and highlight the importance of adequate sunscreen coverage and reapplication when participating in water-based activities. Regular sunscreen application has been shown to reduce the incidence of squamous cell carcinoma and melanoma [9,10] and block the harmful molecular effects of UV radiation on skin cells in vivo [11].

Barriers reported to sunscreen application include concerns over sunscreen esthetics and tactile properties, including a sticky or greasy texture, feeling hot or sweaty, perception that sunscreens cause acne or skin irritation, and dislike of sunscreen appearance [12]. Many cosmetic products are secondary sunscreens with a sun protection factor (SPF) that offers convenience and improved texture and appearance. In Australia, the industry-accepted SPF standard tests primary sunscreens as well as secondary sunscreen products, which are applied at a thickness of 2 mg/cm^2 and rated for SPF from 0 to 50+. For SPF products to be effective, adequate quantities of the product need to be applied with an appropriate frequency of reapplication. There are 2 types of sun protection formulations: (1) physical filters such as titanium dioxide or zinc oxide, which act by scattering sunlight from the skin surface, or (2) chemical filters that transform the energy from the sun into molecular conformational changes [13]. Physical filters cannot be detected with UV photography, and only lotions with chemical filters can be visualized. In addition, some cosmetic products are tinted and contain both chemical and physical filters in their formulations. The physical filters within these products may limit their ability to be visualized. Tinted SPF cosmetics contain a temporary color or pigmentation and can include products such as foundations, lipsticks, and eye shadows.

Objectives

The purpose of this study was to compare UV photography cameras and assess whether these devices can be used as visualization tools for adequate coverage of a range of SPF lotions commonly applied to the face, including sunscreens, moisturizers, and cosmetics.

Methods

This study was conducted in 3 parts: phase 1 was laboratory testing, which involved testing different UV cameras and SPF product coverage; phase 2 was determining whether UV photography could visualize a range of sun protection products self-applied by individuals; and phase 3 was developing a UV webcam and field-testing the device in a public beach setting.

Phase 1: Laboratory Testing of UV Cameras

Commercially available UV cameras were purchased using the purchasing protocol, which involved searching the internet using the terms "UV camera," "sunscreen detector," and "sunscreen camera." A total of 3 devices were identified and purchased for delivery to Australia. The cameras of 2 devices, the Sunscreenr (Vocelight LLC) and Nurugo SPF (Nurugo), attach to Android smartphones and are used in combination with an app. The third device used a digital single-lens reflex (DSLR) camera (Model D5300, Nikon) fitted with a Baader Venus filter (Model Baader Planetarium U-Filter 2", Ultraviolet, ZWL 350 nm).

Participants were eligible to participate if they were aged 18 years or above and were available to attend the university campus. Participants were excluded if they had allergies or were sensitive to sunscreen. The sample size calculation for phase 1 was based on the recommendations from the industry-accepted Sunscreen Standard (AS/NZS 2604:2012), which sets a minimum sample size of 10 participants to assess each sun protection product. Participants were recruited through university email and social media posts. Participants completed a demographic survey and removed any skin care or makeup products from their face and arms using isopropanol wipes and paper towels. Images of the treatment sites (face and forearms where SPF lotions were applied) were captured using the DSLR UV camera and normal photography before any lotions were applied. This was to ensure that there were no SPF lotions on the skin before treatment. The treatment areas were marked by the researchers using plastic cutout rectangles (4□2.5 cm) on the participants' face and both forearms. Each SPF lotion was randomly assigned to a treatment site and applied at concentrations of 2, 1, and 0.4 mg/cm^2 (Figure S1 in Multimedia Appendix 1). The SPF lotions used included (1) sunscreen SPF

50+ (Cancer Council Ultra; active ingredients: homosalate 100 mg/g, octyl salicylate 50 mg/g, butyl methoxydibenzoylmethane 30 mg/g, and octocrylene 80 mg/g), (2) moisturizer secondary sunscreen SPF 50+ (SunSense Moisturizer; active ingredients: bemotrizinol 2%, methylene bis-benzotriazolyl tetramethylbutylphenol 2.5%, and octyl salicylate 5.0%), and (3) moisturizer secondary sunscreen SPF 15+ (Neutrogena Moisturizer; active ingredients: butyl methoxydibenzoylmethane, ethylhexyl methoxycinnamate, ethylhexyl salicylate, and phenylbenzimidazole sulfonic acid). Only SPF lotion products with chemical sunscreen filters were used, as zinc oxide and titanium dioxide cannot be visualized with UV photography. Images were captured immediately after SPF product application (baseline timepoint) and 20 minutes post application (follow-up timepoint) using the 3 UV cameras purchased. UV images of the participants' faces (front, left side, and right side) as well as both forearms were taken at each timepoint.

Image analysis was performed using Image J (National Institutes of Health) [14], and the scale-to-pixel measurement was assigned using the treatment area (4□2.5 cm), with the rectangle tool used to define the region of interest. Image thresholds were set, and the percentage of area with dark pixels (SPF lotion present) were compared with the percentage of area with light pixels (no SPF lotion present) to calculate the percentage of coverage.

Phase 2: Testing UV Photography Using a Range of Sun Protection Products

Part 2a: Observational Study

An observational study was conducted to assess the application of sun protection products of indoor workers. To be eligible, participants had to be aged 18 years or above, a current indoor worker, routinely use products with SPF on their face, and available to visit the researchers to attend both morning and afternoon photo sessions on the same day. Participants were recruited through email, social media, and the Queensland University of Technology workplace health and safety programs. Participants provided consent, completed a baseline questionnaire, and were asked to apply their own SPF products to their face in their usual manner before attending the study visit. To assess if the coverage remained over time, participants were imaged in the morning and then again in the afternoon, with a gap of at least 4 hours between timepoints. A total of 3 UV images of the participants' faces (front, left side, and right side) were taken at each timepoint. Images were captured indoors using a white background and standard lighting, with participants sitting on a stool at a set distance from the camera, and an artificial UV light source (Nurugo) was used for UV illumination. In the afternoon, participants were shown their UV images, and an in-person interview was conducted. During the interview, participants were asked about their level of satisfaction with their UV photography images. The interview questions are listed in Table S1 in Multimedia Appendix 1.

To assess the difference in coverage between the morning and afternoon photo sessions, an automated image analysis method was developed to objectively detect, segment, and quantify the areas of the face within the UV images that were not adequately covered by SPF lotions. Volocity 3D image analysis software (PerkinElmer) was used. A scale-to-pixel measurement was assigned to each image using the ID sticker (19□24 mm), the region of interest tool was imposed, and the find object tool was used to find the percentage of area with dark pixels (SPF lotion present) and compared this with the percentage of area with light pixels (no SPF lotion present). The segmented areas included the nose, cheeks, forehead, and medial canthal area, which were then scored as "yes, adequately protected" or "no, not adequately protected."

Part 2b: Testing Tinted SPF Lotions

Many SPF lotions used by participants in the observational study were tinted products that combined a colored base with SPF protection. Commonly used tinted sun protection products by participants in the observational study were purchased by the researchers for further laboratory testing in 1 volunteer. The 5 products used included (1) Fit Me SPF 18 liquid foundation (*Maybelline*; *active ingredients: octinoxate 7%*), (2) Lasting Radiance SPF 28 liquid foundation (*Rimmel*; *active ingredients: octinoxate*), (3) SkinActive beauty balm (BB) cream SPF 15 (*Garnier*; *active ingredients: octinoxate*), (4) BB cream SPF 15 (*Olay*; *active ingredients: octisalate* and *avobenzone*), and (5) SkinActive BB cream SPF 50+ (*La Roche-Posay*; *active ingredients: homosalate 6.0% w/w, octyl salicylate 5.0% w/w, butyl methoxydibenzoylmethane 5.0% w/w, octocrylene 5.0% w/w, ethylhexyl triazone 4.0% w/w, bemotrizinol 3.0% w/w, drometrizole trisiloxane 3.0% w/w, ecamsule 0.99% w/w*, and *titanium dioxide 0.83% w/w*). The volunteer provided informed consent, completed a demographic survey, and was asked to visit the researchers at the university. At the study visit, the volunteer was asked to remove any skin care or makeup products using isopropanol wipes and then rinse the area using running water and a paper towel. A UV image and normal photography image were taken from the treatment site before application to ensure that no lotions remained on the skin. The participants and research staff were blinded to the brand and SPF strength of the lotion. Lotions were applied to participants' forearms to compare the 5 products at 2, 1, 0.4, and 0.2 mg/cm^2 concentrations each to a 4□2.5 cm area of skin. Tinted sun protection products 4 and 5 were further evaluated at lower concentrations on the face, with applications of 1, 0.6, 0.4, and 0.2 mg/cm^2. Data collection included images captured immediately after application using both the DSLR UV camera and a normal camera (Nikon).

Phases 1 and 2 of the study were approved by the Human Research Ethics Committee of the Queensland University of Technology (number 1800001263) and prospectively registered with the Australian and New Zealand Clinical Trials Register (ACTRN12619000975190; ACTRN12619000145101). The sample size calculation for the phase 2 observational study was based on the recommendations from Lancaster et al [15] of 30 participants, which is widely used in feasibility testing studies.

Phase 3: Development, Safety, and Field-Testing of a UV Webcam

Development

A UV webcam on a large screen was developed for use at public events, which could be used by the public with contactless operation. The UV webcam was developed using a UV transmitting filter (Edmund Optics) and an M12 lens (ArduCam) connected to a printed circuit board for processing electronics and housed within a plastic molding with a 365-nm UV light-emitting diode light source. A high-definition multimedia interface output cable was used to display the image, and a commercially available pressure sensor mat (Radio Parts Pty Ltd) was connected via a custom data acquisition system to report the pressure-sensitive switch information in real time over a USB connection. The pressure sensor mat allowed use data to be collected and stored data locally on a microSD card. The UV webcam functioned with contactless operation and only required the users to stand on the mat for the image to be displayed on the screen. The UV webcam was designed to be plugged into any monitor or display screen with a high-definition multimedia interface connection point and display the image using a plug-and-play approach without requiring any software or an internet connection.

Observational Testing

To check whether the UV webcam was connecting and recording use data from the pressure sensor mat correctly, observational testing was performed in Brisbane, Australia (approximate latitude 27°S, 153°E). A total of 2 volunteers (90 kg and 60 kg) stood on the pressure sensor mat and used the UV camera 10 times, and the time-stamped data collected by the device were then compared with observational data.

Safety Testing

The temperature of the UV webcam device after 2 and 4 hours of continuous operation was recorded using an infrared handheld thermometer (ThermaTwin TN410LCE Infrared Thermometer). The UV radiation emitted by the UV light source was measured using a UV intensity meter (Solar Light Co, model PMA2100) fitted with a digital sensor (Solar Light Co, model PMA2101). The detector head of the sensor was positioned at a distance where a person's face would be placed during use.

Field-Testing

A field study was conducted from November 21 to 27, 2020, in spring in Australia. The UV webcam was deployed to Surfers Paradise beach in Queensland, Australia (approximate latitude 28.0°S, 153.4°E). The UV webcam was placed near the beach entry on the esplanade in a high-traffic area accessed by the public. The UV webcam was deployed at the start of the day until the end of daylight hours, and free SPF 50+ chemical sunscreen was available next to the UV webcam through a touchless automatic dispenser system (Danger Sun Overhead). End users could provide optional feedback if desired using the contact email and phone number provided next to the UV webcam. The deployment of the UV webcam was to assess the functionality and not human subjects' research; therefore, we obtained an institutional ethics review board exemption from the Human Research Ethics Committee of the Queensland University of Technology for this phase of the study.

Weather measurements were collected during the field study. Temperature data were recorded in degrees Celsius for the daily minimum and maximum as well as for observations at 9 AM and 3 PM each day. The temperature data were captured by the Bureau of Meteorology weather station (no.: 040764; Gold Coast Seaway, latitude 28°S, 153°E). The UV radiation data were captured by the Australian Radiation Protection and Nuclear Safety Agency detector (Gold Coast, latitude 28°S, 153°E), with the standard erythemal dose (SED) calculated with daily summaries and hourly observations recorded at 10 AM and noon.

Results

Phase 1: Laboratory Testing of UV Cameras

A total of 10 participants enrolled and completed the laboratory testing phase. The participants were mostly female (8/10, 80%), and 70% (7/10) of the participants had very fair or fair skin (Table S2 in Multimedia Appendix 1). All 3 UV cameras captured well-defined areas when the SPF lotions were applied at concentrations of 2 and 1 mg/cm^2. Figure 1 shows the areas where SPF lotions were applied to the participants' faces, with the dark areas indicating SPF lotions are present.

The quality of the image captured by the DSLR UV camera was the highest of the 3 UV cameras purchased, with an image size of 6000□4000 pixels and a resolution of 300 dpi (dots per inch). The image size captured by the Sunscreenr camera was 1716□1290 pixels at 72 dpi and by the Nurugo SPF camera was 480□640 pixels at 72 dpi. Both the Nurugo SPF and Sunscreenr cameras collected images that had sufficient image quality for an observer to view the images on the small screen of a smartphone.

With the 10 volunteers, the sensitivity of the UV camera devices was also tested using 3 SPF-containing lotions applied at concentrations of 2, 1, and 0.4 mg/cm^2 (Figure S2 in Multimedia Appendix 1). There was perfect agreement (100%) across the UV camera devices when the concentration of the SPF product was high (2 and 1 mg/cm^2; Table 1). The lower 0.4 mg/cm^2 application thickness had less coverage, but there was still strong agreement among the UV camera devices (Table 1).

Figure 1. Comparison of UV photography devices. (A) A digital single-lens reflex (DSLR) UV camera, (B) Nurugo sun protection factor (SPF) camera, and (C) Sunscreenr camera were used to capture images of a SPF 50+ lotion applied to a 4 cm□2.5 cm area at a set concentration on the right cheek (0.4 mg/cm^2), forehead (2 mg/cm^2), and left cheek (1 mg/cm^2).

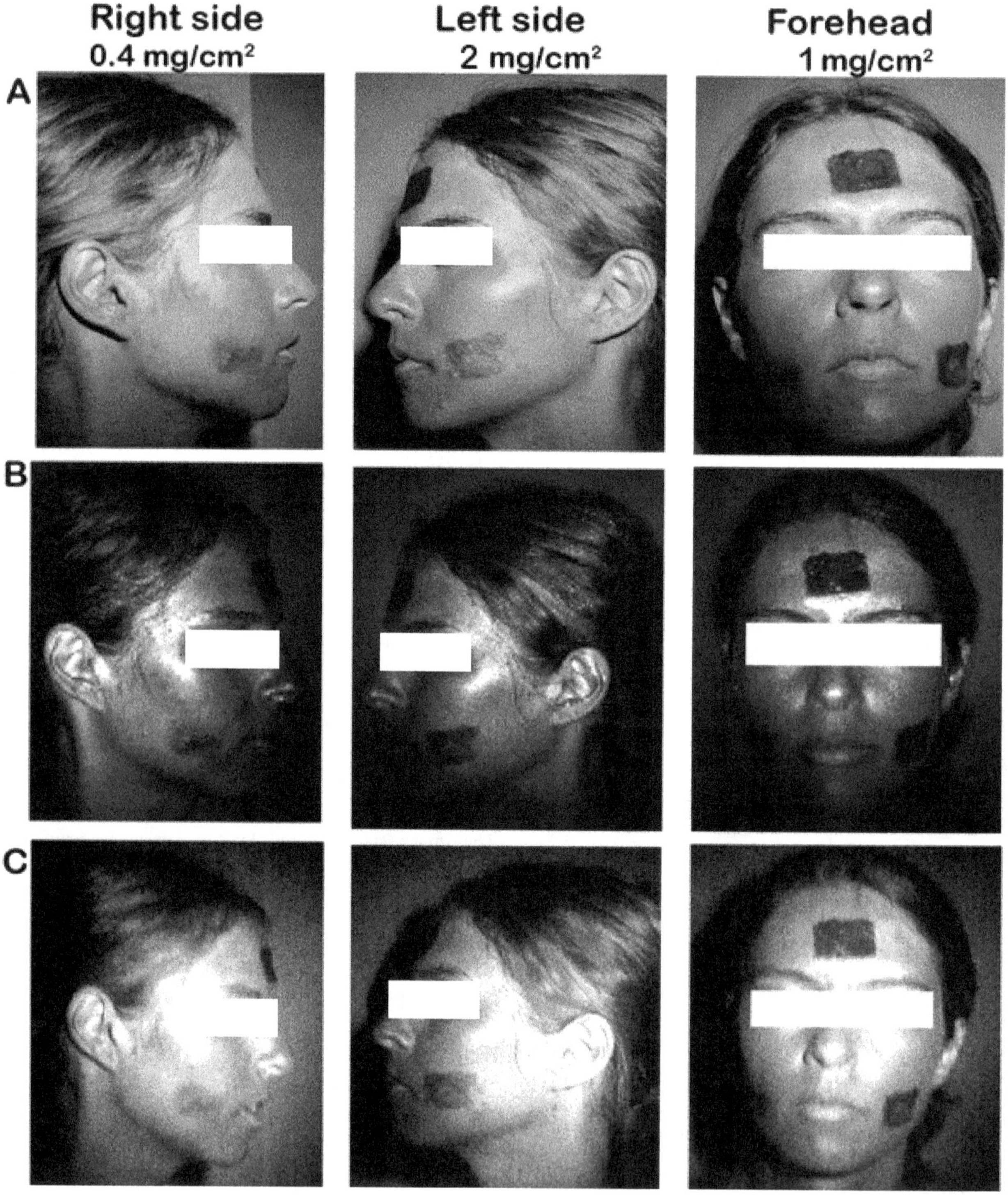

Table 1. The percentage of coverage at each treatment site determined by 3 UV camera devices in 10 volunteers.

Sun protection product	DSLR[a] UV camera (n=10); % (SE)	Sunscreenr UV camera (n=10); % (SE)	Nurugo SPF[b] camera (n=10); % (SE)
Sunscreen SPF 50+ (mg/cm^2)			
2	100 (0)	100 (0)	100 (0)
1	100 (0)	100 (0)	100 (0)
0.4	72 (3.1)	72 (3.1)	73 (3.4)
Moisturizer SPF 50+ (mg/cm^2)			
2	100 (0)	100 (0)	100 (0)
1	100 (0)	100 (0)	100 (0)
0.4	69 (0.2)	68 (1.4)	69 (0.2)
Moisturizer SPF 15+ (mg/cm^2)			
2	100 (0)	100 (0)	100 (0)
1	100 (0)	100 (0)	100 (0)
0.4	69 (0.3)	68 (1.3)	69 (0.3)

[a]DSLR: digital single-lens reflex.

[b]SPF: sun protection factor.

Phase 2: Testing UV Photography Using a Range of Sun Protection Products

Part 2a: Observational Study

A total of 39 participants enrolled and completed the morning photo session, and 2 participants did not return for their afternoon photos. Furthermore, 2 participants wore products that contained only physical active ingredients and were excluded from further analysis (Figure S3 in Multimedia Appendix 1). Overall, 35 participants were included in the analysis.

The participants were mostly females (34/35, 97%), and 63% (22/35) of the participants had very fair or fair skin type (Table S2 in Multimedia Appendix 1). Just over half of the participants had applied 1 SPF-containing product (20/35, 57%), 34% (12/35) of the participants had applied 2 products, and 9% (3/35) of the participants had 3 or more products applied to their faces. The most used type of product was facial moisturizer (22/55, 40%), followed by liquid foundation (17/55, 31%), sunscreen (11/55, 20%), lip balm/lipstick (3/55, 5%), and powder foundation (2/55, 4%). Of the 55 facial products used by the participants, 25% (14/55) were SPF 50+, 53% (29/55) were SPF 15+, 4% (2/55) were below SPF 15, and 18% (10/55) had no SPF rating. A total of 66% (23/35) participants used one or more products that were tinted and contained chemical UV filters as well as varying quantities of titanium dioxide or zinc oxides.

Participants reported high satisfaction with the UV photography images, with 83% (29/35) of participants likely to use UV photography in the future to help guide the application of SPF products, whereas 80% (28/35) of participants would share their UV image with friends or family (Table S2 in Multimedia Appendix 1).

Participants' images captured in the morning showed good coverage of sun protection products on their nose (32/35, 91%), and 80% (28/35) of participants had their cheeks covered, and 71% (25/35) of the participants had their forehead protected. By the afternoon, the coverage of sun protection products had decreased, with only 74% (26/35) of the participants still having good coverage on their nose, 63% (22/35) having their cheeks protected, and 51% (18/35) having their forehead covered. On average, the morning and afternoon photos were taken 4 hours and 37 minutes apart. Commonly missed areas included the medial canthal area (across the eyes), which was missed by 37% (13/35) of the participants in the morning, and by the afternoon, 69% (24/35) of the participants had no sun protection in this area (Figure S4 in Multimedia Appendix 1).

Part 2b: Testing Tinted SPF Lotions

The level of coverage varied greatly between the 5 tinted products, regardless of SPF rating (Figure S5 in Multimedia Appendix 1). Overall, 3 out of the 5 tinted SPF products were barely visible or not visible using UV photography. A review of the product ingredient list revealed that all the 5 products tested listed chemical UV filters as well as varying quantities of titanium dioxide or zinc oxides. UV photography was shown not to be suitable for 3 of the tinted products, as the physical blockers titanium dioxide or zinc oxides may have affected the ability to capture UV images. However, 2 tinted sun protection products were visible using UV photography even at low concentrations. The level of coverage was still high for the SPF 50+ product, yielding a dark area at the treatment site even when applied at 0.2 mg/cm^2 (Figure 2). Although the SPF 15 product had adequate coverage at 1 mg/cm^2, the absorption of UV was reduced at the lower 0.6, 0.4, and 0.2 mg/cm^2 sites (Figure 2).

Figure 2. Tinted cosmetics and sun protection coverage using UV photography. The top panel shows product 4 applied to the cheek at concentrations of 1, 0.6, 0.4, and 0.2 mg/cm^2, and the bottom panel shows product 5 applied at the same concentrations. SPF: sun protection factor.

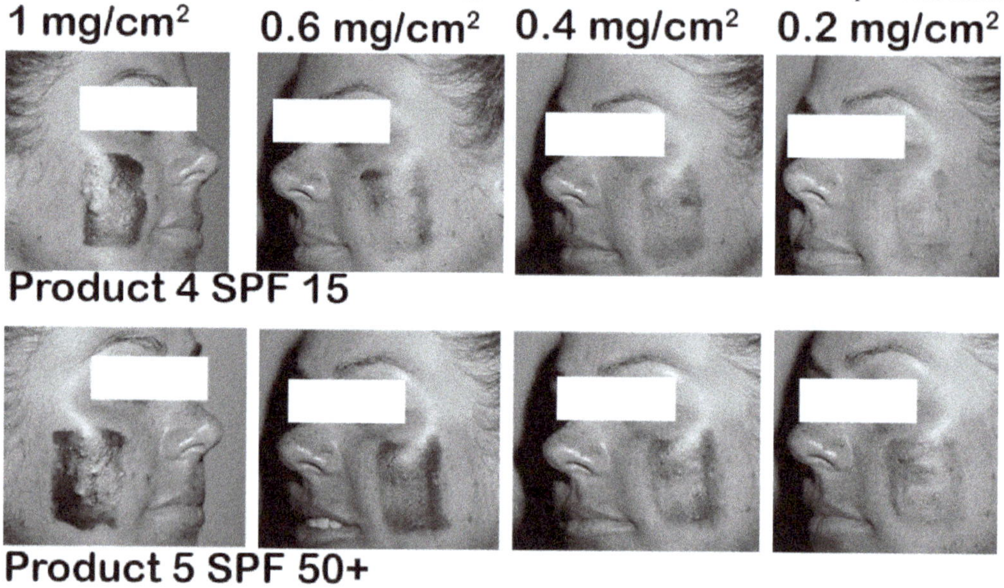

Phase 3: Development, Safety, and Field-Testing of a UV Webcam

Development

The prototype UV webcam was developed to provide personalized feedback about where improvements could be made for sunscreen application (Figure 3).

Figure 3. UV webcam device. The top panel shows the electrical components, which are housed within a plastic box (bottom left panel) and mounted on a monitor connected via a high-definition multimedia interface cable to display UV images (bottom right panel). The darker areas on the face show where sunscreen has been applied.

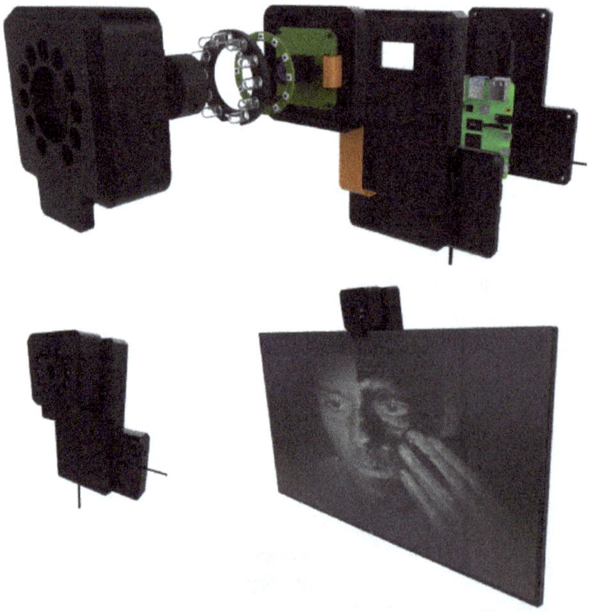

Observational Testing

The UV webcam was able to track use through a pressure-sensitive mat. Testing demonstrated perfect agreement with observed use and device-recorded use, with a κ value of 1.0, and the 95% CI range was 1.0-1.0 (Table 2).

Table 2. Agreement between observed use and UV webcam–recorded use (N=10).

Weight of person using UV webcam (kg)	UV webcam device–reported use, n (%)	
	Yes	No
90 (observed use=10)	10 (100)	0 (0)
60 (observed use=10)	10 (100)	0 (0)

Safety Testing

The prototype unit emits only UV-A irradiation and requires over 7 hours of continuous exposure to equal 15 minutes of midday sun light in Brisbane, Australia. During observational testing and field-testing, no eye or skin irritation was reported or observed using the UV webcam. The temperature of the UV webcam device after 2 and 4 hours of continuous operation was 37.1°C and 37.7°C, respectively.

Field-Testing

The UV webcam recorded data each day and was used 233 times during deployment at the beach location (Figure S6 in Multimedia Appendix 1). The UV radiation exposure level was consistently high, requiring sun protection each day during the field-testing, with daily SEDs ranging from 56 SEDs to 70 SEDs (Table S3 and Figure S7 in Multimedia Appendix 1). The UV index level was above 3 for over 5 hours each day during the field-testing, and no daytime rainfall was recorded (Table S3 in Multimedia Appendix 1). The average daily maximum temperature was 27.6°C (range 18.9-30) during field-testing (Table S3 in Multimedia Appendix 1).

No complaints, adverse events, or concerns were logged from users during the 7 days when the UV webcam was deployed. The UV webcam had sufficient power to function via a USB connection, and the display monitor required a 240-volt power supply.

Discussion

Principal Findings

Our study investigated the use of UV photography as a sun safety educational approach. A total of 3 UV camera systems were tested, and all devices identified the application of a range of SPF 15 to 50+ chemical sunscreens, moisturizers, and cosmetics. The sensitivity of the UV camera devices was shown to be adequate, with SPF-containing products applied at concentrations of 2 and 1 mg/cm^2 clearly visible and SPF-containing products applied at a concentration of 0.4 mg/cm^2 having lower levels of coverage. This study showed that participants were engaged with the personalized feedback approach of UV photography and that a UV webcam connected to a large monitor was used by beachgoers. However, we found that 3 out of the 5 tinted SPF products were not visible using UV photography because of the varying quantities of titanium dioxide and zinc oxides, which limit the sensitivity of UV photography. We recommend the use of UV photography for translucent sun protection lotions, including chemical sunscreens and moisturizers, and found that UV photography is less reliable for tinted products.

Sunscreens and SPF-containing moisturizers or cosmetics are commonly used for sun protection. In Australia, a cohort study of over 40,000 respondents reported that 40% regularly used sunscreen or cosmetics with SPF on their faces [16]. Young adults in a holiday beach setting reported high rates of daily sunscreen use (166/188, 88.3%), and most participants who reported being sunburnt also reported applying sunscreen [17]. Further data also suggest that both adults and children apply far less sunscreen than recommended, resulting in less protection [18,19]. The effectiveness of SPF-containing lotions depends on the application thickness, covering all sun-exposed skin, and regular reapplication [20]. In phase 2, we found that the SPF products had less coverage on the face by the afternoon compared with the morning photo session several hours earlier. Here, we showed that UV photography is a practical, well-liked method to visualize the need for sunscreen reapplication, with most participants indicating that they would use the technology again in the future. An estimated 7220 melanoma cases are attributed to sun exposure in Australia each year, and the effective use of sunscreen could reduce this burden, with health interventions using UV photography offering substantial opportunity for improvement [21].

Strategies to improve sunscreen application are important, as the belief that the whole face or body is protected following an application may increase UV exposure [22]. Previous research using UV photography has found that individuals do not apply sunscreen uniformly across the whole body [18]. A total of 52 participants were asked to apply sunscreen on their whole body, and researchers found that sunscreen application on the front side of the body was better than the back, and females covered their skin better than males [18]. UV photography may assist sunscreen application by providing personalized feedback on missed areas as well as revealing when reapplication is required.

We developed a UV webcam device and deployed it in a high UV environment and found that it was used by beachgoers during the weeklong field test. We chose a beach setting to deploy the UV webcam device because of the high rates of sunburn in these environments. In Queensland, 45% of children reported being sunburnt in the previous 12 months, and 69% of these sunburns happened during a water-based activity [8]. Future research could explore whether beachgoers improve their sunscreen application following personalized feedback from the UV webcam and explore the effect this technology may have on reducing sunburn. Previous research has shown that the benefits of ecological momentary health interventions, which influence behaviors within an environmental context, can improve willingness to change behavior [23].

In addition to visualizing sunscreen coverage, UV photographic imaging has also been shown to be a beneficial tool for assessing skin damage and promoting behavioral change by highlighting the negative effects of the sun on an individual's appearance in sun bed users [24] and young adults [25,26]. To further engage the public, recent strategies by Cancer Council Western Australia have included UV camera imagery to raise awareness of sun damage [27]. UV photography is a valuable public health promotional tool, and it is also a convenient method for use in a research setting. Other methodologies to assess sunscreen application include tape stripping, swabbing of body sites, and laboratory processing of samples using fluorescence spectroscopy, which can be laborious and time-consuming.

A limitation of UV photography imaging is the use of SPF lotions containing physical blockers such as titanium dioxide or zinc oxide, which are not detected. Several tinted foundations use titanium dioxide as an ingredient but have additional chemical filters to reach the stated SPF rating; however, these combination cosmetic products did not perform well in testing, with 3 out of 5 products not being detected by UV photography. Limitations of this study include selection bias, as participants in the observational study were recruited using a convenience sample, and we did not use a random sampling method. Phase 1 and 2 participants were mainly female and therefore may not represent the general population. In phase 2, under the study conditions, participants might have been more cautious than real life and applied SPF lotions more carefully. In phase 3, we did not capture self-reported sunburns or behavioral changes from participants.

Conclusions

Reducing the number of Australians sunburnt each year forms a crucial part of sun safety initiatives, and improving the messaging on the quantity of sunscreen to apply to achieve sufficient coverage as well as commonly missed areas is essential. In this study, we tested a variety of UV cameras and found that UV photography could identify the application of SPF-containing chemical filter sunscreens and moisturizers as well as determine unprotected areas. We found that the participants were engaged with personalized UV photography feedback.

Acknowledgments

The authors would like to thank all the participants for their time. UV radiation measurements were provided by the Australian Radiation Protection and Nuclear Safety Agency UV network, and sunscreen was donated by Danger Sun Overhead during the field-testing phase. This study was funded by the Queensland Government Advance Queensland fund. The sponsors of the study had no role in the study design, collection, analysis, and interpretation of data; in the writing of this manuscript; and in the decision to submit the paper for publication. The corresponding author had full access to all data in the study and the final responsibility for the decision to submit for publication.

Authors' Contributions

EH contributed to conceptualization; funding acquisition; investigation; methodology; project administration; resources; data curation; formal analysis; supervision; visualization; and writing, reviewing, and editing the manuscript. CH contributed to project administration; investigation; formal analysis; and writing, reviewing, and editing the manuscript. HF contributed to the project administration, investigation, and review and editing of the manuscript. SW, JH, and AW contributed to the methodology, investigation, and review and editing of the manuscript.

References

1. Richer V, Kharazmi P, Lee TK, Kalia S, Lui H. Quantifying the visual appearance of sunscreens applied to the skin using indirect computer image colorimetry. Photodermatol Photoimmunol Photomed 2018 Mar;34(2):130-136. [doi: 10.1111/phpp.12361] [Medline: 29080360]
2. Pratt H, Hassanin K, Troughton LD, Czanner G, Zheng Y, McCormick AG, et al. UV imaging reveals facial areas that are prone to skin cancer are disproportionately missed during sunscreen application. PLoS One 2017;12(10):e0185297 [FREE Full text] [doi: 10.1371/journal.pone.0185297] [Medline: 28968413]
3. Martincorena I, Roshan A, Gerstung M, Ellis P, Van LP, McLaren S, et al. Tumor evolution. High burden and pervasive positive selection of somatic mutations in normal human skin. Science 2015 May 22;348(6237):880-886 [FREE Full text] [doi: 10.1126/science.aaa6806] [Medline: 25999502]
4. Baxter JM, Patel AN, Varma S. Facial basal cell carcinoma. Br Med J 2012 Aug 21;345:e5342. [doi: 10.1136/bmj.e5342] [Medline: 22915688]
5. Skin cancer in Australia. Australian Institute of Health and Welfare (AIHW). 2016. URL: https://www.aihw.gov.au/reports/cancer/skin-cancer-in-australia/ [accessed 2019-04-09]
6. Fransen M, Karahalios A, Sharma N, English DR, Giles GG, Sinclair RD. Non-melanoma skin cancer in Australia. Med J Aust 2012 Nov 19;197(10):565-568. [doi: 10.5694/mja12.10654] [Medline: 23163687]
7. Elliott TM, Whiteman DC, Olsen CM, Gordon LG. Estimated healthcare costs of melanoma in Australia over 3 years post-diagnosis. Appl Health Econ Health Policy 2017 Dec;15(6):805-816. [doi: 10.1007/s40258-017-0341-y] [Medline: 28756584]

8. The health of Queenslanders 2020. Report of the Chief Health Officer, Queensland. 2020. URL: https://www.health.qld.gov.au/__data/assets/pdf_file/0019/1011286/cho-report-2020-full.pdf [accessed 2020-12-15]
9. Green AC, Williams GM, Logan V, Strutton GM. Reduced melanoma after regular sunscreen use: randomized trial follow-up. J Clin Oncol 2011 Jan 20;29(3):257-263. [doi: 10.1200/JCO.2010.28.7078] [Medline: 21135266]
10. van der Pols JC, Williams GM, Pandeya N, Logan V, Green AC. Prolonged prevention of squamous cell carcinoma of the skin by regular sunscreen use. Cancer Epidemiol Biomarkers Prev 2006 Dec;15(12):2546-2548 [FREE Full text] [doi: 10.1158/1055-9965.EPI-06-0352] [Medline: 17132769]
11. Hacker E, Boyce Z, Kimlin MG, Wockner L, Pollak T, Vaartjes SA, et al. The effect of MC1R variants and sunscreen on the response of human melanocytes in vivo to ultraviolet radiation and implications for melanoma. Pigment Cell Melanoma Res 2013 Nov;26(6):835-844. [doi: 10.1111/pcmr.12157] [Medline: 23962207]
12. Wang SQ, Virmani P, Lim HW. Consumer acceptability and compliance: the next frontier in sunscreen innovation. Photodermatol Photoimmunol Photomed 2016 Jan;32(1):55-56. [doi: 10.1111/phpp.12211] [Medline: 26409211]
13. Dussert AS, Gooris E, Hemmerle J. Characterization of the mineral content of a physical sunscreen emulsion and its distribution onto human stratum corneum. Int J Cosmet Sci 1997 Jun;19(3):119-129. [doi: 10.1046/j.1467-2494.1997.171707.x] [Medline: 18507639]
14. Schneider CA, Rasband WS, Eliceiri KW. NIH Image to ImageJ: 25 years of image analysis. Nat Methods 2012 Jul;9(7):671-675 [FREE Full text] [doi: 10.1038/nmeth.2089] [Medline: 22930834]
15. Lancaster GA, Dodd S, Williamson PR. Design and analysis of pilot studies: recommendations for good practice. J Eval Clin Pract 2004 May;10(2):307-312. [doi: 10.1111/j.2002.384.doc.x] [Medline: 15189396]
16. Olsen CM, Thompson BS, Green AC, Neale RE, Whiteman DC, QSkin SunHealth Study Group. Sun protection and skin examination practices in a setting of high ambient solar radiation: a population-based cohort study. JAMA Dermatol 2015 Sep;151(9):982-990. [doi: 10.1001/jamadermatol.2015.0739] [Medline: 26039788]
17. Horsham C, Antrobus J, Olsen CM, Ford H, Abernethy D, Hacker E. Testing wearable UV sensors to improve sun protection in young adults at an outdoor festival: field study. JMIR Mhealth Uhealth 2020 Sep 16;8(9):e21243 [FREE Full text] [doi: 10.2196/21243] [Medline: 32936083]
18. Jovanovic Z, Schornstein T, Sutor A, Neufang G, Hagens R. Conventional sunscreen application does not lead to sufficient body coverage. Int J Cosmet Sci 2017 Oct;39(5):550-555. [doi: 10.1111/ics.12413] [Medline: 28699163]
19. Diaz A, Neale RE, Kimlin MG, Jones L, Janda M. The children and sunscreen study: a crossover trial investigating children's sunscreen application thickness and the influence of age and dispenser type. Arch Dermatol 2012 May;148(5):606-612. [doi: 10.1001/archdermatol.2011.2586] [Medline: 22250190]
20. Olsen CM, Wilson LF, Green AC, Biswas N, Loyalka J, Whiteman DC. Prevention of DNA damage in human skin by topical sunscreens. Photodermatol Photoimmunol Photomed 2017 May;33(3):135-142. [doi: 10.1111/phpp.12298] [Medline: 28165636]
21. Olsen CM, Wilson LF, Green AC, Bain CJ, Fritschi L, Neale RE, et al. Cancers in Australia attributable to exposure to solar ultraviolet radiation and prevented by regular sunscreen use. Aust N Z J Public Health 2015 Oct;39(5):471-476 [FREE Full text] [doi: 10.1111/1753-6405.12470] [Medline: 26437734]
22. O'Hara M, Horsham C, Koh U, Janda M. Unintended sunburn after sunscreen application: an exploratory study of sun protection. Health Promot J Austr 2019 Oct 20:533-539. [doi: 10.1002/hpja.301] [Medline: 31631453]
23. Heron KE, Smyth JM. Ecological momentary interventions: incorporating mobile technology into psychosocial and health behaviour treatments. Br J Health Psychol 2010 Feb;15(Pt 1):1-39 [FREE Full text] [doi: 10.1348/135910709X466063] [Medline: 19646331]
24. Gibbons FX, Gerrard M, Lane DJ, Mahler HI, Kulik JA. Using UV photography to reduce use of tanning booths: a test of cognitive mediation. Health Psychol 2005 Jul;24(4):358-363. [doi: 10.1037/0278-6133.24.4.358] [Medline: 16045371]
25. Mahler HI, Kulik JA, Gerrard M, Gibbons FX. Effects of photoaging information and UV photo on sun protection intentions and behaviours: a cross-regional comparison. Psychol Health 2013;28(9):1009-1031. [doi: 10.1080/08870446.2013.777966] [Medline: 23537173]
26. Mahler HI, Kulik JA, Harrell J, Correa A, Gibbons FX, Gerrard M. Effects of UV photographs, photoaging information, and use of sunless tanning lotion on sun protection behaviors. Arch Dermatol 2005 Mar;141(3):373-380. [doi: 10.1001/archderm.141.3.373] [Medline: 15781679]
27. Don't let the sun see your DNA!. Cancer Council Western Australia. 2019. URL: https://www.cancerwa.asn.au/articles/news-2019/dont-let-the-sun-see-your-dna/ [accessed 2020-12-15]

Abbreviations

BB: beauty balm
dpi: dots per inch
DSLR: digital single-lens reflex
SED: standard erythemal dose
SPF: sun protection factor

17

Assessment of Patient Satisfaction with Dermatology Clinics According to Clinic Type: Mixed Methods Study

Jennifer Costigan[1*], MSHI; Sue S Feldman[1*], PhD, MEd, RN; Mark Lemak[2*], MHSA

[1]Department of Health Services Research, School of Health Professions, University of Alabama at Birmingham, Birmingham, AL, United States
[2]University of Alabama at Birmingham Health System, Birmingham, AL, United States
[*]all authors contributed equally

Corresponding Author:
Sue S Feldman, PhD, MEd, RN
Department of Health Services Research
School of Health Professions
University of Alabama at Birmingham
1716 9th Avenue South
SHPB #590K
Birmingham, AL, 35294
United States

Email: suefeldman1009@gmail.com

Abstract

Background: Consumer Assessment of Healthcare Providers and Systems (CAHPS) survey responses are considered significant indicators of the quality of care and patient satisfaction. There is a pressing need to improve patient satisfaction rates as CAHPS survey responses are considered when determining the amount a facility will be reimbursed by the Centers of Medicare and Medicaid each year. Low overall CAHPS scores for an academic medical center's dermatology clinics were anecdotally attributed to clinic type. However, it was unclear whether clinic type was contributing to the low scores or whether there were other factors.

Objective: This study aimed to determine where the efforts of patient satisfaction improvement should be focused for two different types of dermatology clinics (private and rapid access clinics).

Methods: This study used a concurrent mixed methods design. Secondary data derived from the University of Alabama at Birmingham Hospital's Press Ganey website were analyzed for clinic type comparisons and unstructured data were qualitatively analyzed to further enrich the quantitative findings. The University of Alabama at Birmingham Hospital is an academic medical center. The data were analyzed to determine the contributors responsible for each clinic not meeting national benchmarks. Thereafter, a review of these contributing factors was further performed to assess the difference in CAHPS scores between the private and rapid access clinics to determine if clinic type was a contributing factor to the overall scores.

Results: The data sample included 821 responses from May 2017 to May 2018. Overall, when both private clinics and rapid access clinics were viewed collectively, majority of the patients reported stewardship of patient resources as the most poorly rated factor (367/549, 66.8%) and physician communication quality as the most positively rated factor (581/638, 91.0%). However, when private clinics and rapid access clinics were viewed individually, rapid access clinics contributed slightly to the overall lower dermatology scores at the academic medical center.

Conclusions: This study determined that different factors were responsible for lower CAHPS scores for the two different dermatology clinics. Some of the contributing factors were associated with the mission of the clinic. It was suspected that the mission had not been properly communicated to patients, leading to misaligned expectations of care at each clinic.

KEYWORDS

Consumer Assessment of Healthcare Providers and Systems survey scores; patient satisfaction; dermatology; private dermatology clinic; rapid access dermatology clinic; wait time; patient resource stewardship; communication

Introduction

Background

Consumer Assessment of Healthcare Providers and Systems (CAHPS) survey responses are considered significant indicators of the quality of care and patient satisfaction. These scores are derived from a series of standardized patient surveys used to assess patients' experiences and satisfaction with health care in the United States. These surveys include quality measures that patients are most qualified to assess, such as aspects related to communication and interaction with medical staff [1,2].

There is a pressing need to improve patient satisfaction rates as CAHPS scores are considered when determining the amount a facility will be reimbursed by the Centers for Medicare and Medicaid each year [2]. Thus, focusing on improving patient satisfaction can, in turn, help to improve the quality of care and patient outcomes, which are both primary initiatives in health care today.

The overall CAHPS scores for the dermatology clinics of a particular academic medical center (AMC; University of Alabama at Birmingham Hospital) have been unsatisfactory for various measures over the past several years. Anecdotally, the private clinic personnel suspected that the rapid access clinics were contributing to the overall low scores. Private clinics are set up such that patients make appointments in advance with the dermatologist of their choosing. In this environment, they can see the same dermatologist for every appointment. On the other hand, rapid access clinics are set up such that patients can get walk-in or "just-in-time" appointments with the dermatologist or dermatology nurse practitioner on duty. There is some crossover in dermatology clinicians; however, there is no guarantee that the patient can see the clinician of choice in the rapid access clinic environment. Additionally, the rapid access clinics involve a rapid approach. Patients are seen for situational care rather than routine care. For example, ideally, an annual dermatology examination would be scheduled in a private clinic where there is more time per appointment, whereas a newly occurring rash would be seen in a rapid access clinic where there is less time per appointment. This scheduling in the rapid access clinic environment is adopted to accommodate more patients. Assessment of the ambulatory CAHPS scores at a granular level was conducted to identify patterns and specific areas of measure between the two different types of dermatology clinics (private and rapid access) that are impacting the overall CAHPS scores. The overarching question being answered was as follows: Where should the efforts of patient satisfaction improvements be focused in the two different types of dermatology clinics?

CAHPS Survey as a Measure of Patient Experience

CAHPS survey data have been utilized and referenced as direct patient care quality indicators for health care organizations across the United States [1]. The push to move toward a pay-for-performance model and quality-driven health care in the United States has influenced the emergence of such measuring tools and initiatives [3]. According to the Agency for Healthcare Research and Quality, the creator of the CAHPS program, the CAHPS survey is an initiative that was designed to "support investigator-led research to better understand patient experience with health care and develop scientifically valid and feasible strategies and tools to assess patient experience, report survey results, and help organizations use the results to improve the quality of care" [1].

The results of CAHPS measures can effectively bring attention to the shortfalls of health care providers and emphasize the need for improvements in their delivery of quality care. However, there appears to be a gap between understanding the collected data and being able to use and interpret the data to create actionable goals and improvement initiatives [4]. The availability of such data is only valuable if it can be translated and applied to create relevant solutions and to optimize the impact such solutions would have on quality care outcomes for an organization. Thus, determining which care factors and initiatives correlate directly with outcome measures, such as those obtained from CAHPS surveys, remains a challenge in health care today.

Relationship of Data Analysis and Patient Care

Aside from existing challenges, research studies infer that data collection and analysis efforts of patient care and quality measures are highly useful for identifying shortcomings in the delivery of patient care and indicating the importance of continually measuring care plans [5,6]. According to one source, a key element that strengthens patient satisfaction and confidence in clinical care is viewing quality improvement as a constant, iterative, and transparent process [7]. There is also evidence indicating that the publication of care performance data influences quality improvement initiatives to be adopted by hospitals [8]. As such, the awareness of scores being accessible to the public can encourage organizations to be more conscious of their results [8].

Additionally, satisfaction scores are highly useful to identify opportunities for improvement in aspects of patient care. Furthermore, the literature suggests that patient satisfaction should be consistently evaluated and used to assess specific interventions and improvement areas within care practices [5]. For example, in research associated with a Healthcare Information and Management System Society study (HIMSS), measurement of patient satisfaction revealed that providers' perception of their own performance does not always accurately align with patient reality, as approximately 72% of patients responded being extremely or very satisfied with their overall care experience as compared with only 39.7% of providers believing they were extremely or very effective (N=309 and N=204, respectively) [9], suggesting that anecdotal reports may not accurately reflect actual patient satisfaction. This supports the purpose and relevance of the analysis of the dermatology clinics' CAHPS scores. The information contained in patient feedback and surveys can outline the areas in need of improvement and, based on what those areas are, indicate what type of recommendations need to be pursued. The objective of this study was to analyze the ambulatory CAHPS scores at a granular level in order to identify patterns and specific areas of measure in the two different types of dermatology clinics (private and rapid access clinics), which are impacting the overall CAHPS scores.

Methods

Study Design

This study had a concurrent mixed methods design, where the findings from a qualitative analysis were used to enrich the findings from a quantitative analysis. Deidentified secondary data derived from the University of Alabama at Birmingham Hospital's Press Ganey website were analyzed for clinic type comparisons. The data were analyzed to determine the contributors responsible for each clinic not meeting national patient satisfaction benchmarks. Thereafter, these contributing factors were further analyzed to determine the difference in CAHPS scores between the private and rapid access clinics to determine if clinic type was a contributing factor to the overall scores.

Based on the most recent survey template provided, these surveys consist of over 60 different standardized CAHPS questions within 10 different domains, 13 additional nonstandard questions, and a section for additional patient comments that assess patient care experience and satisfaction with their visits to the clinics. The scope of this study required filtering of the dataset by dermatology. In order to separate the private clinics and rapid access clinics from the larger dataset, a holistic week-long schedule was assessed, and it outlined the times of operation and staffing for the dermatology clinics and provided the necessary information for comparison of the survey data by clinic type, which was conducted further in the analysis.

The data sample included 821 responses from May 24, 2017 through May 24, 2018. All data were analyzed using Microsoft Excel (Microsoft Corporation, Redmond, Washington, USA) and Tableau (Salesforce, Mountain View, California, USA) for visualization. This study was conducted at the University of Alabama at Birmingham Hospital (approval number: #300003087).

Analysis of the data was performed in three rounds. Round I (quantitative) identified which CAHPS measures and criteria consistently scored the lowest across all clinics and appeared as the greatest contributors to the department's annual CAHPS scores. This round also tried to determine whether the rapid access clinics scores alone were the sole reason why the dermatology scores were low. Round II (quantitative) examined differences between the private and rapid access clinics. Round III (qualitative) took a more granular approach to further investigate the nonstandard quality measures and unstructured patient comments. Figure 1 illustrates the research process from data collection to the integration of findings.

Figure 1. Mixed methods research design populated with results and the integration of those results. CAHPS: Consumer Assessment of Healthcare Providers and Systems.

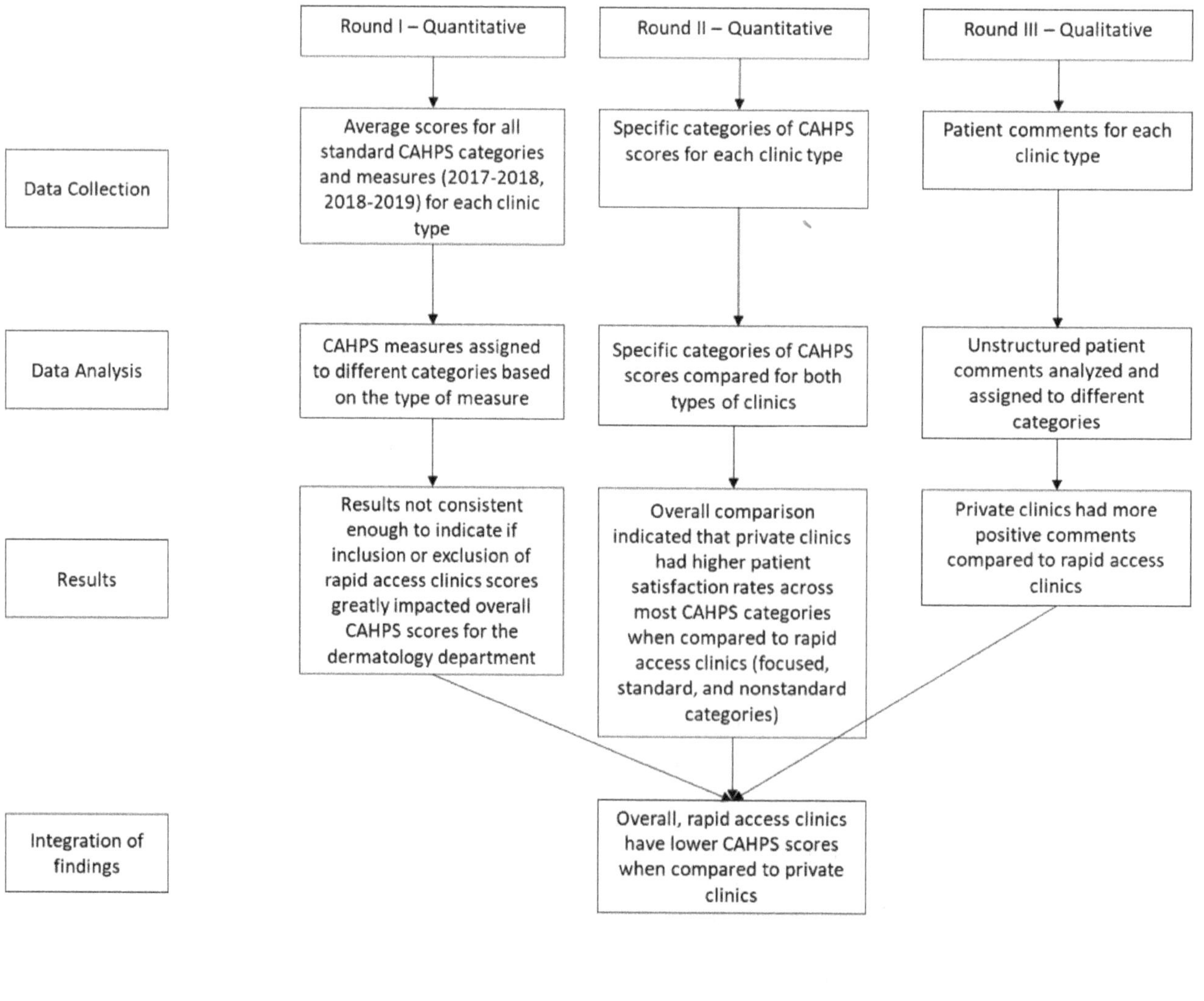

Quantitative Data Analysis

Round I: Contributors to the Annual CAHPS Score

The process for Round I of the analysis involved extracting the average scores for all standard CAHPS categories and measures for the most recent year, which included survey data of only the private clinics (2018-2019), and the prior year, which included survey data for both the rapid access and private clinics (2017-2018), for comparison.

Comparing CAHPS scores between these two years helped to show the impact of omitting rapid access survey data on dermatology clinics' ratings, which was done in 2018-2019. The measures were then ranked from best to worst based on the average values for both years to determine which categories and individual measures had the most opportunities for improvement. This data review helped to highlight the primary areas in need of attention while also providing insights on specific themes or components of care that may be generally lacking among the clinics.

The format in which the data are presented in Press Ganey-generated reports is not ideal for in-depth analysis and requires substantial restructuring. For example, each measure is separated into different sections in the comma separated value (csv) file, with individual sets of rows and columns for each response.

In order to create standard response categories across measures for a more analysis-friendly format, the different response types were grouped together based on their equivalence to another response. For example, "no" and "never" responses were combined into one response subgroup "no/never," whereas "yes, definitely," "yes," and "always" categories were compiled into the response subgroup "yes, definitely/yes/always." CAHPS questions also included "yes, somewhat/sometimes" and "usually" as responses, but for the purpose of this analysis, only the highest and lowest response categories ("no/never" and "yes, definitely/yes/always") were used for comparison. A sample of the data in restructured format is presented in Table 1.

Table 1. Restructured data from Press Ganey survey responses.

CAHPS[a] measure (2017-2018)	Category	Sample size, n	No/never, n (%)	Yes, definitely/yes/always, n (%)
Recommend this provider office	Global	776	16 (2.1)	706 (91.0)
Provider explains in a way you understand	Physician communication quality	777	14 (1.8)	724 (93.2)
Provider listens carefully to you	Physician communication quality	776	18 (2.3)	723 (93.2)
Provider talks with you about a problem/concern	Physician communication quality	775	94 (12.1)	681 (87.9)
Provider gives easy to understand instructions	Physician communication quality	681	8 (1.2)	628 (92.2)
Provider knows important information/medical history	Physician communication quality	775	32 (4.1)	647 (83.5)
Provider shows respect for what you say	Physician communication quality	775	7 (0.9)	734 (94.7)
Provider spends enough time with you	Physician communication quality	777	16 (2.1)	710 (91.4)
Clerks/receptionists are helpful	Office staff quality	776	19 (2.4)	673 (86.7)
Clerks treat you with courtesy/respect	Office staff quality	775	3 (0.4)	718 (92.6)

[a]CAHPS: Consumer Assessment of Healthcare Providers and Systems.

Round II: CAHPS Score by Clinic Type

When using Press Ganey data for an organization's specific needs, such as differentiating clinics, a process must be used to merge the data in ways other than the original intent when the survey was developed. For example, our organization's need was to compare two clinics; however, the survey, in its original form, does not allow for this type of comparison. In this section, we detail the process for readers who have interest in duplicating this or a similar study at their organization. Press Ganey does not readily distinguish clinic types. Therefore, the only way to separate data by clinic type was to cross-analyze the Press Ganey data with a physician schedule tracking sheet. The physician schedule tracking sheet facilitated identification of clinics, as well as physicians associated with certain outcomes that could not be determined solely by the CAHPS data. The clinic schedule included days of the week and times of the day (am vs pm) specific physicians work in the private and rapid access clinics, whereas the CAHPS scores in Press Ganey can be viewed by visit date/time. Using the clinic schedules for comparisons with the data available in Press Ganey, we could match the clinic type with the corresponding CAHPS data.

For example, in order to divide the datasets by clinic type, four separate reports had to be pulled from Press Ganey and complied accordingly using schedule and physician criteria included in the schedule. The first report consisted of average patient satisfaction rates for Monday, Wednesday, and Thursday, which were unfiltered to sort out the first section of private clinic data.

The second report then consisted of patient satisfaction scores for Tuesday and Friday (am appointments only). To separate the remaining data for only the private clinics, a third report was used to extract scores for Tuesday and Friday (pm appointments), which included only those providers who met patients on these specific days. Finally, the fourth report was extracted for only rapid access data, which included patient satisfaction scores for Tuesday and Friday (pm appointments only), and a filter was applied to exclude the providers of the private clinics (pm) for these specific days. This process had to be completed for each time specific data point (standard CAHPS measures, nonstandard quality measures, and patient comments) and was separated by clinic type.

Qualitative Data Analysis

Round III: Unstructured Patient Comments

A third round of analysis took a more granular approach to further investigate patient comments. The use of unstructured text comments required an additional data preparation step, in that they had to be assigned to standard groups that could allow for comparison. The preparation for these comments consisted of reviewing all patient comments for both types of dermatology clinics from 2017-2018 and categorizing them into response type themes as follows: positive, negative, indifferent, and not applicable. For example, a comment "I appreciated the receptionist helping me make my next appointment" was categorized as positive. By contrast, a comment "I waited 3 months for my appointment, only to have it cancelled by the doctor the week beforehand" was categorized as negative. The "positive" and "negative" categorized comments were then further categorized into subthemes based on aspects of care to which they were most frequently related. The subthemes included medical needs not met or questions not answered; lack of or delay with results or records; long wait or slow processing; appointment rushed or barely saw the doctor; lack of communication, direction, or follow up; medical staff rude, impersonal, or did not listen; difficult to schedule timely appointment or appointment cancelled by the doctor; check in process frustrating, receptionist unhelpful, or lack of assistance; and general or other. Thereafter, the data were processed through the same organizational approach described in Round I.

Results

Results Structure

Results are presented in the following order: demographics, contributors to CAHPS scores (Round I), results of nonstandard quality measures of CAHPS scores by clinic type (Round II), and unstructured patient data (Round III).

CAHPS Survey Respondents' Demographic Data

As shown in Table 2, just over half of the respondents were female (464/821, 56.5%), an overwhelming majority were white (650/821, 83.0%), and most were between 50 and 79 years old (589/821, 71.0%). Moreover, a vast majority had some college education (670/821, 87.2%).

Table 2. Survey respondents' demographics (N=821).

Characteristic	Value, n (%)
Gender	
Female	464 (56.5%)
Male	357 (43.5%)
Ethnicity	
White	650 (83.0%)
African American	93 (11.9%)
Asian	7 (0.9%)
Hispanic/Latino	5 (0.7%)
Hawaiian/Pacific Islander	2 (0.3%)
American Indian/Alaska Native	3(0.4%)
Other	13 (1.7%)
Age (years)	
0-17	8 (1.0%)
18-34	79 (9.6%)
35-49	86 (10.5%)
50-64	254 (30.9%)
65-79	335 (40.8%)
80 or older	59 (7.2%)
Education	
Eight grade or lower	7 (0.9%)
Some high school	12 (1.6%)
High school graduate	80 (10.4%)
Some college	195 (25.4%)
Four-year college graduate	183 (23.8%)
Greater than 4 years of college	292 (38.0%)

Quantitative Data Analysis Results

Round I: Contributors to the Annual CAHPS Score

As mentioned in the Methods, the annual CAHPS scores were first analyzed with and without the rapid access clinics included. The negative responses (no/never) are shown in Figure 2 and the positive responses (yes, definitely/yes/always) are shown in Figure 3. Both figures represent the comparison of "no/never" and "yes, definitely/yes/always" response rates overall (all weekdays) across CAHPS categories between the year with rapid access clinic scores (2017-2018) and the year without rapid access clinics scores (2018-2019). On examining Figure 2, stewardship of patient resources indicates, among other things, whether clinicians consider the needs of patients when making therapy, medication, or referral recommendations. For this variable, it was found that 66.8% (367/549) of respondents said "no/never" with the inclusion of rapid access clinics as compared with 70.9% (783/1104) of respondents without the inclusion of rapid access clinics, indicating that the data without the rapid access clinics were worse. Another example is how well providers communicate with patients, which is shown in Figure 2 as "physician communication quality," indicating how effective is provider communication with patients. For this variable, it was found that 2.1% (13/638) of respondents said "no/never" with the inclusion of rapid access clinics (meaning communication was poor) as compared with 2.2% (27/1227) of respondents without the inclusion of rapid access clinics, indicating that the data without the rapid access clinics were worse, and thus, the data were worse for private clinics.

Figure 3 shows the positive responses while using the same quality measures. With regard to stewardship of patient resources, involving whether providers consider the needs of patients, 33.2% (182/549) of respondents said "yes, definitely/yes/always" with the inclusion of rapid access clinics as compared with 29.1% (321/1104) of respondents without the inclusion of rapid access clinics, indicating that a greater percentage thought that their needs were considered in data that included the rapid access clinics. Similarly, with regard to physician communication, 91.0% (581/638) of respondents with the inclusion of rapid access clinics answered "yes, definitely/yes/always" as compared with 90.6% (1112/1227) of respondents without the inclusion of rapid access clinics.

Considering Figures 2 and 3, there does not appear to be a wide variance between most of the measures. One exception is "access to specialists." On assessing the data that included the rapid access clinics (Figure 2), 0.0% of respondents reported "no/never" access to specialists, indicating that specialists are accessible. However, on assessing the data that did not include the rapid access clinics (ie, private clinics only; Figure 2), 10.0% (122/1224) of respondents reported "no/never" access to specialists, indicating that specialists were not accessible. The variance is much wider in Figure 3, which presents the positive responses while using the same quality measures. With regard to access to specialists, Figure 3 demonstrates that 66.7% (2/3) of respondents said "yes, definitely/yes/always" with the inclusion of the rapid access clinics as compared with 20.0% (1/5) of respondents without the inclusion of the rapid access clinics, indicating that more respondents felt that there was access to specialists with inclusion of the rapid access clinics.

Figure 2. Negative responses with and without the rapid access clinics.

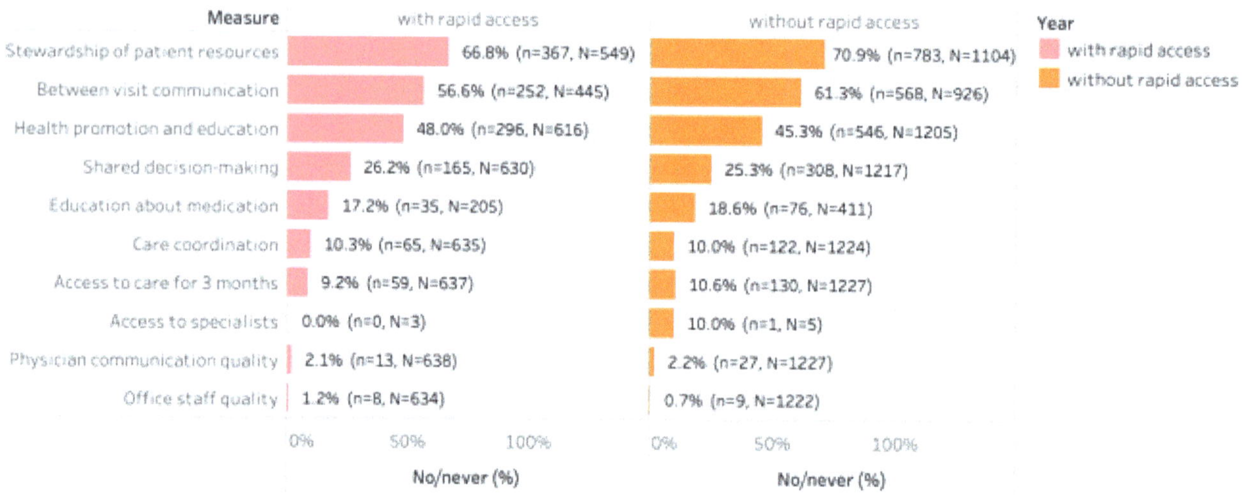

Figure 3. Positive responses with and without the rapid access clinics.

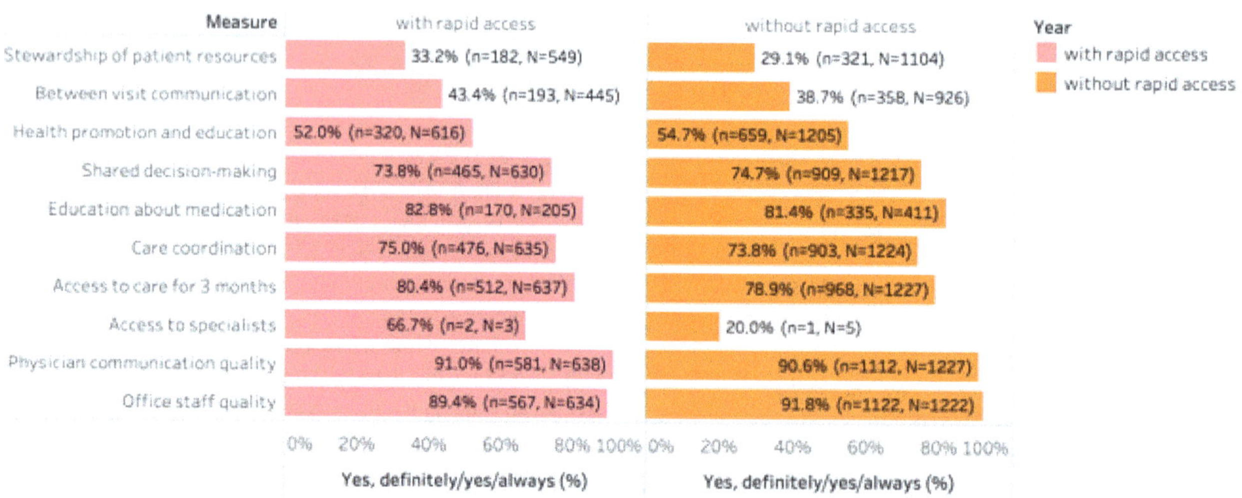

Figures 4 and 5 present comparisons of "no/never" and "yes, definitely/yes/always" response rates for Tuesday and Friday (rapid access clinic days) across CAHPS categories for the year with rapid access clinic scores (2017-2018) and the year without rapid access clinic scores (2018-2019). These results suggest the same conclusions as those involving data for all weekdays. It appears that there was also a slight increase in negative response ratings and a slight decrease in positive response ratings for several of the categories. However, in the case of both results, there were also some CAHPS categories that had an increase in the positive response average and a decrease in the negative response average. Essentially, the results are not consistent enough to indicate whether the inclusion or exclusion of rapid access clinic scores greatly impacted the dermatology clinics' CAHPS scores as a whole. However, these results consistently showed that CAHPS scores for the "stewardship of patient resources" category was higher for the negative response rate (Figure 4), indicating that in the rapid access clinics, patients reported better stewardship of patient resources. Unexpectedly, both with and without inclusion of the rapid access clinics did not receive any responses (positive or negative) for the "access to specialists" category (Figures 4 and 5). Figure 4 shows that when the rapid access clinics were included, there was better consideration for patient resources.

It was noted earlier that the rapid access clinics only operated on Tuesday and Friday afternoons. However, the data in Figure 3 considered the entire day because comparisons were performed between two separate years (one including and the other excluding rapid access clinic data). Therefore, if the data were compared between the two years by Tuesday and Friday (pm), there would have been no rapid access clinic data available according to the criteria for 2018-2019. Using the data of the entire day for the weekdays when the rapid access clinics operated allowed us to observe the impact of excluding rapid access data for those particular days and the results associated with the private clinics alone for the most current year (2018-2019).

Figure 4. Negative responses with and without the rapid access clinics on Tuesday and Friday only. N/A: not applicable.

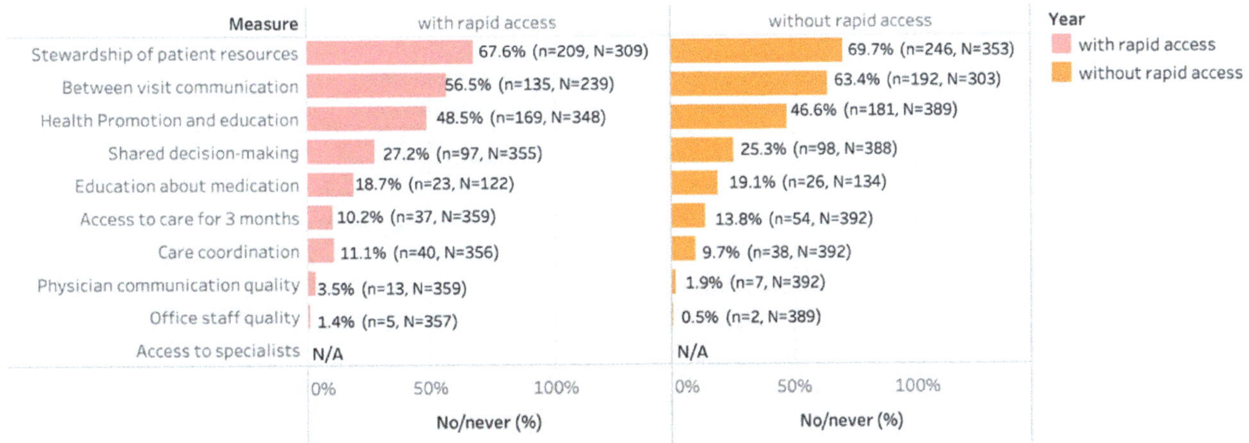

Figure 5. Positive responses with and without the rapid access clinics on Tuesday and Friday only. N/A: not applicable.

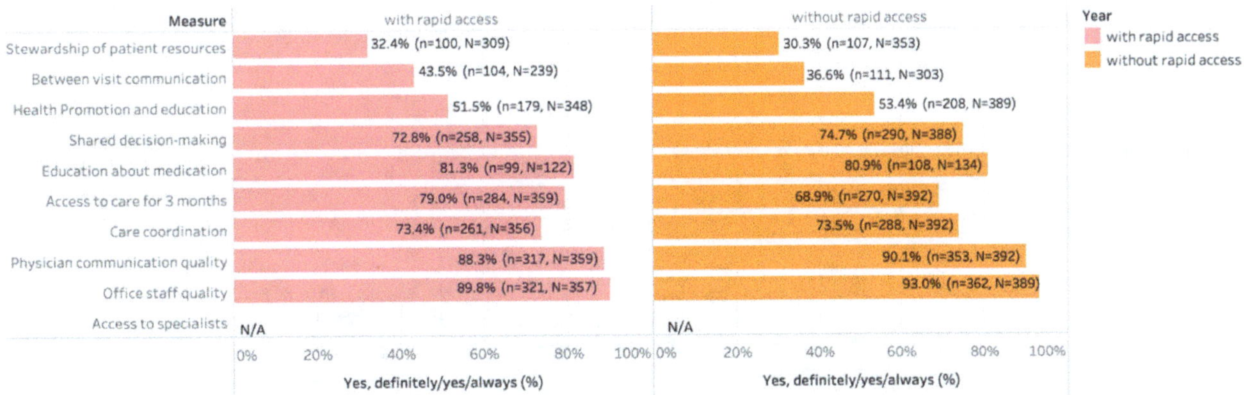

Round II: Data Review by Clinic Type

We show the results relative to how well the private clinics and rapid access clinics scored on average across all CAHPS categories in Figure 6. Thereafter, we show more granular results of the focus measures by clinic, with the results of the private clinics presented in Figure 7 and those of the rapid access clinics presented in Figure 8.

The focus measures were the measures that targeted physician communication quality, standard measures as well as additional measures based on relevance to care quality, and the potential for improvement relative to the effort for change management. All CAHPS categories were used in the first comparison, rather than selecting just those related to the focus measures, in order to conduct a general comparison of all CAHPS categories according to clinic type. In other words, Figure 6 shows the higher level CAHPS categories/domains that were measured. Each of these categories/domains had a set of related CAHPS measures. The categories/domains relevant to the focus measures chosen for analysis are indicated in Figure 6. These focus measures are further assessed in Figures 7 and 8.

The results of the overall CAHPS scores by clinic type, as depicted in Figure 6, showed that the private clinics had higher patient satisfaction rates across most CAHPS categories when compared with the rapid access clinics. When looking further at the focus measures by clinic type (Figures 7 and 8), most of the measures were higher for the private clinics as compared with the rapid access clinics, although some measures were only slightly higher.

We present the findings for focus measures in the private clinics and rapid access clinics in Figures 7 and 8, respectively. On comparing the two clinic types, the results showed that the private clinics scored higher in most areas. The rapid access clinics scored higher in "appointment for care right away," "talk with provider about prescription," "provider gives written medical instructions," and "talk with provider about problem/concern." These findings make sense when considering the nature of the rapid access clinics as a situational environment where a patient shows up with or without an appointment, has a targeted conversation with the provider about typically a singular problem or concern, gets a prescription or some other type of instruction, and leaves.

Figure 6. Consumer Assessment of Healthcare Providers and Systems survey score by clinic type. The asterisks indicate the categories/domains relevant to the focus measures chosen for analysis. N/A: not applicable.

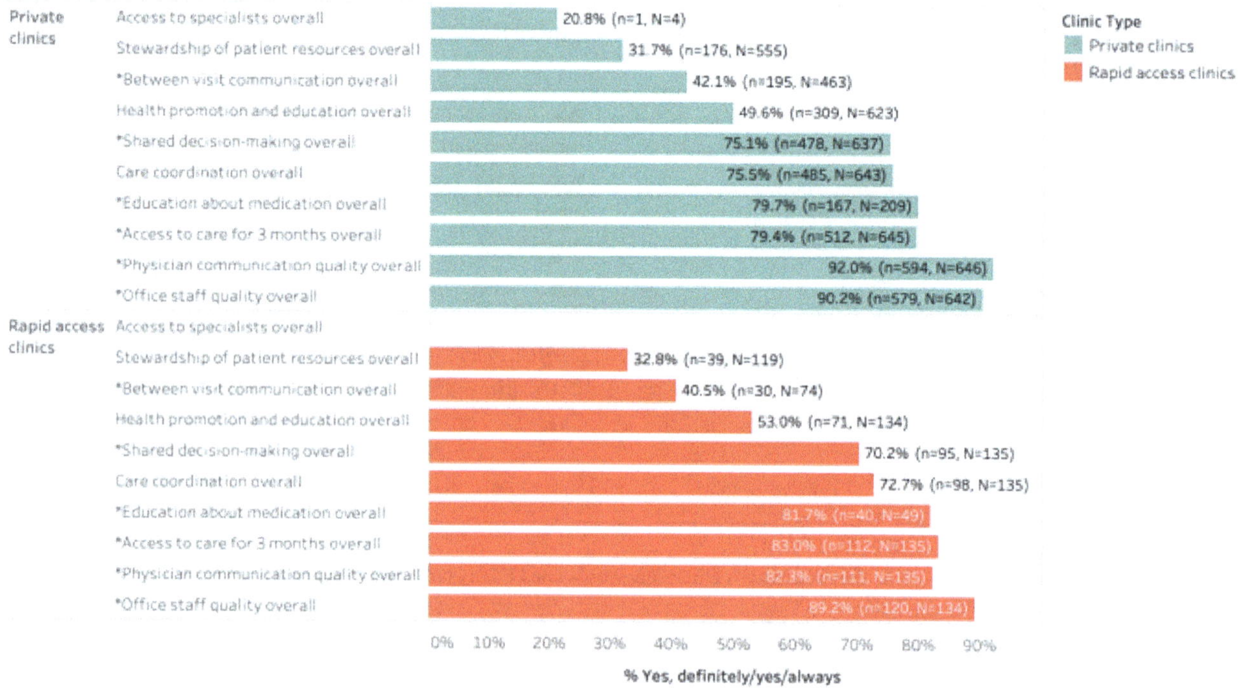

Private clinics
Access to specialists overall
20.8% (n=1, N=4)
Stewardship of patient resources overall
31.7% (n=176, N=555)
*Between visit communication overall
42.1% (n=195, N=463)
Health promotion and education overall
49.6% (n=309, N=623)
*Shared decision-making overall
75.1% (n=478, N=637)
Care coordination overall
75.5% (n=485, N=643)
*Education about medication overall
79.7% (n=167, N=209)
*Access to care for 3 months overall
79.4% (n=512, N=645)
*Physician communication quality overall
92.0% (n=594, N=646)
*Office staff quality overall
90.2% (n=579, N=642)
Rapid access clinics
Access to specialists overall
Stewardship of patient resources overall
32.8% (n=39, N=119)
*Between visit communication overall
40.5% (n=30, N=74)
Health promotion and education overall
53.0% (n=71, N=134)
*Shared decision-making overall
70.2% (n=95, N=135)
Care coordination overall
72.7% (n=98, N=135)
*Education about medication overall
81.7% (n=40, N=49)
*Access to care for 3 months overall
83.0% (n=112, N=135)
*Physician communication quality overall
82.3% (n=111, N=135)
*Office staff quality overall
89.2% (n=120, N=134)
0% 10% 20% 30% 40% 50% 60% 70% 80% 90%
% Yes, definitely/yes/always
Clinic Type
Private clinics
Rapid access clinics

Figure 7. Focus measures for the private clinics.

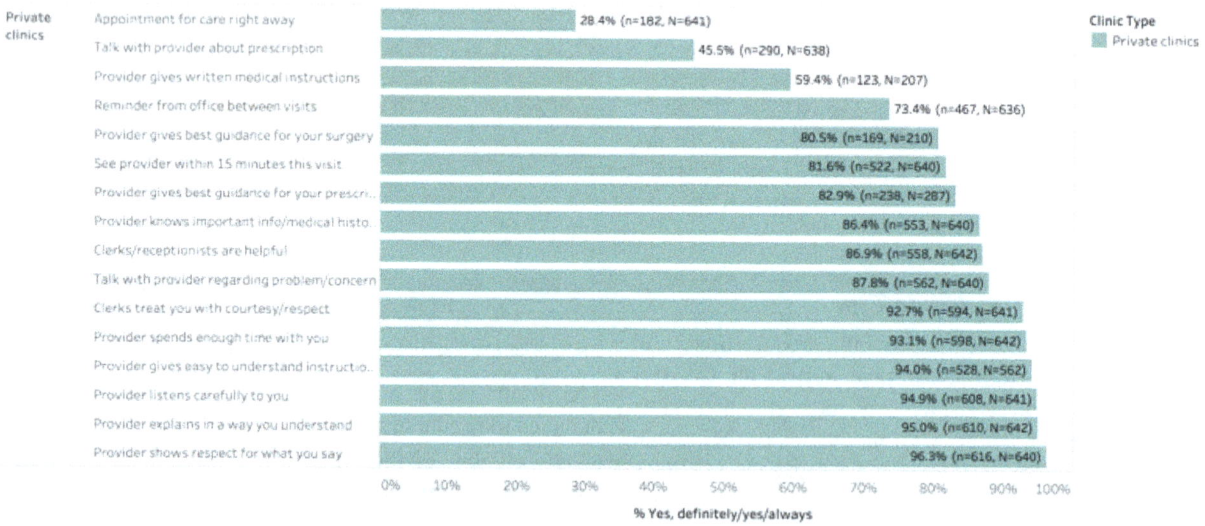

Figure 8. Focus measures for the rapid access clinics.

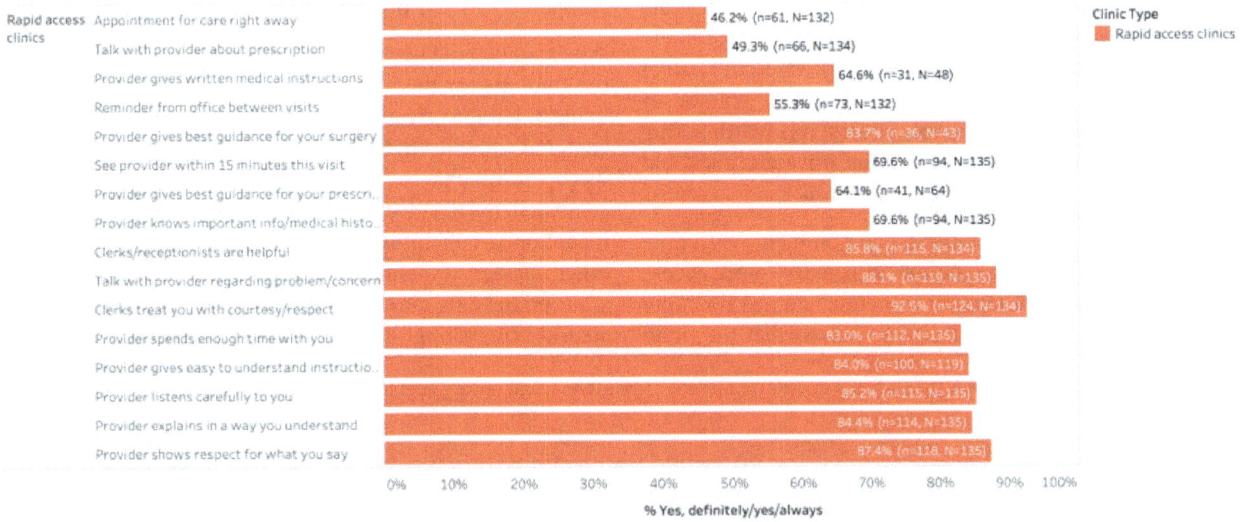

We present the findings for nonstandard focus measures by clinic type in Figure 9. The results showed that the private clinics scored higher than the rapid access clinics. The marginal difference in patient satisfaction between the two clinic types was 12%-15%. Although the primary goal was to find a pattern in patient satisfaction between the clinic types, it can be noted that there is room for improvement in both private and rapid access clinics regarding these measures.

Figure 9. Nonstandard focus measures by clinic type. Asterisks indicate the categories/domains relevant to the focus measures chosen for analysis.

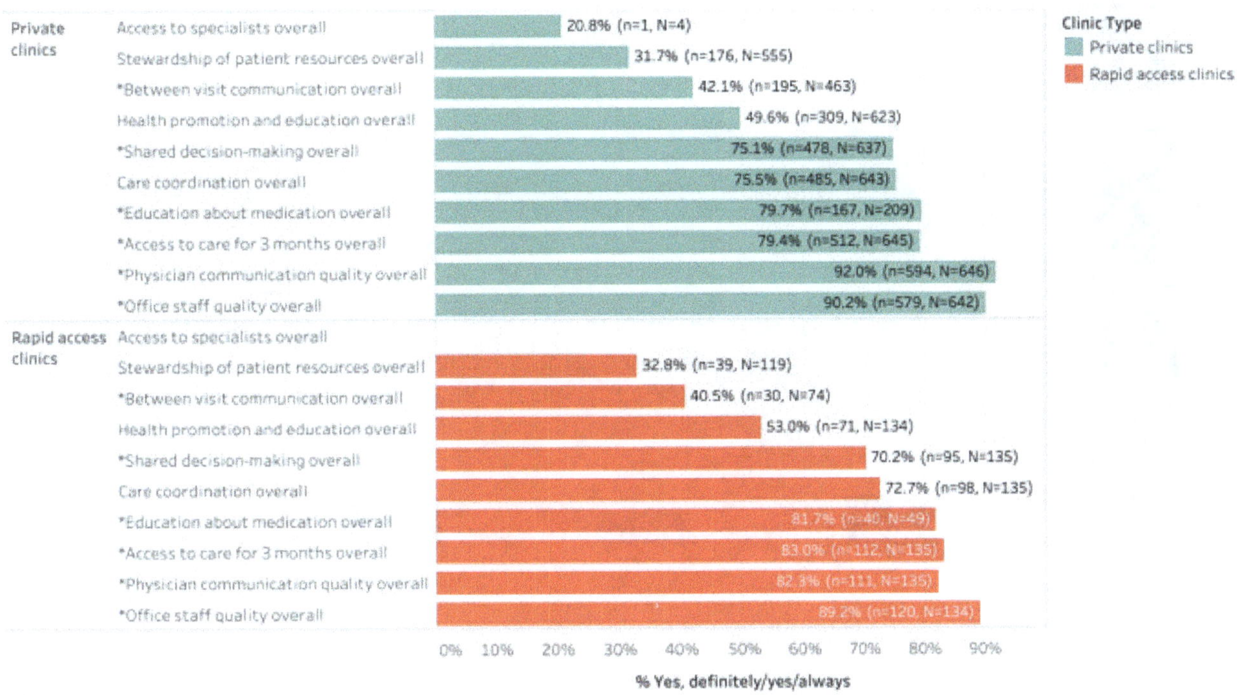

Qualitative Data Analysis Results

Round III: Nonstandard Quality Measures and Patient Comments

We obtained the results of analyzing unstructured patient comments by clinic type. As listed in the Methods, the subthemes included the following: medical needs not met or questions not answered; lack of or delay with results or records; long wait or slow processing; appointment rushed or barely saw the doctor; lack of communication, direction, or follow-up; medical staff rude, impersonal, or did not listen; difficult to schedule timely appointment or appointment cancelled by the doctor; check in process frustrating, receptionist unhelpful, or lack of assistance; and general or other.

Figure 10 shows all patient comments by clinic type. It was found that the private clinics had a much higher rate of positive comments as compared with the rapid access clinics. On breaking down the amount each clinic type contributed to the overall comments for the positive, negative, indifferent, and not applicable categories, the private clinics appeared to contribute the most to each category. However, this finding is most likely influenced by the fact that there are more private clinics that run throughout the week and therefore a greater volume of comments associated with the private clinics. It is worth noting that there were 4454 comments from the private clinics and only 830 comments from the rapid access clinics.

We also assessed the distribution of the comments by clinic type within the sample (ie, the number of negative rapid access comments out of the total number of comments [N] for rapid access only; Figure 10). This analysis showed that the rapid access clinics had a greater makeup of negative comments as compared with the private clinics.

We expanded the negative comments by clinic, and we present the findings for the private clinics and rapid access clinics in Table 3. For the private clinics, the top three negative comments centered around "medical staff rude, impersonal, or did not listen," "difficult to schedule timely appointment or appointment cancelled by the doctor," and "check in process frustrating, receptionist unhelpful, or lack of assistance." The "general or other" category included a variety of comments that did not appropriately fit into any other category (eg, singular words, such as "frustrating" and "disappointing," without any context).

Figure 10. Patient comments by clinic (distributed in positive, negative, indifferent, and not applicable categories).

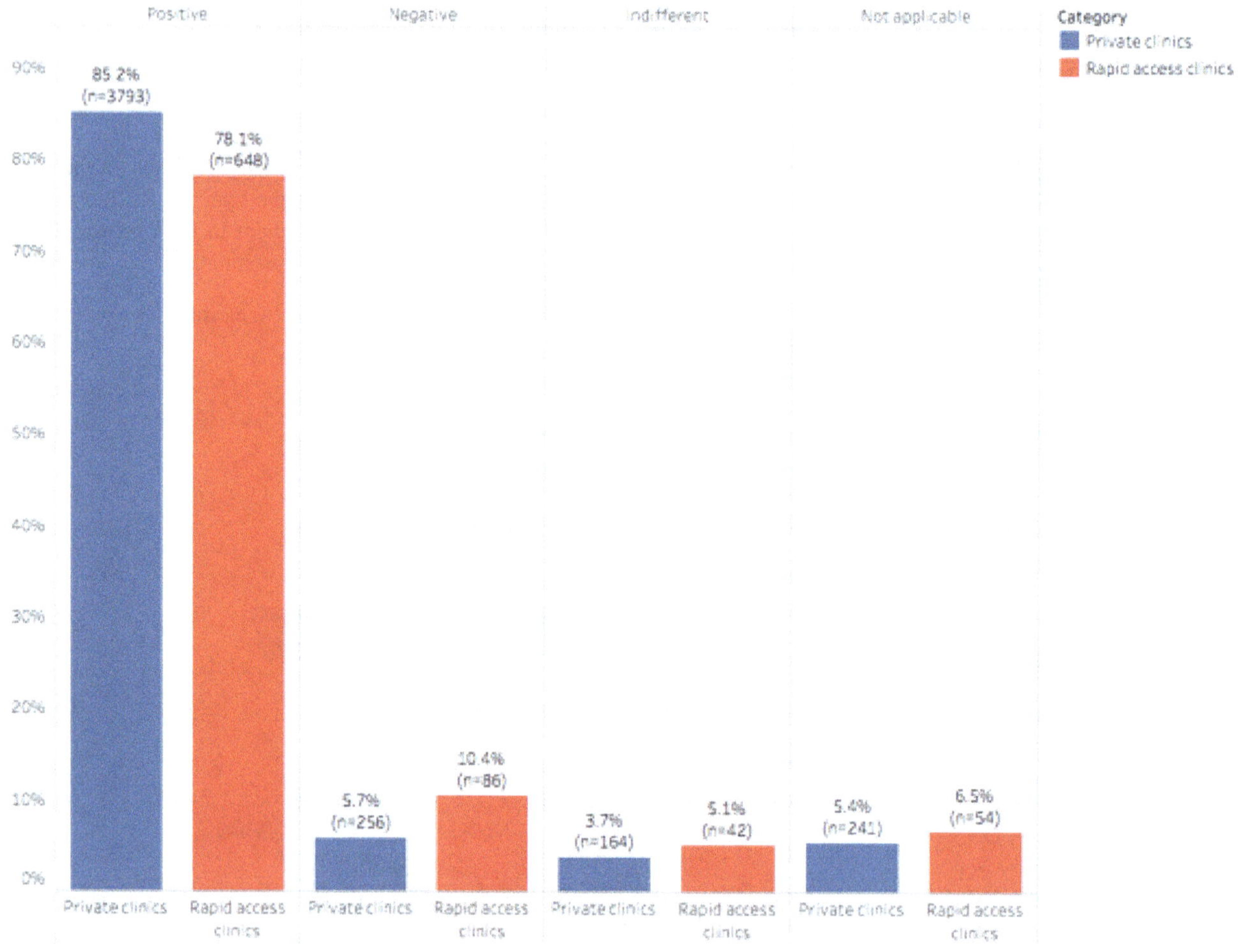

Table 3. Patient negative comments in the private clinics and rapid access clinics.

Comments	Private clinics (N=256), n (%)	Rapid access clinics (N=86), n (%)
Medical needs not met or questions not answered	13 (5.1%)	7 (8.1%)
Lack of or delay with results/records	15 (5.9%)	2 (2.3%)
Long wait or slow processing	18 (7.0%)	14 (16.3%)
Appointment rushed or barely saw the doctor	21 (8.2%)	12 (14.0%)
Lack of communication, direction, or follow-up	25 (9.8%)	11 (12.8%)
Medical staff rude, impersonal, or did not listen	28 (10.9%)	15 (17.4%)
Difficult to schedule timely appointment or appointment canceled by the doctor	32 (12.5%)	5 (5.8%)
Check in process frustrating, receptionist unhelpful, or lack of assistance	37 (14.5%)	4 (4.7%)
General or other	67 (26.2%)	16 (18.6%)

Discussion

Principal Findings

This study assessed two distinct dermatology clinics and their individual and collective contributions to CAHPS scores for the Dermatology Department at an AMC to answer the question, "Where should the efforts of patient satisfaction improvements be focused for the two different types of dermatology clinics?" This study utilized a concurrent mixed methods approach (Figure 1) to answer this question.

The clinics consisted of private clinics (patients make appointments in advance with the dermatologist of their choosing and likely see the same dermatologist with whom they have established a relationship) and rapid access clinics (patients can get walk-in or just-in-time appointments with a dermatologist or dermatology nurse practitioner on duty).

The quantitative data analysis showed that when only private clinic data were collected, there was a slight increase in the negative response rate and a slight decrease in the positive response rate across many categories, perhaps indicating that the contribution of rapid access CAHPS scores to the overall scores may be underestimated [2]. When individual clinic data were expanded, the majority of reviewed CAHPS measures had lower satisfaction for the rapid access clinics (9%-17%) as compared with the private clinics. The exception was "talk with provider about problem/concern," for which the rate was 0.34% higher in the rapid access clinics when compared with the private clinics. Although some of these differences in scores were not substantial, they were consistent enough across the CAHPS categories and measures to give a thought to the individual clinic contribution.

To elaborate further on the qualitative data analysis, the value of patient comments cannot be underestimated as they provide straightforward and insightful feedback from patients. The comments directly express dermatology patients' perceptions of their care while specifically indicating areas in need of improvement, as well as satisfactory aspects of the clinics. As such, consistent with the literature suggesting continued review of CAHPS scores, a frequent review of these comments could contribute to and increase the richness of aggregated data [5,7].

Both quantitative and qualitative data analyses were performed in this study with the goal of the qualitative data analysis findings enriching the quantitative data analysis findings. Integration of the quantitative and qualitative findings from this study suggests that the rapid access clinics contributed to low overall CAHPS scores, but the contribution was not radical. Qualitative analysis of patient comments elaborated the results of quantitative findings, showing that even when patients know they are in an environment of situational care (ie, a rapid access clinic), they want to spend more time with the clinician, want shorter wait times, and want people to listen. The consideration of these comments provided an additional, valuable, and actionable layer to complement the quantitative findings.

Regardless of the clinic, this study suggested that there is work to be done in regards to how staff or clerks interact with patients, as this aspect was scored low in both clinics. There is also work to be done around communication. Clinicians need to be especially conscientious to avoid speaking to their patients in a frustrated or condescending tone.

The difference between real and perceived wait times presents challenges for even the best clinic environment. A patient's perception relative to the wait time could be altered by providing frequent updates on the wait time so as to provide patients with a more accurate perception of the time they are actually waiting, which may be a smaller window of time as compared to what they perceive without receiving any updates [10]. Overbooking patients can lead to communication issues. If there are too many patients, the clinician may spend less time with each patient, giving the patient a sense of being rushed and not being heard.

There is also work to be done around effectively managing delays in the clinic and getting to the root cause of those delays. If found that delays are caused by patients, it would be helpful to identify patients who are frequently late or who do not show up to the clinic. These particular patients could then be flagged and scheduled in the afternoon for future appointments. Scheduling such patients later in the day would minimize the interference with the clinic schedule and overall patient flow throughout the day [10].

Our findings show that appointments are much more difficult to get in private clinics and patients need to wait a long time to get an appointment with their established provider. This is consistent with the nationwide shortage of dermatologists [11].

Limitations

This study had some limitations that need to be acknowledged. First, the data provided for this analysis by Press Ganey were already summarized, and this limited the statistical approaches that could be applied for further assessment. As such, analysis and result reporting were limited to descriptive statistics rather than more traditional statistical analysis to compare one dataset to another.

Another limitation was related to the survey design. The CAHPS survey does not have a not applicable ("N/A") response available as an option for any of the questions. Subsequently, when any of the questions do not apply to patients, which was stated in patient comments, they are forced to answer "no/never" instead, artificially increasing the negative response rate for certain measures as a result.

Additionally, inconsistent response sample sizes (N) for each of the measures likely contributed to skewed reporting. For example, not every patient completed the survey, and those who completed the survey did not always answer every question available (most likely when questions did not apply). This was verified through a review of the original survey copies that were available through Press Ganey. Several of the sample surveys reviewed were only partially filled out.

Lastly, patient comments were fewer for the rapid access clinics as compared with the private clinics. The investigation of methods to increase comments represents an area of future research for researchers.

Nevertheless, this study provides valuable findings related to the degree of the contribution of individual clinics to CAHPS scores.

Conclusion

This study suggests that clinic type is relevant to patient satisfaction. However, the results also suggest that much of the dissatisfaction could be mitigated with better communication and level-setting expectations. There are gaps in research concerning the relationship between CAHPS scores and specific care factors. The findings and the common patterns between patient satisfaction measures and care components that were discovered through the execution of this analysis provide valuable insights into the drivers of patient satisfaction for not only the AMC's dermatology clinics going forward, but also ambulatory facilities in general.

Future research in this area could investigate physician performance relative to clinic type. Additionally, patient satisfaction by time of the day according to clinic type may provide useful insights into patient satisfaction.

Acknowledgments

The authors would like to thank everyone in the Department of Radiology Oncology and Dermatology at the University of Alabama at Birmingham Health System, who helped to guide the focus of this study. The authors would like to deeply thank Shikha Modi, MBA, PhD candidate, for her tireless formatting of this manuscript to prepare it for publication. The authors acknowledge the detailed feedback of the reviewers, which helped make this a stronger paper.

References

1. Agency for Healthcare Research and Quality. 2018. The CAHPS Program URL: http://www.ahrq.gov/cahps/about-cahps/cahps-program/index.html [accessed 2019-10-08]
2. Centers for Medicare & Medicaid Services. 2019. Consumer Assessment of Healthcare Providers & Systems (CAHPS) URL: https://www.cms.gov/research-statistics-data-and-systems/research/cahps/ [accessed 2019-09-22]
3. Eijkenaar F. Pay for performance in health care: an international overview of initiatives. Med Care Res Rev 2012 Jun;69(3):251-276. [doi: 10.1177/1077558711432891] [Medline: 22311954]
4. Audet A, Davis K, Schoenbaum SC. Adoption of patient-centered care practices by physicians: results from a national survey. Arch Intern Med 2006 Apr 10;166(7):754-759. [doi: 10.1001/archinte.166.7.754] [Medline: 16606812]
5. Merkouris A, Athini E, Hatzimbalasi M, Rovithis M, Papastavrou E. Assessment of patient satisfaction in public hospitals in Cyprus: a descriptive study. Health Science Journal 2013;7(1).
6. Safran DG, Karp M, Coltin K, Chang H, Li A, Ogren J, et al. Measuring patients' experiences with individual primary care physicians. Results of a statewide demonstration project. J Gen Intern Med 2006 Jan;21(1):13-21 [FREE Full text] [doi: 10.1111/j.1525-1497.2005.00311.x] [Medline: 16423118]
7. Renedo A, Marston CA, Spyridonidis D, Barlow J. Patient and Public Involvement in Healthcare Quality Improvement: How organizations can help patients and professionals to collaborate. Public Management Review 2014 Feb 07;17(1):17-34. [doi: 10.1080/14719037.2014.881535]
8. Fung CH, Lim Y, Mattke S, Damberg C, Shekelle PG. Systematic review: the evidence that publishing patient care performance data improves quality of care. Ann Intern Med 2008 Jan 15;148(2):111-123. [doi: 10.7326/0003-4819-148-2-200801150-00006] [Medline: 18195336]

9. HIMSS Analytics. 2019. Patient experience study: shifting consumer demand and health system effort to address patient experience URL: https://enterprise.spectrum.com/insights/resources/reports/patient-experience-study-conducted-by-himss-analytics [accessed 2019-10-09]
10. Press Ganey Associates, Inc. Medical Practice Solutions Starter URL: https://www.premiermedicalhv.com/wp-content/uploads/2013/01/Press-Ganey-Medical-Practice-Solutions-Starter.pdf [accessed 2019-08-28]
11. Glazer AM, Rigel DS. Analysis of Trends in Geographic Distribution of US Dermatology Workforce Density. JAMA Dermatol 2017 May 01;153(5):472-473 [FREE Full text] [doi: 10.1001/jamadermatol.2016.6032] [Medline: 28296988]

Abbreviations

AMC: academic medical center
CAHPS: Consumer Assessment of Healthcare Providers and Systems

18

Trends in Hidradenitis Suppurativa Disease Severity and Quality of Life Outcome Measures

Jalal Maghfour[1*], MD; Torunn Elise Sivesind[2*], BS, MD; Robert Paul Dellavalle[2,3], MSPH, PhD, MD; Cory Dunnick[2], MD

[1]Department of Dermatology, Henry Ford Hospital, Detroit, MI, United States

[2]Department of Dermatology, University of Colorado School of Medicine, Aurora, CO, United States

[3]Dermatology Service, Rocky Mountain Regional Veterans Affairs Medical Center, Aurora, CO, United States

[*]these authors contributed equally

Corresponding Author:
Cory Dunnick, MD
Department of Dermatology
University of Colorado School of Medicine
1665 Aurora Ct
Aurora, CO, 80045
United States

Email: cory.dunnick@cuanschutz.edu

Abstract

Background: Although there has been an increase in the number of randomized controlled trials evaluating treatment efficacy for hidradenitis suppurativa (HS), instrument measurements of disease severity and quality of life (QoL) are varied, making the compilation of data and comparisons between studies a challenge for clinicians.

Objective: We aimed to perform a systematic literature search to examine the recent trends in the use of disease severity and QoL outcome instruments in randomized controlled trials that have been conducted on patients with HS.

Methods: A scoping review was conducted in February 2021. The PubMed, Embase, Web of Science, and Cochrane databases were used to identify all articles published from January 1964 to February 2021. In total, 41 articles were included in this systematic review.

Results: The HS Clinical Response (HiSCR) score (18/41, 44%) was the most commonly used instrument for disease severity, followed by the Sartorius and Modified Sartorius scales (combined: 16/41, 39%). The Dermatology Life Quality Index (18/41, 44%) and visual analogue pain scales (12/41, 29%) were the most commonly used QoL outcome instruments in HS research.

Conclusions: Randomized controlled trials conducted from 2013 onward commonly used the validated HiSCR score, while older studies were more heterogeneous and less likely to use a validated scale. A few (6/18, 33%) QoL measures were validated instruments but were not specific to HS; therefore, they may not be representative of all factors that impact patients with HS.

KEYWORDS

hidradenitis suppurativa; severity of illness index; patient-reported outcome measures; quality of life; treatment outcome; illness index; patient outcomes; disease severity; Sartorius; dermatology; treatment interventions

Introduction

Hidradenitis suppurativa (HS) is a debilitating chronic inflammatory condition that most commonly involves the axilla, inframammary, inguinal, and anogenital regions [1]. HS is characterized by inflamed nodules that generally progress to painful abscesses, sinus tracts, fibrosis, and scarring [2]. HS has been shown to be associated with the increased incidence of metabolic, autoimmune, and psychosocial comorbidities [2]. Although it has been historically difficult to ascertain the exact prevalence of the disease due to underdiagnosis and variations in the estimates among epidemiologic studies, a recent meta-analysis [3] estimated a worldwide prevalence of 0.3% (range 0.2%-0.6%).

Despite the burden of the disease, the treatment of HS is heterogeneous, and effective management has proven difficult; however, new therapies are under investigation. Randomized controlled trials (RCTs) that are investigating these new therapies have used various instruments to quantify HS disease severity and its impact on patients' quality of life (QoL).

It is well established that HS results in significant emotional, social, and psychological burdens on patients [4]. Recent studies have reported on the increased prevalence of anxiety, depression, and suicidality among patients with HS [5]. These psychological conditions are indicative of a poor QoL [6] and highlight the importance of incorporating patient-focused outcome measures in HS research. Both the US Federal Drug Administration and European Medicines Agency have recommended the evidence-based use of patient-reported outcome measures (PROMs) in clinical trials and have emphasized their importance [7]. PROMs are particularly important in chronic debilitating skin diseases, such as HS. In HS research, RCTs have reported objective and subjective outcomes via a diverse assortment of scales and questionnaires, making the compilation of data and comparisons between studies quite difficult. A previously published study identified 30 different outcome instruments in HS research [8] and found that nearly 90% of these instruments had not been validated. Given the role of clinical research in providing evidence to inform clinical decision-making, the standardization of outcome measures is crucial to enabling data comparisons between studies.

The purpose of this study was to investigate trends in disease severity scales and QoL instruments that were used in HS-related RCTs conducted between January 1964 and February 2021 via a systematic search of the literature.

Methods

A scoping review of the literature was conducted in February 2021 by using the following four databases: PubMed, Embase, Web of Science, and Cochrane. To ensure transparency and reproducibility, the literature search was conducted according to the framework established by the PRISMA (Preferred Reporting Items for Systematic Reviews and Meta-Analyses) reporting guidelines [9] and was prospectively registered with PROSPERO. The key search terms were *Hidradenitis Suppurativa*, *acne inversa*, *randomized controlled trial*, *RCT*, *quality of life*, *QoL*, *QOL*, *patient reported outcome measures*, *PROM*, *HS severity*, *severity of HS*, *Sartorius scale*, *Hurley stage*, and *severity of illness index*. Detailed search results are included in Multimedia Appendix 1.

This scoping review included published RCTs that reported disease severity, QoL, or both. Secondary articles (eg, reviews and meta-analyses), case reports and case series, cohort studies, letters to editors, commentaries, and in vivo and in vitro experimental studies were excluded. Two reviewers (JM and TS) independently screened articles to include those that met the defined inclusion criteria, were written in English, and were available as full texts. In total, 111 articles were excluded during title and abstract screening for the following reasons: (1) a non-RCT study design (eg, cohort studies, observational studies, reviews, letters), (2) insufficient data, (3) articles written in languages other than English, and (4) articles that were unavailable in a full-text format. An additional 19 studies were excluded after careful review due to the lack of reporting on disease severity and QoL outcome measures.

Results

Summary of Articles

A total of 171 nonduplicated reports were identified; 60 articles underwent a full-text review, and a total of 41 studies [10-50] were included in this review (Figure 1). For each included RCT, the level of evidence was rated according to the evidence levels established by the Oxford Centre for Evidence-Based Medicine [51].

Figure 1. The search process is depicted by using a flow diagram that was adapted from the PRISMA (Preferred Reporting Items for Systematic Reviews and Meta-Analyses) guidelines.

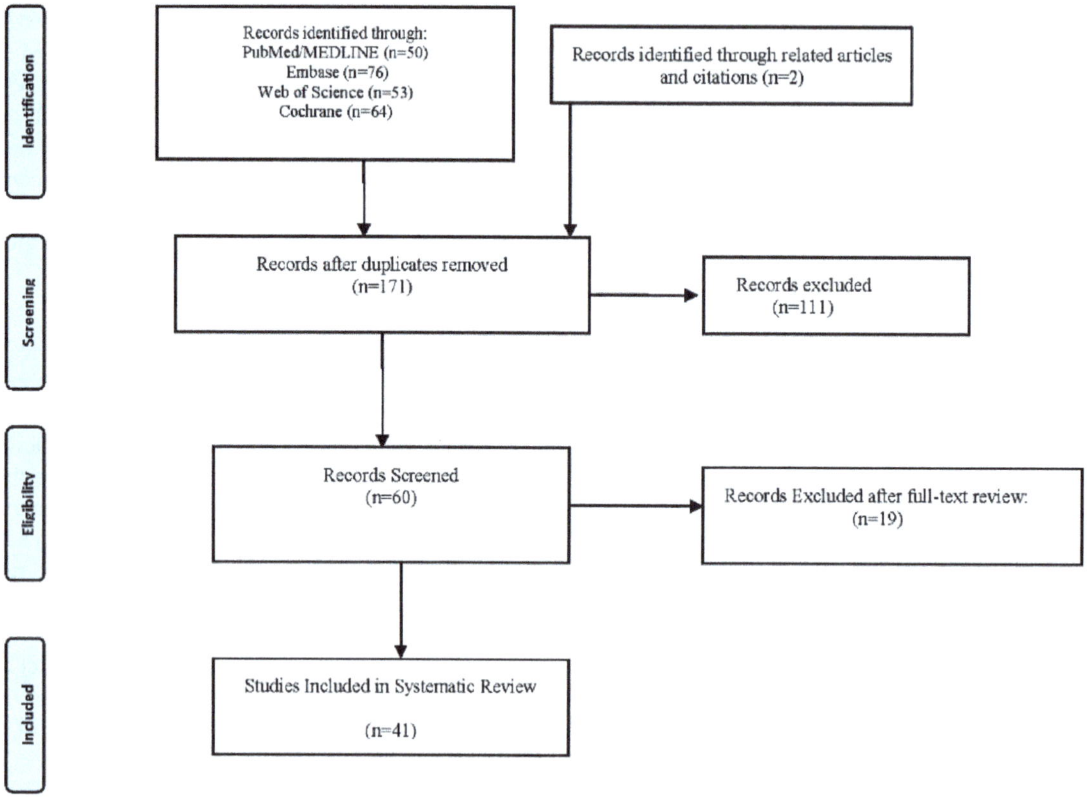

Data Extraction

The following data were extracted: (1) the proportion of RCTs that used disease severity indices or QoL outcome instruments, (2) the total number of and the frequency of use of disease severity scales, and (3) the total number of and the frequency of use of QoL outcome measures.

Study Characteristics

A total of 41 RCTs that were published between 1986 and 2021 were identified; these accounted for a total of 3235 participants. The appraisal of studies via the methods outlined by the Oxford Centre for Evidence-Based Medicine evidence ratings scheme was performed; 17 RCTs qualified as level 1b studies, while the remaining 24 studies were level 2b studies. Summary information for the characteristics of the included studies, including evidence levels, is available in Multimedia Appendix 2. Of the 41 included RCTs, 38 (93%) used disease severity outcome measures, and of these 38 RCTs, 30 (79%) used more than 1 scale to assess disease severity. Additionally, 30 of the 41 studies (73%) included QoL measures; of these 30 studies, 20 studies (67%) assessed more than 1 QoL measure.

Disease Severity Outcome Measures

A total of 25 disease severity outcome measures were identified in this review. The HS Clinical Response (HiSCR) score (19/41, 46%) was the most common instrument used in HS clinical research. HiSCR score use increased from the year 2012 onward. Of the 27 RCTs published since 2012, 18 (67%) used the HiSCR score as an outcome measure (Table 1).

The Sartorius Scale and its modified version—the Modified Sartorius Scale (MSS), which was denoted by some authors as the *Hidradenitis Suppurativa Lesion, Area, Severity Index* (HS-LASI; Sartorius Scale: 7/41, 17%; MSS: 9/41, 22%)—were the second most frequently used instruments for disease severity assessment. The Physician Global Assessment (PGA; 8/41, 20%) was the third most commonly used instrument for disease severity. Only 5 of the 41 RCTs (12%) used the PGA scale that was specific to HS (also known as the HS-PGA). The Hurley stage was primarily used to stratify patients' disease severity prior to enrollment; only 3 studies incorporated the Hurley stage as an outcome measure. A recently developed and validated HS outcome measure—the International HS Severity Scoring System (IHS4)—was identified in a single RCT that was published in 2021 [50].

There were several studies that used inflammatory markers, including C-reactive protein levels, erythrocyte sedimentation rates, and cytokine profiles (7/41, 17%). Further, 1 RCT used noninvasive sonographic imaging to evaluate lesion depth and vascularity (Table 2).

Table 1. The frequency and proportion of disease severity outcome measures.

Disease severity outcome instrument	Studies, n (%)
Hidradenitis Suppurativa Clinical Response[a]	18 (44)
Modified Sartorius Scale[a]; Hidradenitis Suppurativa Lesion, Area, Severity Index; and Modified Hidradenitis Suppurativa Lesion, Area, Severity Index	9 (22)
Physician Global Assessment and evaluation	8 (20)
Sartorius Scale	7 (17)
Hidradenitis Suppurativa Physician Global Assessment[a]	5 (12)
Adverse events	5 (12)
Hurley stage	5 (12)
Abscess and nodule count	5 (12)
Mean improvement in abscesses, fistulae, and nodules	3 (7)
Recurrence	2 (5)
Hidradenitis Suppurativa Severity Index	2 (5)
Time to hidradenitis suppurativa exacerbation	2 (5)
Histological changes	2 (5)
International Hidradenitis Suppurativa Severity Scoring System[a]	1 (2)
Disease Activity Score (visual analogue scale)	1 (2)
Wound healing	1 (2)
Incidence of hidradenitis suppurativa flare	1 (2)
Manchester postinflammatory scar scoring	1 (2)
Hair follicle count	1 (2)
Average number of days to lesion resolution	1 (2)
Investigator and physician assessment	1 (2)

[a]A validated hidradenitis suppurativa scale.

Table 2. Laboratory and noninvasive imaging as outcome measures of disease severity.

Diagnostic and inflammatory markers as outcome measures	Studies, n (%)
C-reactive protein	5 (12)
Erythrocyte sedimentation rate	1 (2)
Cytokine profile	1 (2)
Ultrasound findings (eg, vascularity and the depth of lesions)	1 (2)

QoL Outcome Measures

A total of 18 QoL outcome instruments were identified. These are summarized in Table 3.

The Dermatology Life Quality Index (DLQI) was the most common patient-centered outcome reported in this review (18/41, 44%). A total of 17 studies assessed participants' pain. Pain was primarily measured by using a visual analogue scale (11/41, 27%) or a numerical ranking (6/41, 15%), although 1 study used the HS-related skin pain scale. In total, 5 of the 41 studies (12%) used the Patient/Participant Global Self-Assessment, which measures various parameters, including pain, pruritus, and disease burden. Patients' satisfaction with treatment was assessed in 4 of the 41 studies (10%), and 3 RCTs used the Workers Productivity and Impairment Activity Index-Specific Health Problem (WPAI-SHP). Psychological distress was assessed by 2 of the 41 studies (5%), which incorporated the 9-question Patient Health Questionnaire-9 (PHQ-9) depressive symptom scale as a PROM, and by 1 study that used the Hospital Anxiety and Depression Scale (HADS). The European Qol-5 Dimension (EQ-5D), which includes a domain for the assessment of anxiety and depression, was used in 1 RCT.

Table 3. Frequency and proportion of quality of life outcome measures.

QoL instrument	Frequency of use in studies, n (%)
Dermatology Life Quality Index[a]	18 (60)
Pain using a visual analogue scale	12 (37)
Pain using a numeric rating scale	6 (20)
Patient/Participant Global Assessment and evaluation	6 (20)
Patient satisfaction	4 (10)
Workers Productivity and Impairment Activity Index-Specific Health Problem[a]	3 (10)
Self-reported pruritus	2 (7)
Patient Health Questionnaire-9[a]	2 (7)
European Quality of Life-5 Dimension[a]	1 (3)
Hidradenitis suppurativa–related skin pain	1 (3)
Patient's overall disease severity and impression (visual analogue scale)	1 (3)
Treatment Satisfaction Questionnaire for Medication[a]	1 (3)
Number of self-reported hidradenitis suppurativa flares	1 (3)
Soreness (visual analogue scale)	1 (3)
Self-assessment of disease burden	1 (3)
Hidradenitis suppurativa–related impairment of general health using a visual analogue scale	1 (3)
Change in the number of daily dressings per week	1 (3)
Hospital Anxiety and Depression Scale[a]	1 (3)

[a]A validated quality of life outcome instrument.

Discussion

Principal Findings

HS continues to represent a disease management challenge and result in a substantial disease burden for patients [2]. Our review of 41 RCTs (published in English) identified 25 disease severity measurements (Tables 1 and 2) and 18 QoL instrument scales (Table 3). Overall, we identified a diverse assortment of outcome measures, which may indicate a barrier to their synthesis and translation into clinical practice.

With regard to the validity of the outcome measures identified in our review, both the HS-PGA and HiSCR score have been shown to be valid assessments, with HiSCR being the most extensively validated outcome measure in published RCTs. The two most commonly reported disease severity scales in our study—the HiSCR score and the Sartorius Scale and MSS—differ substantially in their approaches and frames of reference; the HiSCR assesses clinical responses from baseline (namely, a reduction in inflammatory lesion count), and the Sartorius Scale and MSS assess the extent of HS inflammation by counting anatomic regions and the types and numbers of lesions.

The HiSCR score was the only validated scoring system that appeared in the studies reviewed (all reviewed articles: 18/41, 44%; articles reporting disease severity as an outcome: 18/38, 47%), making it the most commonly used validated scale in HS research. The HiSCR score is a validated scoring system that is used to evaluate treatment response, and it has been shown to be reliable in both clinical research and daily practice [24]. Although the minimal clinically important difference for HiSCR scores has not been established, a 50% reduction in the total abscess and nodule count appears to be meaningful to both patients and physicians [33].

Although only 5 RCTs used the HS-PGA, it is important to highlight that it is considered to be a relatively easy scoring system that assesses treatment efficacy in clinical research. Similar to the HiSCR score, it is a dynamic outcome instrument that can be used to monitor disease progression [52]. However, compared to the HiSCR score, the HS-PGA has a lower sensitivity for rapidly identifying changes in HS-specific lesions. For instance, some patients with severe HS-specific lesions can experience clinically important improvements without achieving meaningful reductions in their HS-PGA scores [52].

The Sartorius Scale, which is widely used to assess clinical responses to treatment based on the involved anatomical regions and the number and type of lesions involved (nodules, fistulae, and abscesses), the distance between lesions, and whether normal skin exists between lesions, poses a challenge to results interpretation [53]. In addition to being only partially validated, the Sartorius Scale may be quite time consuming to administer and difficult to replicate in a busy outpatient clinic.

The MSS (or HS-LASI) represents a more streamlined version of the original Sartorius Scale; the MSS includes a reduced number of specific types of lesions and a reduced number of points for each parameter [54]. Although it is simpler than the traditional Sartorius Scale, the MSS (or HS-LASI) remains time-consuming and difficult to interpret in the context of assessing coalescing and large lesions. In this review, we identified 2 RCTs that used the HS-LASI scale [22,27], whereas 11 RCTs used a combination of both the MSS and the traditional Sartorius Scale. The overlap in the naming and content of the Sartorius Scale and its variants, such as the MSS and HS-LASI, can hinder meaningful comparisons between studies and thus create challenges in interpreting data and making informed clinical decisions.

In 2016, Ingram et al [8] found that 90% of outcome measures that are used in HS research are not validated; however, the research landscape appears to be changing. We found that RCTs published from 2014 onward were more likely to use the validated HiSCR scale, while older studies used more diverse outcome measures, of which many had low interobserver reliability [55], and were less likely to have used a validated scale. In 2018, the HS ALLIANCE working group highlighted the need to incorporate validated outcome measures and PROMs in HS research [56]. In 2017, the members of the European HS Foundation demonstrated the validity of a novel instrument—the IHS4 [57]. The IHS4 has been shown to be a dynamic instrument for assessing HS severity and is applicable to both clinical research and daily clinical practice [57]. We found a single, recent RCT (published in 2021) that used the IHS4 as an outcome measure [50].

As with instruments of disease severity assessment, patient-reported QoL measures demonstrate significant heterogeneity and are generally nonspecific [57]. Although the majority of articles (30/41, 73%) discussed the impact of HS on patients' lives, the instruments that were used remain inadequate for capturing the overall impact of disease burden on patients. Of all of the QoL instruments identified in this review, the DLQI appeared in 44% (18/41) of RCTs, making it the most commonly used patient-centered instrument in HS research. The DLQI is a validated instrument that is widely used for an array of dermatologic conditions, such as psoriasis and atopic dermatitis, but is not specific to HS.

In addition to QoL instruments, specific outcomes pertaining to pain assessment are needed. Although the visual analogue pain scale has been validated in clinical research, it is not specific to HS. Despite various treatment options, a recent survey study revealed that inadequate pain management is perceived as an unmet need by both patients and health care providers [58]. Given that pain is associated with psychosocial comorbidities [34], it is essential to develop specific core outcome scales that assess pain management and treatment responses.

In contrast to disease severity outcome measures, we identified 6 validated QoL instruments. These include the DLQI, PHQ-9, HADS, EQ-5D, WPAI-SHP, and Treatment Satisfaction Questionnaire for Medication [59]. However, these are not HS-specific QoL instruments. The emotional, social, and psychological impacts of HS on patients cannot be overstated; while QoL can be measured in various ways, the current QoL instruments that are used in HS research may not adequately capture changes that specifically pertain to the HS population.

In 2018, the first HISTORIC (HS Core Outcomes Set International Collaboration) Delphi study [60] reached a consensus on the following five core domains that are relevant to all types of clinical research: pain, physical signs, HS-specific QoL, global assessment, and the progression of the disease course. HISTORIC Delphi also developed the HS QoL (HiSQOL) scale—an HS-specific QoL instrument [61].

Over the past several years, there has been an increased effort to develop validated, HS-specific QoL outcome instruments, including the aforementioned HiSQOL scale, the HIDRAdisk, and the 44-item HS-QoL questionnaire [61-64]. Promising HS-specific QoL instruments such as these may soon be incorporated in future clinical trial outcome measurements.

Kimball et al [65] introduced the following two specific questionnaires in 2018: the HS Symptom Assessment (HSSA) and the HS Impact Assessment (HSIA). Both the HSSA and HSIA are validated instruments and are considered to be reliable tools for assessing symptoms and the efficacy of HS treatment. We identified no RCTs that used these two instruments for the evaluation of therapeutic interventions for HS.

Ongoing research may soon allow for new technologies to supplement the clinical assessment of HS lesion severity, which relies, in part, on manual palpation–noninvasive imaging techniques such as medial infrared thermography, and may soon aid in the evaluation of disease state and treatment response [66]. The broader adoption of standardized, validated QoL and disease severity measurement tools may allow for the better assessment of the overall impact of disease burden on patients, including the effect of HS on mental health [65], which, in our review, was not well characterized by the limited patient outcome measures reported.

Limitations

The limitations of this review include that it was restricted to published RCTs and that it excluded other types of publications, such as cohort studies, case control studies and case series, and ongoing or current clinical trials, that may provide further insight. We chose to include RCTs exclusively, as it was a priority to assess evidence of the highest level. It is unclear if other studies with less rigorous methods have similar trends in reporting disease severity and QoL outcome measures—an area that remains open for further follow-up studies. None of the included studies in this review involved pediatric participants; therefore, the trends in outcome measures that we identified may not be applicable to this population group. In addition, this review did not explore the utility of HS interventions and therefore cannot add to the body of knowledge regarding treatment efficacy in HS.

Conclusion

This review highlights the heterogeneity of outcome measures that are used in RCTs to assess disease severity and QoL for patients with HS. Among the 41 English RCTs published from 1964 to 2021, the HiSCR score remained the predominant outcome instrument that was used to assess HS disease severity.

The IHS4, which is representative of an expanding number of validated disease severity outcome measures, was used in only 1 RCT among those published from 1964 to 2021. Patient QoL measures remain central to evaluating disease impact and the degree of improvement for patients in clinical studies. PROMs are gaining importance in clinical research and are strongly supported by guidance from both the US Federal Drug Administration and European Medicines Agency. Recently developed instruments with proven validity, such as the HSSA, HSIA, and HiSQOL scale, represent advancements in measuring the QoL outcomes of HS. Our findings underscore the need for standardized outcome measures that are essential for comparability among studies and the improved quality of research evidence.

References

1. Tchero H, Herlin C, Bekara F, Fluieraru S, Teot L. Hidradenitis suppurativa: A systematic review and meta-analysis of therapeutic interventions. Indian J Dermatol Venereol Leprol 2019;85(3):248-257 [FREE Full text] [doi: 10.4103/ijdvl.IJDVL_69_18] [Medline: 30924446]
2. Marvel J, Vlahiotis A, Sainski-Nguyen A, Willson T, Kimball A. Disease burden and cost of hidradenitis suppurativa: a retrospective examination of US administrative claims data. BMJ Open 2019 Sep 30;9(9):e030579 [FREE Full text] [doi: 10.1136/bmjopen-2019-030579] [Medline: 31575575]
3. Phan K, Charlton O, Smith SD. Global prevalence of hidradenitis suppurativa and geographical variation—systematic review and meta-analysis. Biomedical Dermatology 2020 Jan 04;4(1):1-6. [doi: 10.1186/s41702-019-0052-0]
4. Dufour DN, Emtestam L, Jemec GB. Hidradenitis suppurativa: a common and burdensome, yet under-recognised, inflammatory skin disease. Postgrad Med J 2014 Apr;90(1062):216-221; quiz 220 [FREE Full text] [doi: 10.1136/postgradmedj-2013-131994] [Medline: 24567417]
5. Misitzis A, Goldust M, Jafferany M, Lotti T. Psychiatric comorbidities in patients with hidradenitis suppurativa. Dermatol Ther 2020 Jul;33(4):e13541. [doi: 10.1111/dth.13541] [Medline: 32385861]
6. Weigelt MA, Milrad SF, Kirby JRS, Lev-Tov H. Psychosocial impact of hidradenitis suppurativa: a practical guide for clinicians. J Dermatolog Treat 2021 Jun 14:1-8. [doi: 10.1080/09546634.2021.1937483] [Medline: 34060964]
7. Bottomley A, Jones D, Claassens L. Patient-reported outcomes: assessment and current perspectives of the guidelines of the Food and Drug Administration and the reflection paper of the European Medicines Agency. Eur J Cancer 2009 Feb;45(3):347-353. [doi: 10.1016/j.ejca.2008.09.032] [Medline: 19013787]
8. Ingram JR, Hadjieconomou S, Piguet V. Development of core outcome sets in hidradenitis suppurativa: systematic review of outcome measure instruments to inform the process. Br J Dermatol 2016 Aug;175(2):263-272. [doi: 10.1111/bjd.14475] [Medline: 26873867]
9. Liberati A, Altman DG, Tetzlaff J, Mulrow C, Gøtzsche PC, Ioannidis JPA, et al. The PRISMA statement for reporting systematic reviews and meta-analyses of studies that evaluate healthcare interventions: explanation and elaboration. BMJ 2009 Jul 21;339:b2700 [FREE Full text] [doi: 10.1136/bmj.b2700] [Medline: 19622552]
10. Mortimer PS, Dawber RP, Gales MA, Moore RA. A double-blind controlled cross-over trial of cyproterone acetate in females with hidradenitis suppurativa. Br J Dermatol 1986 Sep;115(3):263-268. [doi: 10.1111/j.1365-2133.1986.tb05740.x] [Medline: 2944534]
11. Miller I, Lynggaard CD, Lophaven S, Zachariae C, Dufour DN, Jemec GBE. A double-blind placebo-controlled randomized trial of adalimumab in the treatment of hidradenitis suppurativa. Br J Dermatol 2011 Aug;165(2):391-298. [doi: 10.1111/j.1365-2133.2011.10339.x] [Medline: 21457202]
12. Lee RA, Dommasch E, Treat J, Sciacca-Kirby J, Chachkin S, Williams J, et al. A prospective clinical trial of open-label etanercept for the treatment of hidradenitis suppurativa. J Am Acad Dermatol 2009 Apr;60(4):565-573 [FREE Full text] [doi: 10.1016/j.jaad.2008.11.898] [Medline: 19185954]
13. Yildiz H, Senol L, Ercan E, Bilgili ME, Abuaf OK. A prospective randomized controlled trial assessing the efficacy of adjunctive hyperbaric oxygen therapy in the treatment of hidradenitis suppurativa. Int J Dermatol 2016 Feb;55(2):232-237. [doi: 10.1111/ijd.12936] [Medline: 26267600]
14. Kimball AB, Kerdel F, Adams D, Mrowietz U, Gelfand JM, Gniadecki R, et al. Adalimumab for the treatment of moderate to severe Hidradenitis suppurativa: a parallel randomized trial. Ann Intern Med 2012 Dec 18;157(12):846-855. [doi: 10.7326/0003-4819-157-12-201212180-00004] [Medline: 23247938]
15. Gottlieb A, Menter A, Armstrong A, Ocampo C, Gu Y, Teixeira HD. Adalimumab treatment in women with moderate-to-severe hidradenitis suppurativa from the placebo-controlled portion of a phase 2, randomized, double-blind study. J Drugs Dermatol 2016 Oct 01;15(10):1192-1196. [Medline: 27741335]
16. Vossen ARJV, van Huijkelom MAPC, Nijsten TEC, Bakker EWP, van der Zee HH, van Doorn MBA, et al. Aggravation of mild axillary hidradenitis suppurativa by microwave ablation: Results of a randomized intrapatient-controlled trial. J Am Acad Dermatol 2019 Mar;80(3):777-779. [doi: 10.1016/j.jaad.2018.06.032] [Medline: 29940205]
17. Giamarellos-Bourboulis EJ, Pelekanou E, Antonopoulou A, Petropoulou H, Baziaka F, Karagianni V, et al. An open-label phase II study of the safety and efficacy of etanercept for the therapy of hidradenitis suppurativa. Br J Dermatol 2008 Mar;158(3):567-572. [doi: 10.1111/j.1365-2133.2007.08372.x] [Medline: 18076705]

18. Vossen ARJV, van Doorn MBA, van der Zee HH, Prens EP. Apremilast for moderate hidradenitis suppurativa: Results of a randomized controlled trial. J Am Acad Dermatol 2019 Jan;80(1):80-88. [doi: 10.1016/j.jaad.2018.06.046] [Medline: 30482392]
19. Grimstad Ø, Kvammen B, Swartling C. Botulinum toxin type B for hidradenitis suppurativa: A randomised, double-blind, placebo-controlled pilot study. Am J Clin Dermatol 2020 Oct;21(5):741-748 [FREE Full text] [doi: 10.1007/s40257-020-00537-9] [Medline: 32761500]
20. Azim AAA, Salem RT, Abdelghani R. Combined fractional carbon dioxide laser and long-pulsed neodymium : yttrium-aluminium-garnet (1064 nm) laser in treatment of hidradenitis suppurativa; a prospective randomized intra-individual controlled study. Int J Dermatol 2018 Sep;57(9):1135-1144. [doi: 10.1111/ijd.14075] [Medline: 29907956]
21. Wilden S, Friis M, Tuettenberg A, Staubach-Renz P, Wegner J, Grabbe S, et al. Combined treatment of hidradenitis suppurativa with intense pulsed light (IPL) and radiofrequency (RF). J Dermatolog Treat 2021 Aug;32(5):530-537. [doi: 10.1080/09546634.2019.1677842] [Medline: 31609667]
22. Xu LY, Wright DR, Mahmoud BH, Ozog DM, Mehregan DA, Hamzavi IH. Histopathologic study of hidradenitis suppurativa following long-pulsed 1064-nm Nd:YAG laser treatment. Arch Dermatol 2011 Jan;147(1):21-28. [doi: 10.1001/archdermatol.2010.245] [Medline: 20855672]
23. Grant A, Gonzalez T, Montgomery MO, Cardenas V, Kerdel FA. Infliximab therapy for patients with moderate to severe hidradenitis suppurativa: a randomized, double-blind, placebo-controlled crossover trial. J Am Acad Dermatol 2010 Feb;62(2):205-217. [doi: 10.1016/j.jaad.2009.06.050] [Medline: 20115947]
24. Fajgenbaum K, Crouse L, Dong L, Zeng D, Sayed C. Intralesional triamcinolone may not be beneficial for treating acute hidradenitis suppurativa lesions: A double-blind, randomized, placebo-controlled trial. Dermatol Surg 2020 May;46(5):685-689. [doi: 10.1097/DSS.0000000000002112] [Medline: 31490300]
25. Zouboulis CC, Okun MM, Prens EP, Gniadecki R, Foley PA, Lynde C, et al. Long-term adalimumab efficacy in patients with moderate-to-severe hidradenitis suppurativa/acne inversa: 3-year results of a phase 3 open-label extension study. J Am Acad Dermatol 2019 Jan;80(1):60-69.e2. [doi: 10.1016/j.jaad.2018.05.040] [Medline: 29860040]
26. Kanni T, Argyropoulou M, Spyridopoulos T, Pistiki A, Stecher M, Dinarello CA, et al. MABp1 targeting IL-1α for moderate to severe hidradenitis suppurativa not eligible for adalimumab: A randomized study. J Invest Dermatol 2018 Apr;138(4):795-801 [FREE Full text] [doi: 10.1016/j.jid.2017.10.030] [Medline: 29129600]
27. Tierney E, Mahmoud BH, Hexsel C, Ozog D, Hamzavi I. Randomized control trial for the treatment of hidradenitis suppurativa with a neodymium-doped yttrium aluminium garnet laser. Dermatol Surg 2009 Aug;35(8):1188-1198. [doi: 10.1111/j.1524-4725.2009.01214.x] [Medline: 19438670]
28. Tzanetakou V, Kanni T, Giatrakou S, Katoulis A, Papadavid E, Netea MG, et al. Safety and efficacy of anakinra in severe hidradenitis suppurativa: A randomized clinical trial. JAMA Dermatol 2016 Jan;152(1):52-59. [doi: 10.1001/jamadermatol.2015.3903] [Medline: 26579854]
29. Buimer MG, Ankersmit MFP, Wobbes T, Klinkenbijl JHG. Surgical treatment of hidradenitis suppurativa with gentamicin sulfate: a prospective randomized study. Dermatol Surg 2008 Feb;34(2):224-227. [doi: 10.1111/j.1524-4725.2007.34041.x] [Medline: 18093197]
30. Jemec GB, Wendelboe P. Topical clindamycin versus systemic tetracycline in the treatment of hidradenitis suppurativa. J Am Acad Dermatol 1998 Dec;39(6):971-974. [doi: 10.1016/s0190-9622(98)70272-5] [Medline: 9843011]
31. Adams DR, Yankura JA, Fogelberg AC, Anderson BE. Treatment of hidradenitis suppurativa with etanercept injection. Arch Dermatol 2010 May;146(5):501-504. [doi: 10.1001/archdermatol.2010.72] [Medline: 20479297]
32. Highton L, Chan WY, Khwaja N, Laitung JKG. Treatment of hidradenitis suppurativa with intense pulsed light: a prospective study. Plast Reconstr Surg 2011 Aug;128(2):459-466. [doi: 10.1097/PRS.0b013e31821e6fb5] [Medline: 21788837]
33. Kimball AB, Okun MM, Williams DA, Gottlieb AB, Papp KA, Zouboulis CC, et al. Two phase 3 trials of adalimumab for hidradenitis suppurativa. N Engl J Med 2016 Aug 04;375(5):422-434. [doi: 10.1056/NEJMoa1504370] [Medline: 27518661]
34. Scheinfeld N, Sundaram M, Teixeira H, Gu Y, Okun M. Reduction in pain scores and improvement in depressive symptoms in patients with hidradenitis suppurativa treated with adalimumab in a phase 2, randomized, placebo-controlled trial. Dermatol Online J 2016 Mar 16;22(3):13030/qt38x5922j [FREE Full text] [doi: 10.5070/d3223030360] [Medline: 27136622]
35. Jemec GBE, Sundaram M, Pinsky B, Shu L, Okun M, Bao Y. Adalimumab improves treatment satisfaction with medication (TS-M) in patients with moderate to severe hidradenitis suppurativa (HS) in a 12-week randomized controlled trial (PIONEER II). J Am Acad Dermatol 2015 May;72(5):AB39. [doi: 10.1016/j.jaad.2015.02.167]
36. Kimball A, Zouboulis C, Armstrong A, Korman N, Crowley J, Lynde C, et al. Safety and efficacy of adalimumab in patients with moderate to severe hidradenitis suppurativa: Results from first 12 weeks of PIONEER I, a phase 3, randomized, placebo-controlled trial. J Am Acad Dermatol 2015 May;72(5):AB60. [doi: 10.1016/j.jaad.2015.02.251]
37. Kimball AB, Sobell JM, Zouboulis CC, Gu Y, Williams DA, Sundaram M, et al. HiSCR (Hidradenitis Suppurativa Clinical Response): a novel clinical endpoint to evaluate therapeutic outcomes in patients with hidradenitis suppurativa from the placebo-controlled portion of a phase 2 adalimumab study. J Eur Acad Dermatol Venereol 2016 Jun 22;30(6):989-994 [FREE Full text] [doi: 10.1111/jdv.13216] [Medline: 26201313]
38. Kimball A, Prens E, Bechara F. Novel anti-IL17 antibody (CJM112) reduces inflammation of hidradenitis suppurativa patients in a placebo-controlled trial. Experimental Dermatology 2019;28:33.

39. Kimball AB, Jemec GBE, Brooks DM, Gu Y, Teixeira HD. Progression of hidradenitis suppurativa: Outcomes of placebo-treated patients in a phase 3, randomized, placebo-controlled trial (PIONEER II). J Am Acad Dermatol 2016 May;74(5):AB68. [doi: 10.1016/j.jaad.2016.02.270]
40. Armstrong A, Pinsky B, Sundaram M, Gu Y, Williams D, Bao Y. HUMIRA improves health-related quality of life (HRQoL) in patients with moderate to severe hidradenitis suppurativa (HS): results from the first 12 weeks of PIONEER I. Journal of Investigative Dermatology 2014 Sep;134:S34.
41. Armstrong A, Pinsky B, Sundaram M, Shu L, Okun M, Bao Y. Adalimumab improves health-related quality of life (HRQoL) in patients with moderate to severe hidradenitis suppurativa (HS): Results from the first 12 weeks of PIONEER II. J Am Acad Dermatol 2015 May;72(5):AB38. [doi: 10.1016/j.jaad.2015.02.166]
42. Gottlieb A, Menter A, Armstrong A, Ocampo C, Gu Y, Teixeira HD. Adalimumab Treatment in Women With Moderate-to-Severe Hidradenitis Suppurativa from the Placebo-Controlled Portion of a Phase 2, Randomized, Double-Blind Study. J Drugs Dermatol 2016 Oct 01;15(10):1192-1196. [Medline: 27741335]
43. Gulliver W, Bachelez H, Paek SY, Qureshi A, Geng Z, Mulder G. Concomitant antibiotic use in patients with moderate-to-severe hidradenitis suppurativa who were treated with adalimumab or placebo in a phase 3 study (PIONEER II). J Am Acad Dermatol 2017 Jun;76(6):AB81. [doi: 10.1016/j.jaad.2017.04.329]
44. Okun M, Yang M, Sundaram M, Gu Y. Validation of the hidradenitis suppurativa clinical response as a clinical endpoint for hidradenitis suppurativa treatment evaluation. J Am Acad Dermatol 2013 Apr;68(4):AB68. [doi: 10.1016/j.jaad.2012.12.281]
45. Fadel MA, Tawfik AA. New topical photodynamic therapy for treatment of hidradenitis suppurativa using methylene blue niosomal gel: a single-blind, randomized, comparative study. Clin Exp Dermatol 2015 Mar;40(2):116-122. [doi: 10.1111/ced.12459] [Medline: 25262788]
46. Mrowietz U, Williams D, Sundaram M, Wang Y. Adalimumab improves health-related quality of life and work productivity in patients with hidradenitis suppurativa: Results from a placebo-controlled phase II trial. J Am Acad Dermatol 2012 Apr;66(4):AB42. [doi: 10.1016/j.jaad.2011.11.184]
47. Giamarellos-Bourboulis E, Henneberg J, Otto I. IFX-1 in patients with moderate to severe hidradenitis suppurativa/acne inversa (HS): Baseline characteristics of a double-blind, randomized phase 2B dose-finding study (SHINE). Experimental Dermatology 2019;28:25-26.
48. Giamarellos-Bourboulis EJ, Sobell J, Ryan C, Wolkenstein PJ, Geng Z, Mulder GD. Infection-free clinical response among patients with hidradenitis suppurativa who were treated with adalimumab: Results from two phase 3 studies. Wounds 2017 Nov;29(11):E98-E102 [FREE Full text] [Medline: 29166256]
49. Andersen PL, Riis PT, Thorlacius L, Sigsgaard V, Nielsen CW, Chafranska L, et al. [Intense pulsed light treatment for hidradenitis suppurativa: a within-person randomized controlled trial]. Eur J Dermatol 2020 Dec 01;30(6):723-729. [doi: 10.1684/ejd.2020.3920] [Medline: 33300880]
50. Schultheis M, Staubach P, Nikolakis G, Grabbe S, Ruckes C, von Stebut E, et al. LAight® therapy significantly enhances treatment efficacy of 16 weeks of topical clindamycin solution in Hurley I and II hidradenitis suppurativa: Results from period A of RELIEVE, a multicenter randomized, controlled trial. Dermatology 2021 Sep 14:1-11. [doi: 10.1159/000518540] [Medline: 34535610]
51. Burns PB, Rohrich RJ, Chung KC. The levels of evidence and their role in evidence-based medicine. Plast Reconstr Surg 2011 Jul;128(1):305-310 [FREE Full text] [doi: 10.1097/PRS.0b013e318219c171] [Medline: 21701348]
52. Marzano AV, Chiricozzi A, Giovanardi G, Argenziano G, Bettoli V, Bianchi L, et al. Creation of a severity index for hidradenitis suppurativa that includes a validated quality-of-life measure: the HIDRAscore. J Eur Acad Dermatol Venereol 2020 Aug;34(8):1815-1821 [FREE Full text] [doi: 10.1111/jdv.16328] [Medline: 32119143]
53. Sartorius K, Lapins J, Emtestam L, Jemec GBE. Suggestions for uniform outcome variables when reporting treatment effects in hidradenitis suppurativa. Br J Dermatol 2003 Jul;149(1):211-213. [doi: 10.1046/j.1365-2133.2003.05390.x] [Medline: 12890229]
54. Sartorius K, Emtestam L, Jemec GBE, Lapins J. Objective scoring of hidradenitis suppurativa reflecting the role of tobacco smoking and obesity. Br J Dermatol 2009 Oct;161(4):831-839. [doi: 10.1111/j.1365-2133.2009.09198.x] [Medline: 19438453]
55. Sartorius K, Killasli H, Heilborn J, Jemec GBE, Lapins J, Emtestam L. Interobserver variability of clinical scores in hidradenitis suppurativa is low. Br J Dermatol 2010 Jun;162(6):1261-1268. [doi: 10.1111/j.1365-2133.2010.09715.x] [Medline: 20184581]
56. Zouboulis CC, Bechara FG, Dickinson-Blok JL, Gulliver W, Horváth B, Hughes R, et al. Hidradenitis suppurativa/acne inversa: a practical framework for treatment optimization - systematic review and recommendations from the HS ALLIANCE working group. J Eur Acad Dermatol Venereol 2019 Jan;33(1):19-31 [FREE Full text] [doi: 10.1111/jdv.15233] [Medline: 30176066]
57. Zouboulis CC, Tzellos T, Kyrgidis A, Jemec GBE, Bechara FG, Giamarellos-Bourboulis EJ, European Hidradenitis Suppurativa Foundation Investigator Group. Development and validation of the International Hidradenitis Suppurativa Severity Score System (IHS4), a novel dynamic scoring system to assess HS severity. Br J Dermatol 2017 Nov;177(5):1401-1409. [doi: 10.1111/bjd.15748] [Medline: 28636793]

58. Willems D, Hiligsmann M, van der Zee HH, Sayed CJ, Evers SMAA. Identifying unmet care needs and important treatment attributes in the management of hidradenitis suppurativa: A qualitative interview study. Patient 2021 Aug 09:1-12 [FREE Full text] [doi: 10.1007/s40271-021-00539-7] [Medline: 34368925]
59. Vellaichamy G, Braunberger TL, Jones JL, Peacock A, Nahhas AF, Hamzavi IH. Patient-reported outcomes in hidradenitis suppurativa. G Ital Dermatol Venereol 2019 Apr;154(2):137-147 [FREE Full text] [doi: 10.23736/S0392-0488.18.06021-2] [Medline: 30375207]
60. Thorlacius L, Ingram JR, Villumsen B, Esmann S, Kirby JS, Gottlieb AB, HIdradenitis SuppuraTiva cORe outcomes set International Collaboration (HISTORIC). A core domain set for hidradenitis suppurativa trial outcomes: an international Delphi process. Br J Dermatol 2018 Sep;179(3):642-650 [FREE Full text] [doi: 10.1111/bjd.16672] [Medline: 29654696]
61. Zouboulis CC, Chernyshov PV. Hidradenitis suppurativa-specific, patient-reported outcome measures. J Eur Acad Dermatol Venereol 2021 Jul;35(7):1420-1421. [doi: 10.1111/jdv.17306] [Medline: 34139050]
62. Peris K, Lo Schiavo A, Fabbrocini G, Dini V, Patrizi A, Fusano M, et al. HIDRAdisk: validation of an innovative visual tool to assess the burden of hidradenitis suppurativa. J Eur Acad Dermatol Venereol 2019 Apr;33(4):766-773 [FREE Full text] [doi: 10.1111/jdv.15425] [Medline: 30633405]
63. Thorlacius L, Esmann S, Miller I, Vinding G, Jemec GBE. Development of HiSQOL: A Hidradenitis Suppurativa-Specific Quality of Life Instrument. Skin Appendage Disord 2019 Jun;5(4):221-229 [FREE Full text] [doi: 10.1159/000496234] [Medline: 31367600]
64. McLellan C, Sisic M, Oon HH, Tan J. Preliminary validation of the HS-QoL: A quality-of-life measure for hidradenitis suppurativa. J Cutan Med Surg 2018;22(2):142-146. [doi: 10.1177/1203475417736281] [Medline: 28992738]
65. Kimball AB, Sundaram M, Banderas B, Foley C, Shields AL. Development and initial psychometric evaluation of patient-reported outcome questionnaires to evaluate the symptoms and impact of hidradenitis suppurativa. J Dermatolog Treat 2018 Mar;29(2):152-164. [doi: 10.1080/09546634.2017.1341614] [Medline: 28608738]
66. Elkin K, Daveluy S, Avanaki K. Review of imaging technologies used in hidradenitis suppurativa. Skin Res Technol 2020 Jan;26(1):3-10. [doi: 10.1111/srt.12772] [Medline: 31595571]

Abbreviations

DLQI: Dermatology Life Quality Index
EQ-5D: European Quality of Life-5 Dimension
HADS: Hospital Anxiety and Depression Scale
HiSCR: Hidradenitis Suppurativa Clinical Response
HiSQOL: Hidradenitis Suppurativa Quality Of Life
HISTORIC: Hidradenitis Suppurativa Core Outcomes Set International Collaboration
HS: hidradenitis suppurativa
HSIA: Hidradenitis Suppurativa Impact Assessment
HS-LASI: Hidradenitis Suppurativa Lesion, Area, Severity Index
HSSA: Hidradenitis Suppurativa Symptom Assessment
IHS4: International Hidradenitis Suppurativa Severity Scoring System
MSS: Modified Sartorius Scale
PGA: Physician Global Assessment
PHQ-9: Patient Health Questionnaire-9
PRISMA: Preferred Reporting Items for Systematic Reviews and Meta-Analyses
PROM: patient-reported outcome measure
QoL: quality of life
RCT: randomized controlled trial
WPAI-SHP: Workers Productivity and Impairment Activity Index-Specific Health Problem

19

Conflicts of Interest Among Authors of Systematic Reviews and Meta-Analyses Investigating Interventions for Melanoma

Zane Rulon[1*], BSc; Kalyn Powers[2*], BSPS; J Michael Anderson[1*], BSc; Michael Weaver[3], MSc; Austin Johnson[1], BSc; Micah Hartwell[1], PhD; Matt Vassar[1], PhD

[1]Center for Health Sciences, Oklahoma State University, Tulsa, OK, United States

[2]College of Pharmacy, Southwestern Oklahoma State University, Weatherford, OK, United States

[3]College of Osteopathic Medicine, Kansas City University of Medicine and Biosciences, Joplin, OK, United States

[*]these authors contributed equally

Corresponding Author:
J Michael Anderson, BSc
Center for Health Sciences
Oklahoma State University
1111 W 17th St N
Tulsa, OK, 74107
United States

Email: jande31@okstate.edu

Abstract

Background: Previous studies have highlighted the potential influence that industry relationships may have on the outcomes of medical research.

Objective: We aimed to determine the prevalence of author conflicts of interest (COIs) in systematic reviews focusing on melanoma interventions, as well as to determine whether the presence of these COIs were associated with an increased likelihood of reporting favorable results and conclusions.

Methods: This cross-sectional study included systematic reviews with or without meta-analyses focusing on interventions for melanoma. We searched MEDLINE and Embase for eligible systematic reviews published between September 1, 2016, and June 2, 2020. COI disclosures were cross-referenced with information from the CMS (Centers for Medicare & Medicaid Services) Open Payments database, Dollars for Profs, Google Patents, the United States Patent and Trademark Office, and previously published COI disclosure statements. Results were quantified using descriptive statistics, and relationships were evaluated by Fisher exact tests.

Results: Of the 23 systematic reviews included in our sample, 12 (52%) had at least one author with a COI. Of these 12 reviews, 7 (58%) reported narrative results favoring the treatment group and 9 (75%) reported conclusions favoring the treatment group. Of the 11 systematic reviews without a conflicted author, 4 (36%) reported results favoring the treatment group and 5 (45%) reported conclusions favoring the treatment group. We found no significant association between the presence of author COIs and the favorability of results (P=.53) or conclusions (P=.15).

Conclusions: Author COIs did not appear to influence the outcomes of systematic reviews regarding melanoma interventions. Clinicians and other readers of dermatology literature should be cognizant of the influence that industry may have on the nature of reported outcomes, including those from systematic reviews and meta-analyses.

KEYWORDS

conflicts of interest; industry sponsorship; melanoma; cross-sectional analysis; systematic review; meta-analysis

Introduction

According to the US Centers for Disease Control and Prevention [1], there were over 77,000 new cases of melanoma annually between 2012 and 2016, with an incidence rate of 21.8 per 100,000. During the same period, 9000 individuals died from melanoma each year. The estimated annual cost of melanoma treatment in the United States for people over 65 years old was estimated to be US $390 million in 2010 [1]. Due to the prevalence of melanoma and the cost of treatment, improved treatment strategies and novel interventions are critically needed. Well-conducted systematic reviews—considered the highest level of evidence (level 1a) [2]—are routinely used for developing guidelines, assessing novel treatments, and informing clinical decision making [3]. The two most recent clinical practice guidelines from the American Society of Clinical Oncology—Systemic Therapy for Melanoma and Sentinel Lymph Node Biopsy for Melanoma—both include systematic reviews to support their recommendations [4,5]. These guidelines influence physician decision making and patient care. Any bias in the systematic reviews can affect the validity of the data presented.

When appraising results of systematic reviews, it is important to consider whether the authors have industry ties or other conflicts of interest (COIs), as these competing interests may introduce bias that can have downstream effects on patient care [6]. The field of dermatology is not exempt from potential bias from industry ties. For example, dermatologists received more than US $34 million in industry payments in 2014 [7]. Further, Feng et al [8] reported that 73% of all dermatologists accepted industry payments. Considering the nonnegligible presence of industry in the field of dermatology, efforts to increase the transparency of these clinician-industry relationships have been made in hopes of mitigating industry bias within the field.

With the goal of minimizing potential bias, the Physician Payments Sunshine Act was passed in 2010, which requires all physicians to publicly disclose their corroboration with pharmaceutical and medical industries [9]. Since then, further improvements have been made to induce disclosures of industry ties. One such improvement was the creation of the publicly accessible CMS (Centers for Medicare & Medicaid Services) Open Payments database [7], which catalogs all financial relationships between US physicians and industry. According to a study by Young et al [10], nearly two-thirds of people surveyed rated transparency as somewhat or very important; however, nearly 90% of the same subjects had never heard of the CMS Open Payments database. These findings demonstrate that this tool is grossly underutilized by the patient population. With access to these records, Tringale et al [11] found that 48% of physicians accepted payments, totaling US $2.4 billion in one year. Further investigations have found that these relationships among US-based physicians and industry may act as a nidus for COIs [12-16].

While recognition of these relationships is increasing, little literature exists on the pervasiveness of financial and nonfinancial COIs among authors of systematic reviews and meta-analyses [17-19]. While financial relationships are often considered the most influential contributors to possible COIs, other potential conflicts may arise from personal, academic, and intellectual factors [20]. Any COIs among authors of systematic reviews regarding melanoma treatments have the potential to affect patient care and, thus, warrant evaluation [21-23].

To our knowledge, no study has assessed COIs among this group of authors. In this analysis, we strive to identify the nature and types of COIs, both disclosed and undisclosed, of authors of systematic reviews on melanoma therapies. Additionally, we aim to evaluate whether an association exists between sponsorship of systematic reviews and the results and conclusions reported.

Methods

Overview

To enhance the transparency and reproducibility of our work, we have provided our study materials, methods, and protocol on Open Science Framework [24]. While drafting this manuscript, we followed the PRISMA (Preferred Reporting Items for Systematic Reviews and Meta-Analyses) guidelines [25] and Murad and Wang's guidelines for reporting meta-epidemiological methodology [26].

Search Strategy

We searched MEDLINE (Ovid) and Embase (Ovid) on June 2, 2020, for systematic reviews with or without meta-analyses specific to the treatment of melanoma. Our exact search string can be found in Multimedia Appendix 1.

Screening

Two authors (ZR and KP) screened search returns by title and abstract in a duplicate, masked manner. After title and abstract screening, full texts were screened according to the eligibility criteria described below. Discrepancies were resolved by a group consensus meeting, with third-party adjudication, if necessary.

Eligibility Criteria

To be included, articles must have (1) been considered a systematic review or meta-analysis according to the PRISMA-P (PRISMA for Protocols) definition [27]; (2) been a head-to-head comparison of a specific intervention, or combination of interventions, to another intervention or to a placebo or standard of care; (3) been specific to the treatment of melanoma; (4) been published between the dates of September 1, 2016, and June 2, 2020; (5) been published in English; and (6) synthesized data from human participants. The dates of inclusion were based on the International Committee of Medical Journal Editors (ICMJE) recommendation, which states that authors should disclose COIs that occurred 36 months prior to journal submission [28]. By including systematic reviews published after September 1, 2016, we were able to cross-reference reported payments on the CMS Open Payments database—which went live in September 2013—in the 36 months prior to the dates of publication of the systematic reviews within our sample to ensure compliance with ICMJE's COI disclosure policy.

Training

Before the study began, investigators received an online training overview. Training included details regarding the study design, objectives, protocol, materials, and data extraction from one systematic review as an example. This training session is available online for reference [24].

Data Extraction

The same investigators (ZR and KP) who performed study screening also completed data extraction in a masked, duplicate fashion using a pilot-tested Google Form. The full texts of the included studies were analyzed for general study characteristics, including the following: (1) PubMed identification number and/or DOI (Digital Object Identifier), (2) name of journal, (3) date of publication, (4) author names, (5) treatment interventions being compared, (6) affiliations for the first and last authors, (7) funding source, (8) complete COI statement, (9) whether the systematic review or meta-analysis addressed risk of bias (RoB), (10) the verbatim RoB statement, (11) whether a systematic review author was also an author on one or more of the primary studies included in the review (yes or no), (12) the total number of self-cited primary studies, (13) whether an overall pooled effect estimate was calculated (yes or no), (14) the statistical significance of the pooled effect estimate, and (15) whether narrative results and conclusions favored the treatment or comparison group (eg, placebo, standard of care, or control). For the purpose of our study, *conclusion* was defined as the combined discussion and conclusion sections of the review.

Favorability of Narrative Results and Conclusions

Narrative results and conclusions were deemed as *favorable*, *unfavorable*, or *mixed or inconclusive*. While appraising the results section, *favorable* was assigned when only positive results were reported. *Unfavorable* was assigned when only negative results were reported. *Mixed or inconclusive* was assigned if both positive and negative results were reported. While appraising the conclusion, *favorable* was assigned when authors stated or implied favorability of the intervention group over the comparator group. *Unfavorable* was assigned when authors stated or implied favorability of the comparator group over the intervention group. *Mixed or inconclusive* was assigned if the conclusion section did not meet criteria for *favorable* or *unfavorable* (eg, reporting negative population outcome but positive subgroup analysis).

Identification of Undisclosed COIs

Our search for undisclosed COIs was undertaken using the stepwise strategy outlined in Figure 1. We used a similar search strategy used by Mandrioli et al [29], with slight modifications. These modifications included the use of additional databases: the CMS Open Payments database, Dollars for Profs, and the United States Patent and Trademark Office (USPTO). Multimedia Appendix 2 describes each database. All authors were searched for within these databases for undisclosed COIs, regardless of disclosure status. To ensure the accuracy of data collection, MW used the Python programming language (Python Software Foundation) to create database-specific search strings for the USPTO, Google Patents, and PubMed. If results from the patent searches could not be definitively linked to the author in question, we erred on the side of caution and did not consider this as an undisclosed COI. Based on recommendations for COI disclosure offered by the ICMJE, we limited our search of PubMed to include studies published in the 36 months prior to the date of the systematic review included in our sample. Author COI disclosure statements from the PubMed search results were cross-referenced with the COI disclosure statement found in the systematic review from our sample to determine if previously published studies included additional COIs not disclosed in the systematic review from our sample. In the event that more than 10 records were returned from our PubMed search, each investigator (ZR and KP) individually assigned random numbers to the records and screened the first 10 randomized records for an undisclosed COI. This stepwise search process was continued until an undisclosed COI was discovered, at which point the search was terminated and the author was considered to have an undisclosed COI [29].

Figure 1. Stepwise search for undisclosed conflicts of interest (COIs) among systematic review authors.

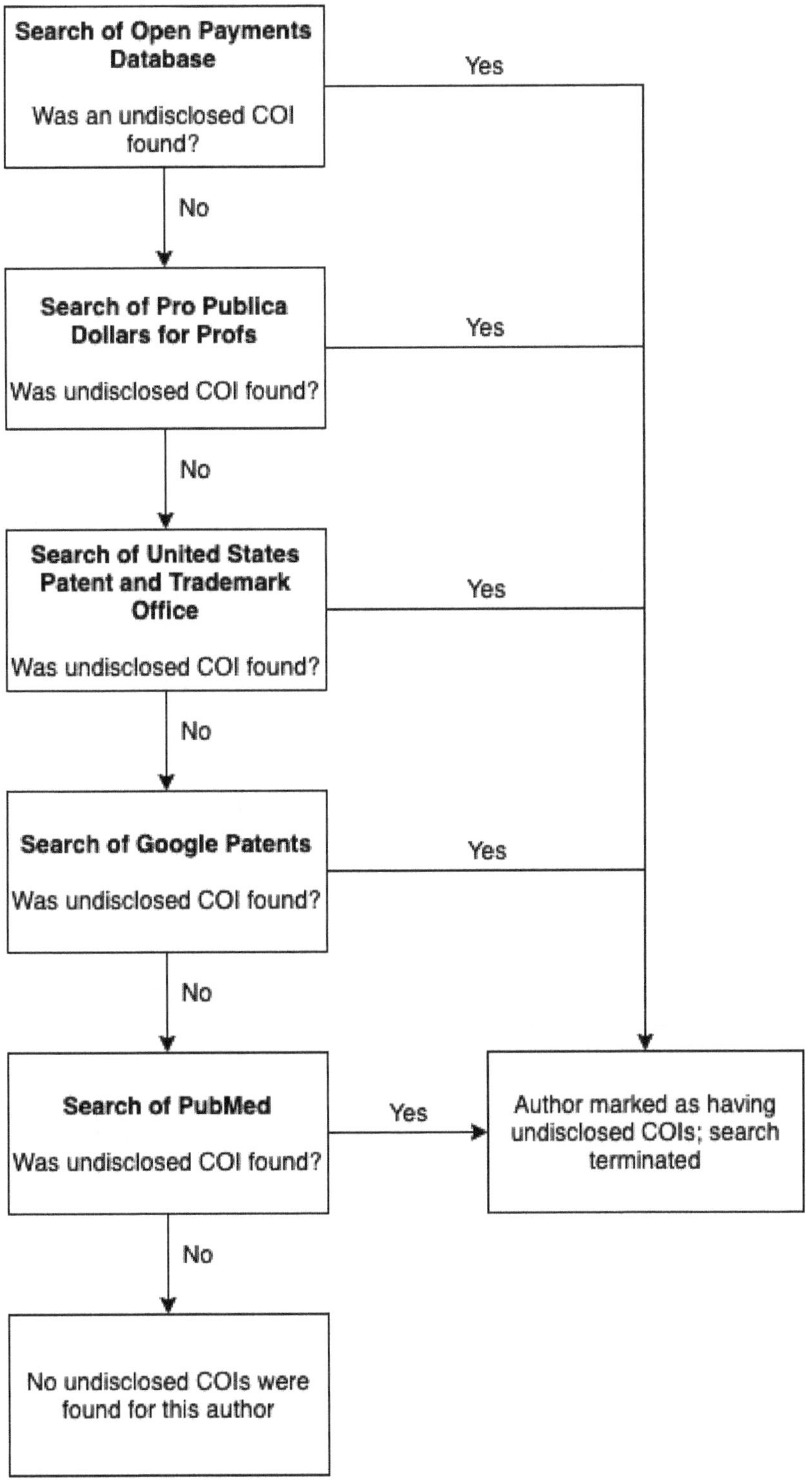

RoB Evaluation

We used the Cochrane Collaboration's criteria to assess the risk of funding bias in the included systematic reviews, as well as the four items used by Mandrioli et al [29]. Overall RoB was determined using the following criteria: (1) selection for inclusions and exclusions was explicit and *well-defined* and could be replicated by others, (2) the study inclusion method involved two or more assessors selecting studies, (3) search strategies were comprehensive, and (4) studies controlled for methodological differences that may introduce bias. We considered the RoB to be high if fewer than three items received a satisfactory *yes* answer.

Statistical Analysis

Results were calculated and reported as descriptive statistics. Relationships between systematic review characteristics and outcomes were evaluated by Fisher exact tests, when possible. Stata 16.1 (StataCorp, LLC) was used for all analyses.

Results

Overview

Our search of MEDLINE and Embase yielded 2388 records. A total of 2312 records were excluded after title and abstract screening. Full-text screening led to the exclusion of an additional 53 records. A total of 23 systematic reviews with or without meta-analyses investigating treatment interventions for melanoma were included (Figure 2).

Figure 2. PRISMA (Preferred Reporting Items for Systematic Reviews and Meta-Analyses) flowchart for included studies.

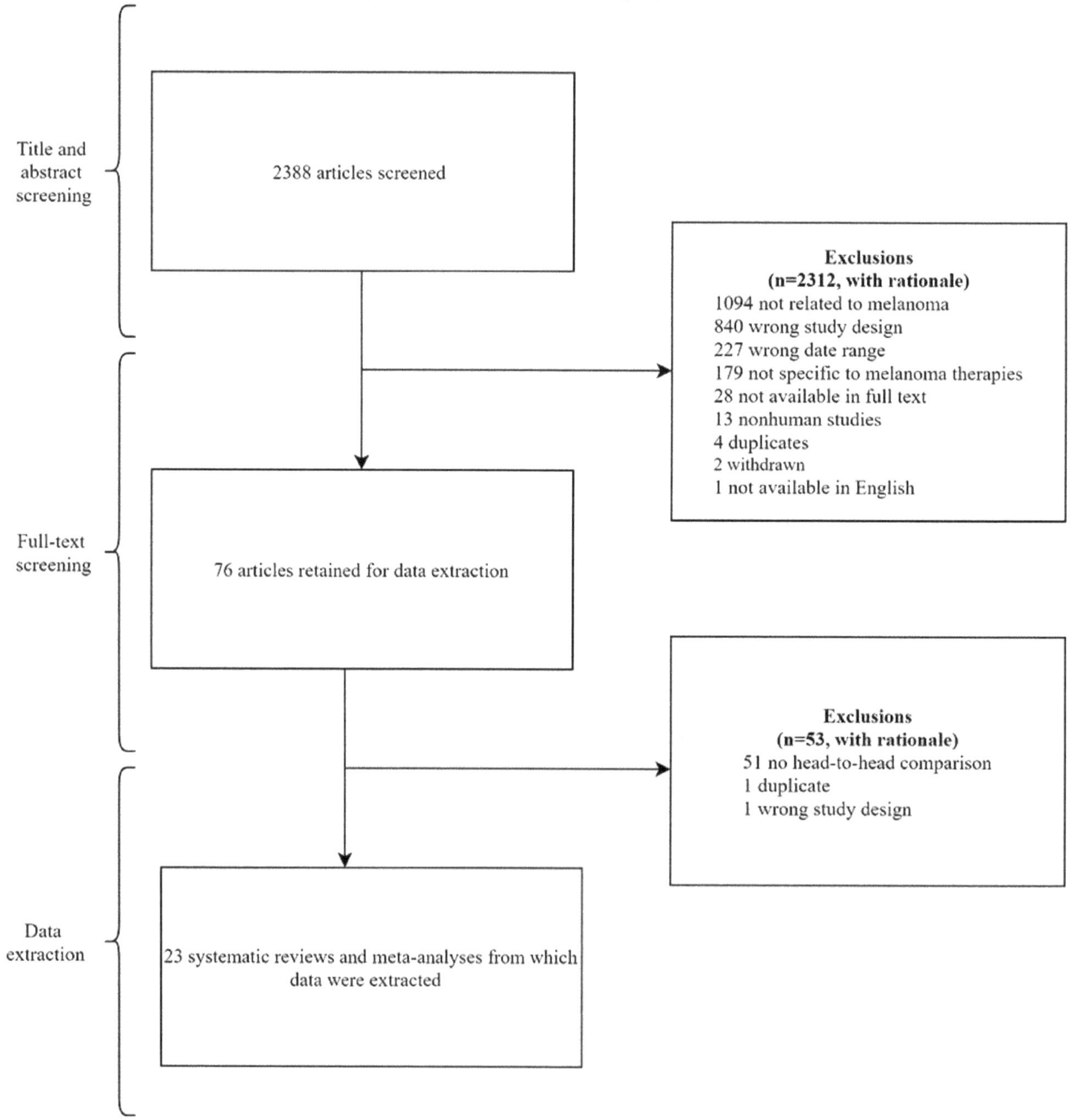

Systematic Review Characteristics

The 23 systematic reviews included in our final sample were conducted by 120 authors and published within 21 journals. Systematic reviews investigated pharmacologic interventions (8/23, 35%), surgical interventions (7/23, 30%), or a multidisciplinary treatment approach (8/23, 35%). Of the 23 systematic reviews, 19 (83%) reported that none of the authors had a COI, 2 (9%) reported that at least one author had a COI, and 2 (9%) failed to provide a COI disclosure statement. Only 1 systematic review out of 23 (4%) was found to have a high RoB. Additional study characteristics are provided in Table 1.

Table 1. Characteristics of systematic reviews.

Characteristic and form response	Value (N=23), n (%)
Journal	
International Immunopharmacology	3 (13)
Annals of Oncology	1 (4)
Anticancer Research	1 (4)
Cancer Medicine	1 (4)
Cancers	1 (4)
Cutaneous and Ocular Toxicology	1 (4)
European Journal of Cancer (Oxford, England: 1990)	1 (4)
European Journal of Surgical Oncology	1 (4)
Head & Neck	1 (4)
American Journal of Rhinology & Allergy	1 (4)
JAMA Network Open	1 (4)
Journal of Dermatological Treatment	1 (4)
Journal of Oncology	1 (4)
Journal of the American Academy of Dermatology	1 (4)
Journal of the European Academy of Dermatology and Venereology	1 (4)
OncoTargets and Therapy	1 (4)
Oncotarget	1 (4)
Technology in Cancer Research & Treatment	1 (4)
The British Journal of Surgery	1 (4)
The Journal of Laryngology and Otology	1 (4)
The Laryngoscope	1 (4)
Accuracy of author conflict of interest (COI) disclosure statement (N=120 authors)	
No COI found	95 (79)
All COIs completely disclosed in systematic review	20 (17)
Incomplete COI disclosure (found to have disclosed and undisclosed)	5 (4)
Intervention type	
Drug	8 (35)
Multiple	8 (35)
Surgical technique or intervention	7 (30)
Affiliation of first author	
Public academic institution	16 (69)
Government	4 (17)
Private academic institution	3 (13)
Affiliation of last author	
Public academic institution	17 (74)
Government	3 (13)
Private academic institution	3 (13)
Source of funding	
No funding received	8 (35)
Public	8 (35)
No statement present	6 (26)

Characteristic and form response	Value (N=23), n (%)
University	1 (4)
COI statement	
All authors report no COIs	19 (83)
One or more authors report a COI	2 (9)
No COI statement present	2 (9)
Self-citation of primary studies	
Yes, included one or more self-cited primary studies	4 (17)
No, did not include self-cited primary studies	19 (83)

Author Characteristics and Completeness of COI Disclosures

Of the 120 authors, 25 (20.8%) were found to have a COI, either disclosed, undisclosed, or both. Of these 25 authors, 20 (80%) reported no COI within the review's disclosure statement but were found to have an undisclosed COI. The remaining 5 authors out of 25 (20%) disclosed one or more COI but were found to have an additional undisclosed COI that was omitted from the COI disclosure statement (Table 1).

Relationship Between COI and Favorability of Results and Conclusions

Of the 12 systematic reviews with one or more authors with a COI, 7 (58%) reported narrative results favoring the treatment group and 9 (75%) reported conclusions favoring the treatment group. Of the 11 systematic reviews with no conflicted authors, 4 (36%) reported results favoring the treatment group and 5 (46%) reported conclusions favoring the treatment group. Our results showed no statistically significant association between author COIs and the favorability of results (*P*=.53) or conclusions (*P*=.15) (Table 2).

Table 2. Association between favorability of results and conclusions, risk of bias, and conflicts of interest (COIs) among systematic review authors.

Review outcomes	COIs among systematic review authors, n (%)		*P* value[a]
	No COIs (n=11)	COIs (n=12)	
Favorability of results			.53
Results favor treatment group	4 (36)	7 (58)	
Results are mixed or inconclusive	1 (9)	0 (0)	
Results favor placebo or control group	6 (55)	5 (42)	
Favorability of discussion and conclusions			.15
Discussion favors treatment group	5 (45)	9 (75)	
Discussion is mixed or inconclusive	0 (0)	0 (0)	
Discussion favors placebo or control group	6 (55)	3 (25)	
Risk of bias: high	0 (0)	1 (8)	.52

[a]*P* values were calculated from Fisher exact tests.

Relationship Between Sponsorship and Favorability of Results and Conclusions

Of the 23 systematic reviews, 9 (39%) received funding support, 8 (35%) did not receive funding support, and 6 (26%) did not provide a funding statement. Of the 9 reviews receiving nonindustry support, 3 (33%) reported results favoring the treatment group and 3 (33%) reported conclusions favoring the treatment group (Table 3). Because our sample did not include a single industry-funded systematic review, we could not assess for a relationship between industry sponsorship and the favorability of review results and conclusions.

Table 3. Association between favorability of results and conclusions, risk of bias, and systematic review sponsorship.

Review outcomes	Funding details, n (%)			
	Industry (n=0)	Nonindustry (n=9)	No funding received (n=8)	No statement listed (n=6)
Favorability of results				
Results favor treatment group	0 (0)	6 (67)	3 (38)	2 (33)
Results are mixed or inconclusive	0 (0)	0 (0)	0 (0)	1 (17)
Results favor placebo or control group	0 (0)	3 (33)	5 (62)	3 (50)
Favorability of discussion and conclusions				
Discussion favors treatment group	0 (0)	8 (88)	3 (37)	3 (50)
Discussion is mixed or inconclusive	0 (0)	0 (0)	0 (0)	0 (0)
Discussion favors placebo or control group	0 (0)	1 (11)	5 (62)	3 (50)
Risk of bias				
High risk of bias	0 (0)	1 (11)	0 (0)	0 (0)
Low risk of bias	0 (0)	8 (89)	8 (100)	6 (100)

Relationship Between RoB, Industry Sponsorship, and COIs

Only 1 of the 23 systematic reviews (4%) was found to have a high RoB. This systematic review received nonindustry support and was conducted by one or more authors with at least one COI. Because only 1 systematic review had a high RoB, we were unable to determine whether high RoB influenced the nature of review results and conclusions.

Discussion

Principal Findings

The results of our study indicate that COIs are a regular, often incompletely disclosed, occurrence in systematic reviews investigating melanoma interventions. Roughly one-half of the included systematic reviews were authored by at least one author with a potential COI. Additionally, one-fifth of the systematic review authors did not fully disclose all potential COIs. Previous work using the CMS Open Payments database to detail physician-industry relationships found variable rates of undisclosed COIs among clinical practice guidelines authors in multiple disciplines [30-33]. For example, undisclosed COIs were found to be present for 45% (22/49) of authors in dermatology [30], 6% (3/49) of authors in otolaryngology [31], 31% (23/74) of authors in orthopedics [32], and 20% (20/54) of authors in urology [33]. Similarly, of the 9 authors from our sample who were found on the CMS Open Payments database, all had at least one undisclosed COI that was omitted from the systematic review COI disclosure statement. In an assessment of the association between COIs and results, conclusions, and methodological quality, Hansen et al [34] found that systematic reviews with a COI were more likely to have favorable conclusions than those without a COI. Although our analysis failed to identify a similar association between author COIs and review outcomes, the high rates of undisclosed COIs among authors included in our sample highlight the need for more complete COI disclosure. Inconsistency in the completeness of COI disclosure is evident, and one potential explanation may be a lack of adherence to a comprehensive, more uniform disclosure guideline.

Complete disclosure of COIs is a widespread issue, and the lack of standardization of disclosure requirements between journals could partially explain the high rate of undisclosed COIs in our sample. For example, a study by Zhu and Sun [35] found that only 31% of medical journals mentioned a COI policy, 7% required a COI statement, and 4% standardized the COI submissions form. In addition to the inconsistent presence of journal COI disclosure policies, journals often fail to clearly outline expectations regarding COI disclosure requirements, making it difficult or impossible to establish what COI information should be disclosed. For instance, a 2007 study by Ancker and Flanagin [36] determined that only 68% of journals provided examples of what may be perceived as a potential COI and only 46% of journals explicitly defined the term. The same authors reported, upon initial attempts, that they were only able to locate COI disclosure policies for 33% of "high-impact, peer-reviewed" journals. Results from studies such as these highlight that, even when COI disclosure policies are present, authors are often left to determine for themselves what information should be disclosed at the time of manuscript submission.

Resnik and Elliott [37] reached a similar conclusion concerning the potential influence of financial biases on the design and interpretation of the study. These authors highlighted the difficulties in judging a study on scientific merit alone and presented methods to take financial relationships into account, without crudely discrediting the results of the study. To help address financial bias in medical literature, we recommend an initiative to develop a similar database to the CMS Open Payments database that would centralize potential COIs, financial and otherwise, and include all stakeholders in academic medicine (eg, clinicians, researchers, editors, funders, and peer reviewers), as well as research stakeholders with non-US–based affiliations.

Furthermore, we encourage readers to consider COIs when interpreting the results of systematic reviews. Analyses designed to define the prevalence of undisclosed and disclosed COIs in medical literature may increase awareness and emphasis on the issues surrounding COIs and lead to more standardized disclosure policies, such as an ICMJE COI form expanded to a global scale [20]. Perhaps a more comprehensive and enforced implementation of a standardized COI form would decrease the chances of potential COIs remaining undisclosed. Even though complete COI disclosure may be a step in the right direction, it can be difficult to interpret the degree of influence these COIs have on the procedures and results of a study. Maharaj [38] attempted to solve this issue by developing a COI scale that provides a numerical score for a study based on the potential bias risk from the disclosed COIs. Scales similar to that of Maharaj could be used as a means to compare the degree of influence that disclosed COIs have in a systematic review [38]. These measures may aid in improving transparency and accessibility in medical research, dermatological and otherwise.

Our study had several strengths. The design of our analysis maximized our ability to locate and confirm potential undisclosed COIs. Our protocol was established a priori and was published for reference on Open Science Framework with other materials and protocol amendments to increase transparency and reproducibility. Data extraction was carried out as recommended by the Cochrane Handbook [39]. Prior to the study, investigators received training to account for any differences in investigational analysis, data extraction was standardized using pilot-tested Google Forms, and a search string–generating program was used to promote search uniformity. Limitations of our study include a small sample size and difficulty verifying authors with common names on patent websites. In addition, our sample lacked industry-sponsored systematic reviews, thereby preventing further analysis into the role that industry may have on the nature of reported results and conclusions. Taken together, COIs and industry sponsorship may affect the favorability of study outcomes, but the source of the discrepancy in favorability between systematic reviews with COIs and those without remains unclear [8,30,40].

Conclusions

COIs are common, yet often incompletely disclosed, in systematic reviews investigating melanoma interventions. However, our results suggest that the presence of author COIs did not influence the favorability of reported outcomes of melanoma systematic reviews. Future investigations are needed to more fully evaluate the influence that COIs and industry sponsorship may have on the nature and direction of results and conclusions within published dermatology literature.

References

1. Centers for Disease Control and Prevention. Melanoma Incidence and Mortality, United States–2012–2016. USCS Data Brief, no. 9. Atlanta, GA: Centers for Disease Control and Prevention, US Department of Health and Human Services; 2019 Jul. URL: https://www.cdc.gov/cancer/uscs/about/data-briefs/no9-melanoma-incidence-mortality-UnitedStates-2012-2016.htm [accessed 2020-07-01]
2. OCEBM Levels of Evidence Working Group. The Oxford 2011 Levels of Evidence. Oxford, UK: Oxford Centre for Evidence-Based Medicine; 2011. URL: https://www.cebm.ox.ac.uk/resources/levels-of-evidence/ocebm-levels-of-evidence [accessed 2020-01-13]
3. McGowan J, Sampson M. Systematic reviews need systematic searchers. J Med Libr Assoc 2005 Jan;93(1):74-80 [FREE Full text] [Medline: 15685278]
4. Seth R, Messersmith H, Kaur V, Kirkwood JM, Kudchadkar R, McQuade JL, et al. Systemic therapy for melanoma: ASCO guideline. J Clin Oncol 2020 Nov 20;38(33):3947-3970. [doi: 10.1200/JCO.20.00198] [Medline: 32228358]
5. Wong SL, Faries MB, Kennedy EB, Agarwala SS, Akhurst TJ, Ariyan C, et al. Sentinel lymph node biopsy and management of regional lymph nodes in melanoma: American Society of Clinical Oncology and Society of Surgical Oncology clinical practice guideline update. J Clin Oncol 2018 Feb 01;36(4):399-413. [doi: 10.1200/JCO.2017.75.7724] [Medline: 29232171]
6. Forsyth SR, Odierna DH, Krauth D, Bero LA. Conflicts of interest and critiques of the use of systematic reviews in policymaking: An analysis of opinion articles. Syst Rev 2014 Nov 18;3:122 [FREE Full text] [doi: 10.1186/2046-4053-3-122] [Medline: 25417178]
7. Open Payments Data - CMS. URL: https://openpaymentsdata.cms.gov/ [accessed 2020-06-27]
8. Feng H, Wu P, Leger M. Exploring the industry-dermatologist financial relationship: Insight from the Open Payment data. JAMA Dermatol 2016 Dec 01;152(12):1307-1313. [doi: 10.1001/jamadermatol.2016.3037] [Medline: 27706478]
9. Kirschner NM, Sulmasy LS, Kesselheim AS. Health policy basics: The Physician Payment Sunshine Act and the Open Payments program. Ann Intern Med 2014 Oct 07;161(7):519-521. [doi: 10.7326/M14-1303] [Medline: 25069795]
10. Young PD, Xie D, Schmidt H. Towards patient-centered conflicts of interest policy. Int J Health Policy Manag 2018 Feb 01;7(2):112-119 [FREE Full text] [doi: 10.15171/ijhpm.2017.128] [Medline: 29524935]
11. Tringale KR, Marshall D, Mackey TK, Connor M, Murphy JD, Hattangadi-Gluth JA. Types and distribution of payments from industry to physicians in 2015. JAMA 2017 May 02;317(17):1774-1784 [FREE Full text] [doi: 10.1001/jama.2017.3091] [Medline: 28464140]
12. Drazen JM. Revisiting the commercial-academic interface. N Engl J Med 2015 May 07;372(19):1853-1854. [doi: 10.1056/NEJMe1503623] [Medline: 25946285]

13. Marshall DC, Jackson ME, Hattangadi-Gluth JA. Disclosure of industry payments to physicians: An epidemiologic analysis of early data from the Open Payments program. Mayo Clin Proc 2016 Jan;91(1):84-96 [FREE Full text] [doi: 10.1016/j.mayocp.2015.10.016] [Medline: 26763512]
14. Ahn R, Woodbridge A, Abraham A, Saba S, Korenstein D, Madden E, et al. Financial ties of principal investigators and randomized controlled trial outcomes: Cross sectional study. BMJ 2017 Jan 17;356:i6770 [FREE Full text] [doi: 10.1136/bmj.i6770] [Medline: 28096109]
15. Bauchner H, Fontanarosa PB, Flanagin A. Conflicts of interests, authors, and journals: New challenges for a persistent problem. JAMA 2018 Dec 11;320(22):2315-2318. [doi: 10.1001/jama.2018.17593] [Medline: 30422174]
16. Checketts J, Vassar M. Financial relations between leaders of US medical societies and industry. BMJ 2020 May 27;369:m1811. [doi: 10.1136/bmj.m1811] [Medline: 32461247]
17. Hurley MP, Stafford RS, Lane AT. Characterizing the relationship between free drug samples and prescription patterns for acne vulgaris and rosacea. JAMA Dermatol 2014 May;150(5):487-493 [FREE Full text] [doi: 10.1001/jamadermatol.2013.9715] [Medline: 24740450]
18. Sams WM, Freedberg IM. The dermatology-industry interface: Defining the boundaries. J Am Acad Dermatol 2000 Sep;43(3):550-554. [doi: 10.1067/mjd.2000.107502] [Medline: 10954674]
19. Williams H, Naldi L, Paul C, Vahlquist A, Schroter S, Jobling R. Conflicts of interest in dermatology. Acta Derm Venereol 2006;86(6):485-497 [FREE Full text] [doi: 10.2340/00015555-0191] [Medline: 17106594]
20. Recommendations for the Conduct, Reporting, Editing, and Publication of Scholarly Work in Medical Journals. International Committee of Medical Journal Editors. URL: http://www.icmje.org/recommendations/ [accessed 2019-12-09]
21. Lavis JN. How can we support the use of systematic reviews in policymaking? PLoS Med 2009 Nov;6(11):e1000141 [FREE Full text] [doi: 10.1371/journal.pmed.1000141] [Medline: 19936223]
22. Bekelman JE, Li Y, Gross CP. Scope and impact of financial conflicts of interest in biomedical research: A systematic review. JAMA 2003;289(4):454-465. [doi: 10.1001/jama.289.4.454] [Medline: 12533125]
23. Lundh A, Lexchin J, Mintzes B, Schroll JB, Bero L. Industry sponsorship and research outcome. Cochrane Database Syst Rev 2017 Feb 16;2:MR000033. [doi: 10.1002/14651858.MR000033.pub3] [Medline: 28207928]
24. Rulon Z, Powers K, Anderson M, Weaver M, Hartwell M, Vassar M. Conflicts of interest among authors of systematic reviews regarding the treatment of melanoma. Open Science Framework. 2020 Jul. URL: https://osf.io/rp5md/ [accessed 2020-07-03]
25. PRISMA for systematic review protocols (PRISMA-P). PRISMA. 2015. URL: http://prisma-statement.org/Extensions/Protocols.aspx [accessed 2020-07-20]
26. Murad MH, Wang Z. Guidelines for reporting meta-epidemiological methodology research. Evid Based Med 2017 Aug;22(4):139-142 [FREE Full text] [doi: 10.1136/ebmed-2017-110713] [Medline: 28701372]
27. Moher D, Shamseer L, Clarke M, Ghersi D, Liberati A, Petticrew M, PRISMA-P Group. Preferred reporting items for systematic review and meta-analysis protocols (PRISMA-P) 2015 statement. Syst Rev 2015 Jan 01;4:1 [FREE Full text] [doi: 10.1186/2046-4053-4-1] [Medline: 25554246]
28. Disclosure of interest: ICMJE disclosure form. International Committee of Medical Journal Editors. URL: http://www.icmje.org/disclosure-of-interest/ [accessed 2020-07-20]
29. Mandrioli D, Kearns CE, Bero LA. Relationship between research outcomes and risk of bias, study sponsorship, and author financial conflicts of interest in reviews of the effects of artificially sweetened beverages on weight outcomes: A systematic review of reviews. PLoS One 2016;11(9):e0162198 [FREE Full text] [doi: 10.1371/journal.pone.0162198] [Medline: 27606602]
30. Checketts JX, Sims MT, Vassar M. Evaluating industry payments among dermatology clinical practice guidelines authors. JAMA Dermatol 2017 Dec 01;153(12):1229-1235 [FREE Full text] [doi: 10.1001/jamadermatol.2017.3109] [Medline: 29049553]
31. Horn J, Checketts JX, Jawhar O, Vassar M. Evaluation of industry relationships among authors of otolaryngology clinical practice guidelines. JAMA Otolaryngol Head Neck Surg 2018 Mar 01;144(3):194-201 [FREE Full text] [doi: 10.1001/jamaoto.2017.2741] [Medline: 29270633]
32. Checketts JX, Cook C, Vassar M. An evaluation of industry relationships among contributors to AAOS clinical practice guidelines and appropriate use criteria. J Bone Joint Surg Am 2018 Jan 17;100(2):e10. [doi: 10.2106/JBJS.17.00184] [Medline: 29342070]
33. Carlisle A, Bowers A, Wayant C, Meyer C, Vassar M. Financial conflicts of interest among authors of urology clinical practice guidelines. Eur Urol 2018 Sep;74(3):348-354. [doi: 10.1016/j.eururo.2018.04.023] [Medline: 29747945]
34. Hansen C, Lundh A, Rasmussen K, Hróbjartsson A. Financial conflicts of interest in systematic reviews: Associations with results, conclusions, and methodological quality. Cochrane Database Syst Rev 2019 Aug 05;8:MR000047 [FREE Full text] [doi: 10.1002/14651858.MR000047.pub2] [Medline: 31425611]
35. Zhu J, Sun J. Conflicts of interest disclosure policies among Chinese medical journals: A cross-sectional study. PLoS One 2019;14(7):e0219564 [FREE Full text] [doi: 10.1371/journal.pone.0219564] [Medline: 31287849]
36. Ancker JS, Flanagin A. A comparison of conflict of interest policies at peer-reviewed journals in different scientific disciplines. Sci Eng Ethics 2007 Jun;13(2):147-157. [doi: 10.1007/s11948-007-9011-z] [Medline: 17717729]

37. Resnik DB, Elliott KC. Taking financial relationships into account when assessing research. Account Res 2013;20(3):184-205 [FREE Full text] [doi: 10.1080/08989621.2013.788383] [Medline: 23672544]
38. Maharaj SVM. A new method for scoring financial conflicts of interest. Int J Occup Environ Health 2015;21(1):49-52 [FREE Full text] [doi: 10.1179/2049396714Y.0000000097] [Medline: 25633929]
39. Higgins JPT, Thomas J, Chandler J, Cumpston M, Li T, Page MJ, et al, editors. Cochrane Handbook for Systematic Reviews of Interventions. 2nd edition. Hoboken, NJ: Wiley-Blackwell; 2019.
40. Perlis CS, Harwood M, Perlis RH. Extent and impact of industry sponsorship conflicts of interest in dermatology research. J Am Acad Dermatol 2005 Jun;52(6):967-971. [doi: 10.1016/j.jaad.2005.01.020] [Medline: 15928613]

Abbreviations

CMS: Centers for Medicare & Medicaid Services
COI: conflict of interest
DOI: Digital Object Identifier
ICMJE: International Committee of Medical Journal Editors
PRISMA: Preferred Reporting Items for Systematic Reviews and Meta-Analyses
PRISMA-P: Preferred Reporting Items for Systematic Reviews and Meta-Analyses for Protocols
RoB: risk of bias
USPTO: United States Patent and Trademark Office

20

Applying an Author-Weighted Scheme to Identify the Most Influential Countries in Research Achievements on Skin Cancer

Tsair-Wei Chien[1], MBA; Hsien-Yi Wang[2,3], MD; Feng-Jie Lai[1,4], MD

[1]Department of Dermatology, Chi-Mei Medical Center, Tainan, Taiwan
[2]Department of Nephrology, Chi-Mei Medical Center, Tainan, Taiwan
[3]Department of Sports Management, Chia-Nan University of Pharmacy and Science, Tainan, Taiwan
[4]Center for General Education, Southern Taiwan University of Science and Technology, Tainan, Taiwan

Corresponding Author:
Feng-Jie Lai, MD
Department of Dermatology
Chi-Mei Medical Center
#901, Chung Hwa Road
Yung Kung District
Tainan
Taiwan

Email: smile@mail.chimei.org.tw

Abstract

Background: Skin cancers are caused by the development of abnormal cells that can invade or spread to other parts of the body. The countries whose authors contribute the most amount of articles on skin cancer to academia is still unknown.

Objective: The objectives of this study are to apply an author-weighted scheme (AWS) to quantify the credits for coauthors on an article byline and allocate the author weights to the country-level credits in articles.

Methods: On July 20, 2019, we obtained 16,804 abstracts published since 1938, based on a keyword search of "skin cancer" in PubMed. The author names, countries/areas, and journals were recorded. International author collaborations on skin cancer were analyzed based on country-level credits in articles. We aimed to do the following: (1) present country distribution for the first authors and the most popular journals, (2) show choropleth maps to highlight the most influential countries, and (3) draw scatter plots based on the Kano model to characterize the features of country-level research achievements. We programmed Excel Visual Basic for Applications (Microsoft Corp) routines to extract data from PubMed. Google Maps was used to display graphical representations.

Results: Our results suggest that researchers in the United States have published most frequently, accounting for 30.37% (5103), while Germany accounts for 7.34% (1234), followed by Australia (997, 5.93%). The top three continents for the proportion of published articles are North America, Europe, and Asia, accounting for 32.29%, 31.71%, and 10.41%, respectively.

Conclusions: This study offers an objective picture of the representativeness and evolution of international research on the topic of skin cancer. The research approaches used here have the potential to be applied to other areas besides skin cancer.

KEYWORDS

choropleth map; author-weighted scheme; Google Maps; x-index; skin cancer; journal impact factor

Introduction

Skin cancers are tumors that arise mostly from the skin due to the development of abnormal cells that invade or spread to other parts of the body [1]. There are three main types of skin cancers: basal cell skin cancer, squamous cell skin cancer, and melanoma [2]. Skin cancers often appear as a painless raised area of skin with small blood vessels running over it but may present with an ulcer [2]; they may be caused by exposure to ultraviolet radiation from the sun [3].

Ultraviolet exposure has increased partly due to a thinner ozone layer [4,5]. Between 20% and 30% of melanomas develop from moles [6]. People with light skin are at higher risk as are people with reduced immune function [2,7] from taking immunosuppressant medications or through infection with HIV [8,9]. Skin cancer is the most common form of cancer, accounting for at least 40% of cases globally [8,10]. In 2012, melanoma occurred in 232,000 people worldwide and resulted in 55,000 deaths [6]. Australia and New Zealand have the highest rates of melanoma in the world [6]. Which countries have contributed the most to research on skin cancer based on author publications and quality of research is unknown.

We were motivated to investigate which countries contributed the most to research on skin cancer and how much authors from Australia and New Zealand have contributed to the current body of knowledge.

Given the multidisciplinary aspect of skin cancer research, it is necessary to gather specialists in medicine, pathology, and biomedical science to ensure collaboration through resource sharing, exchange of ideas, knowledge dissemination, and information acquisition. No researcher has investigated scientific collaborations on skin cancer, particularly using a fair author-weighted scheme (AWS) for quantifying coauthor contributions to their articles. As such, country-level research achievements are required to evaluate and compare whether AWS has been applied.

Some researchers have applied visualization approaches to interpreting their study results, notably in genetic research, which was identified as the primary collaborative field [11]. However, the pattern of data display was a static JPG format picture, unlike the dynamic dashboard on Google Maps. The dashboard allows readers to see more detail on research topics by using the zoom-in/zoom-out functionality [12-14]. Furthermore, all coauthors in an article sharing equal credits is problematic and unfair. Quantifying coauthor contributions has been proposed in the literature [15,16], but few published articles were applicable in the past. Similarly, country-level research achievements cannot be fairly obtained if the AWS has not been adopted.

It is also unknown whether the United States and Europe still dominate publication output in science [17,18] using the x-index [19] to measure, even though Australia and New Zealand have the highest rates of melanoma in the world [6]. The bibliometric x-index [19] (Figure 1), newly proposed in 2018, has a twofold implication. One is citation-oriented and another productivity-oriented. A graphical representation is required to complement the x-index and disclose the deeper insights and knowledge of the attribute toward the influential, the productive, or the neutral (or, say, one-dimensional performance in the Kano model) [19,20], which can be displayed by using the Kano model [21]. The five elements (ie, scatter plots based on the Kano model, x-index as the bubble, citations on the y-axis, publications on the x-axis, and the AWS) are worthy to carry out and demonstrate in this study.

The objectives of this study are to apply an AWS to quantify the credits for coauthors on an article byline and allocate the author weights to the country-level credits in articles. Three tasks will be achieved: (1) presenting country distribution for the first authors and the most popular journals, (2) showing choropleth maps to highlight the most influential countries, and (3) drawing scatter plots based on the Kano model to characterize the features of country-level research achievements.

Figure 1. Equation for the x-index.

$\sqrt{\max(i \times c_i)}$, where all c_i are sorted by article citations in descending order and i denotes the number of the individual author's publications

Methods

Data Source

We searched the PubMed database using the title keywords "skin cancer" on July 20, 2019. The search terms were the string "skin cancer" [Title/Abstract] AND ("1900" [Date-Publication]: "2018" [Date-Publication]); the process can be seen in a YouTube video [22]. A total of 17,975 articles published between 1945 and 2018 were extracted. Among these, 16,878 identified the nation/area of the first author (Figure 2).

We made an Excel Visual Basic for Applications (Microsoft Corp) module to handle the data. All downloaded abstracts met the requirement for the type of journal article. Others, like those marked with "Published Erratum," "Editorial," "conference abstracts," "commentary," or those that did not name the author's nation, were excluded from this study. Ethical approval was not necessary for this study as no human subjects or personal data were involved.

Figure 2. Flow diagram of study selection.

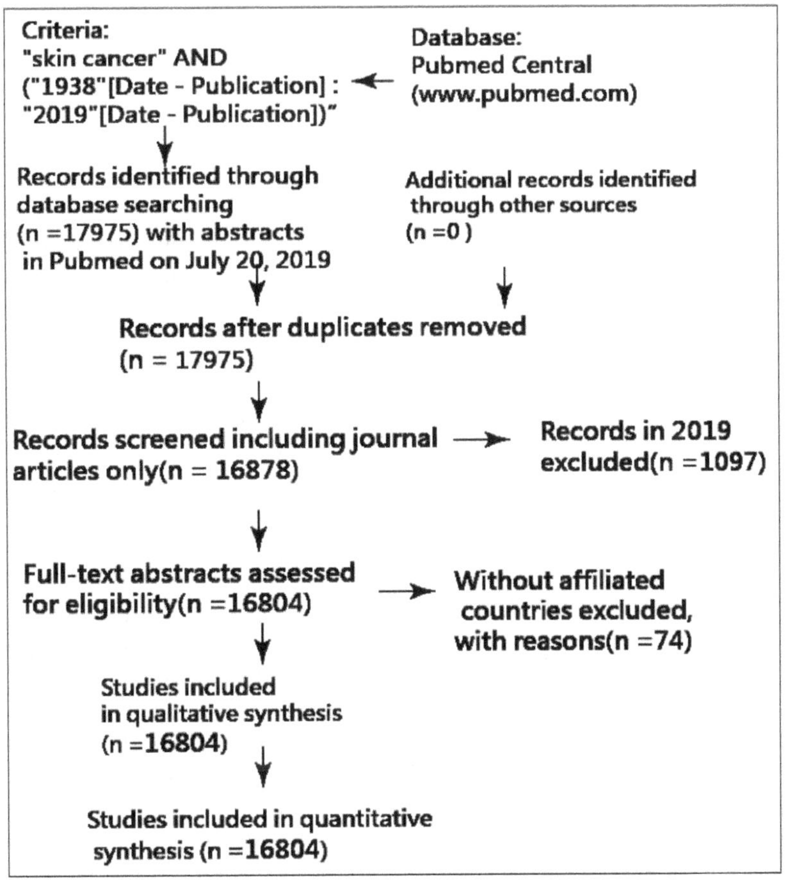

Seven Elements Used for Displaying Study Results

The seven elements are as follows:

1. Scatter plots were based on the Kano model.
2. Bubbles were sized by the x-index and colored by the types of research achievements.
3. Citations used for computing the x-index for countries were replaced with the journal impact factors (JIFs) published by inCites Journal Citation Reports (Clarivate Analytics) 2018. The JIFs were shown on the y-axis on the scatter plot mentioned above.
4. The number of publications for countries/areas was located on the x-axis.
5. We applied the AWS [23,24] as below.
6. See Figure 3, where the powers (m) as the ordered author name (m) on the article from m–1 to 0, the author number is m–1, more importance is given to the first (=exp[m–1], primary) and the last (=exp[m–1]_ as the corresponding or supervisory authors. We assume that the others (the middle authors) have made smaller contributions to their articles. The sum of all authors in an article byline equals 1.0.
7. The trend of publications for countries/areas was computed by the correlation coefficients using the correl(A,B) function in Excel (Microsoft Corp), where A denotes the series from 2009 to 2018 and B represents the outputs across the 10 years.

Figure 3. Author-weighted scheme equation.

$$W_m = \frac{\exp(\gamma_m)}{\sum_{m=0}^{m-1} \exp(\gamma_m)} = \frac{(2.27)^{\gamma_m}}{\sum_{m=0}^{m-1} \exp(\gamma_m)}$$

Tasks to Reach the Study Goal

Country-Level and Journal-Based Publications on Skin Cancer in the Past

We applied two contingency tables to represent the country distribution for the first authors and the most popular journals.

Choropleth Maps to Highlight the Most Influential Countries

A choropleth map was used to highlight the most influential countries/areas where authors were affiliated. The country-level citations were replaced by the JIF as seen in Figure 4, where the author weight came from Figure 1 and the total weights on an article for a country (*h*) are determined by the country-level weights on the article (*i*). The x-index (Figure 1) [19] was used to denote the research achievements for a country by the steps:

(1) sorting the country-based C_{hi} in Figure 4 and (2) determining the number of publications at i and the responding c_i. The countries were dispersed with bubbles sized by x-index and colored by the types of research achievements using the Kano model to display.

Figure 4. The equation used for computing the country-level citations.

$$C_{hi} = \sum_{m=0}^{m-1}(W_{h\epsilon m} \times c_i)$$

Scatter Plots to Characterize Types of Country Research Achievements

The scatter plot was based on the Kano model, which classified members on the plot into three types: the attribute toward the influential, the productive, or the neutral (or, say, one dimension along at the 45-degree line in the Kano model) [19,20].

Creating Dashboards on Google Maps

The x-index was yielded by author-made modules in Excel (Microsoft Corp). We created pages of HTML used for Google Maps. All relevant information on the entities (ie, countries or states in the United States) can be linked to dashboards on Google Maps.

Results

Distribution of Publications by Author-Affiliated Countries and Areas

Multimedia Appendix 1 presents 16,804 papers that included author-affiliated countries/areas. It is evident that researchers in the United States have published most frequently, accounting for 30.37% (5103), while German scholars account for 7.34% (1234), followed by Australia (997, 5.93%). The trend in the number of publications is presented at the bottom right (=1.0) of Multimedia Appendix 1, indicating a continuously increasing trend observed in this study. The three countries with the highest trends are Italy (0.98), China (0.97), and Germany (0.93).

The top three continents for the proportion of published articles are North America, Europe, and Asia, accounting for 32.29%, 31.71%, and 10.41%, respectively. Australia and New Zealand in the Oceania continent account for a mere 6.46% (see Multimedia Appendix 1), far behind the three continents of North America, Europe, and Asia.

Figure 5 displays a choropleth map based on the publications and first authors. Overall, the most influential countries/areas are the United States and Germany in Europe. Further information is available on the Google map [25] by clicking on each bubble. Another choropleth map (Figure 6) is also based on the publications and first authors in the United States as shown on the Google map [26]. We see that the three states with the highest x-indexes are California, Massachusetts, and New York.

Figure 5. Choropleth map presenting the most productive countries and areas of articles on skin cancer since 1938 (n=16,804).

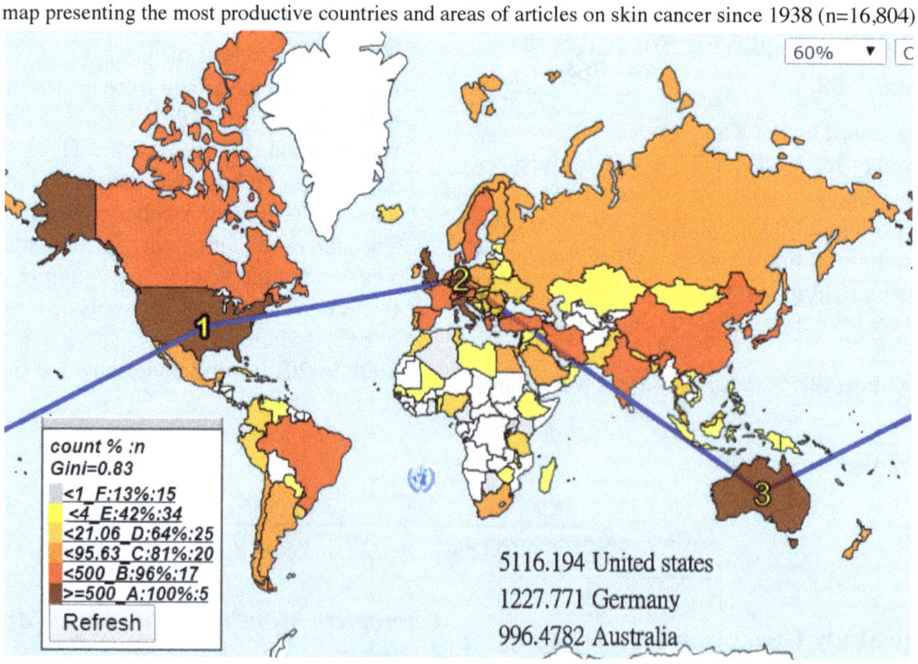

Figure 6. Choropleth map presenting the most productive states in the United States for articles on skin cancer since 1938 (n=5103).

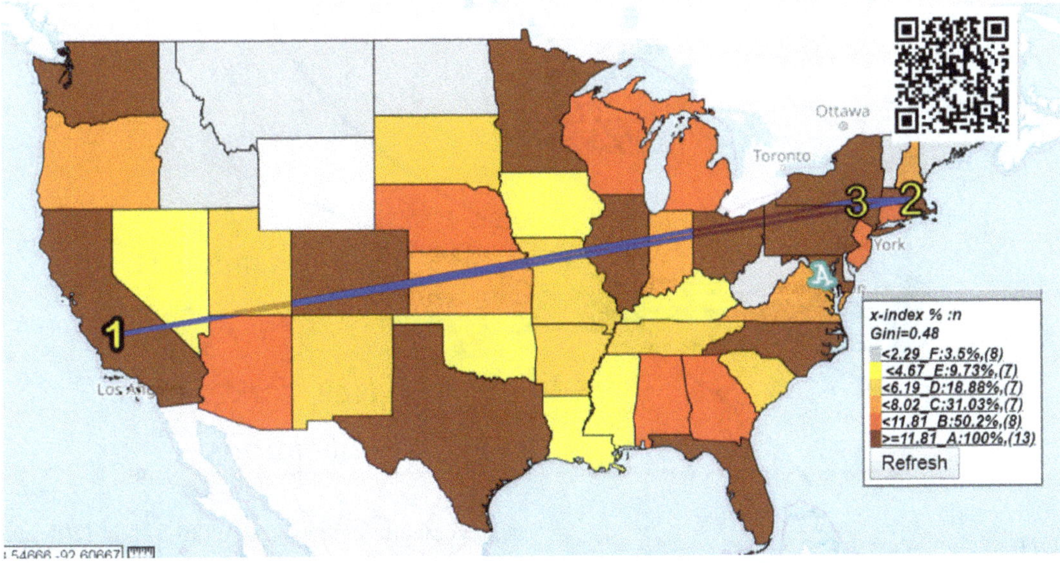

Published Papers in Journals

The top 20 journals with the highest numbers of publications on skin cancer are shown in Multimedia Appendix 2. The journals publishing the most articles on skin cancer are Journal of the American Academy of Dermatology, British Journal of Dermatology, and Journal of Investigative Dermatology. Journal of the European Academy of Dermatology and Venereology and JAMA Dermatology presented highly positive increases (>0.90 in trend) in the publication of papers on skin cancer (last column in Multimedia Appendix 2).

Scatter Plots to Characterize the Type of Country Research Achievements

Using the x-index [19] (Figure 1) makes it hard to discriminate the characteristics toward the influential, the productive, or the neutral. We applied the scatter plots based on the Kano model that can be easily used to identify the type for the country of interest.

We can see the United States is productivity-oriented and others are influence-oriented (Figure 7). As for states in the United States (Figure 8), both California and New York are productive. Massachusetts is neutral, and Minnesota is the influential type. Interested readers can scan the QR code in the figures for details about the name of the country (or state) on the dashboards.

Figure 7. Using the x-index to evaluate the achievements on skin cancer for different countries.

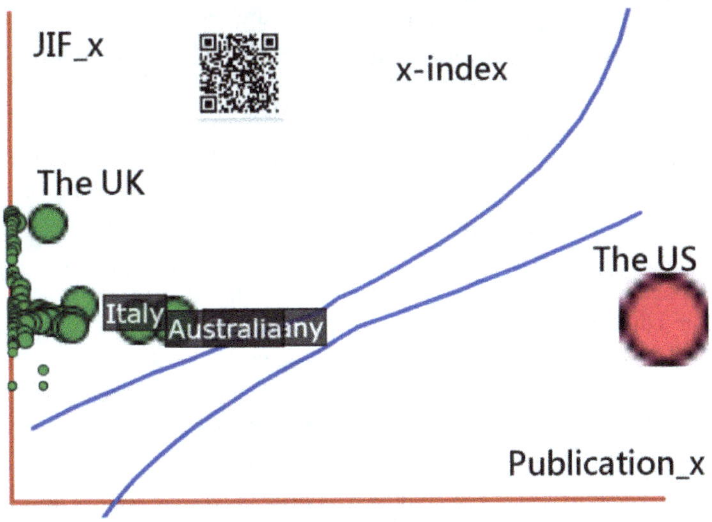

Figure 8. Using the x-index to evaluate the achievements on skin cancer for the United States.

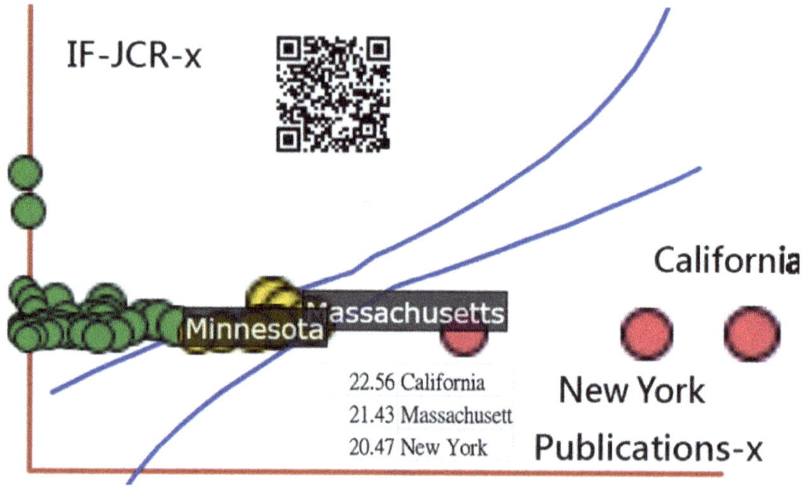

Discussion

Principal Findings

The research question in this study was to disclose the country-level research achievements on the topic of skin cancer. The AWS was particularly applied to quantify the credits for coauthors on articles and allocate the weights to the countries/areas using the equations in Figure 1 and Figure 3. Three tasks were achieved and illustrated: (1) the top three most productive countries are the United States, Germany, and Australia based on the countries to which the first authors are affiliated, (2) the journal with the most frequent publications is Journal of the American Academy of Dermatology, and (3) the top three influential countries are similar to the productive results. The correlation coefficient is 0.86 between the two indices (ie, the x-indexes and the number of publications [Multimedia Appendix 1]) around the 116 countries/areas, and the three types of entities in Figure 7 and 8 are toward the productive, the influential, and the neutral, respectively, using the Kano model to classify.

Previous research has investigated coauthor collaboration using social network analysis [27-29]. Our research using AWS weights is similar to the computation of degree centralities based on the weights between two entities in social network analysis but markedly different as we employ unique visual representations displayed on Google Maps. The application of this visual allows us to compare countries through bubbles in color and size. If the entity bubble is clicked on, the country information will appear on the map. This animated dashboard has been used in applications in other scientific fields to demonstrate entity characteristics [12,23,24].

A total of 16,804 abstracts were identified when searching PubMed on the keywords "skin cancer" on July 20, 2019. No previous literature uses the seven elements mentioned in Methods to present relevant knowledge to readers or dynamically applies Google Maps as we did in this study. Scientific publication is one of the objective measurements to evaluate the achievements of a medical specialty or discipline as we did in Multimedia Appendix 1. Numerous scientometrics have been proposed to measure author-level research achievements, such as h, g, e [30-32], h′ [20], and R- and AR indexes [32]. The drawback is those indices ignoring the AWS for quantifying coauthors' contributions in articles, not to mention the country-weighted scheme we applied in Figure 3. It is worth combining the seven elements and Google Maps to provide knowledge and information to the readership of journals in the future.

Strengths and Limitations

One strength of this study is the sophisticated use of Google Maps and in-text links for each topic [33-35]. Readers can manipulate the links independently to better understand author collaboration. The depiction of distribution by nation in figures is a useful feature to understand the research achievements on skin cancer. As it is said, a picture is worth a thousand words, so we hope future studies can report other types of information to readers using the Google application programing interface.

There are several limitations to this study. First, caution should be taken when interpreting and generalizing findings beyond this type of research, as data were extracted exclusively from PubMed.

Second, although the data were extracted from PubMed and carefully handled, the original download may have included errors, which may affect the resulting reports in this study.

Third, the formula (Figure 1) used in this study is also a special case of the general AWS model [23,24]. Any change in the parameters (eg, m in Figure 3) might present different weights for authors. Similarly, the assumption of corresponding (or supervisory) authors being the last authors might be challenged. Any parameters changed in our proposed formula would affect the computations of the metric.

Fourth, the data extracted from PubMed is different from other major citation databases such as the Scientific Citation Index (Clarivate Analytics) and Scopus (Elsevier). The results of the most influential countries/areas might be different if other databases were applied.

Fifth, the x-index [19] (Figure 1) is computed by both citations and publications. Replacing citations with the JIF to represent the quality of articles is another limitation. Although paper impact (ie, citations) and journal impact (ie, JIF) on researchers' performance are frequently related [36-39], applying citations to the x-index is recommended in future studies if citations for each article can be obtained.

Conclusion

In conclusion, this study offers an objective picture of the representativeness and evolution of international research on the topic of skin cancer by employing Google Maps to present results. We chose visualization technology to analyze country-level research achievements on skin cancer. As a result, researchers will be able to produce effective research diagrams on Google Maps, improve the efficiency of research work, and provide in-depth insight into the relationships among countries/areas and the types of their research achievements based on the Kano model. The results can provide readers with insight into the evolution of the skin cancer in publications across time and countries/areas.

Acknowledgments

We thank Coding Language Service for providing medical writing services on the manuscript.

Authors' Contributions

TWC conceived and designed the study, HYW interpreted the data, and FJL monitored the process and the manuscript. TWC drafted the manuscript. All authors read the manuscript and approved the final manuscript.

References

1. National Cancer Institute. Defining cancer URL: https://www.cancer.gov/about-cancer/understanding/what-is-cancer [accessed 2019-10-10]
2. National Cancer Institute. Skin cancer treatment URL: https://www.cancer.gov/types/skin/hp/skin-treatment-pdq#section/all [accessed 2019-10-10]
3. Gallagher RP, Lee TK, Bajdik CD, Borugian M. Ultraviolet radiation. Chronic Dis Can 2010;29 Suppl 1:51-68. [Medline: 21199599]
4. Maverakis E, Miyamura Y, Bowen MP, Correa G, Ono Y, Goodarzi H. Light, including ultraviolet. J Autoimmun 2010 May;34(3):J247-J257 [FREE Full text] [doi: 10.1016/j.jaut.2009.11.011] [Medline: 20018479]
5. Fabbrocini G, Triassi M, Mauriello MC, Torre G, Annunziata MC, De Vita V, et al. Epidemiology of skin cancer: role of some environmental factors. Cancers (Basel) 2010 Nov 24;2(4):1980-1989 [FREE Full text] [doi: 10.3390/cancers2041980] [Medline: 24281212]
6. McGuire S, World Health Organization, International Agency for Research on Cancer. World Cancer Report 2014. Adv Nutr 2016 Mar;7(2):418-419 [FREE Full text] [doi: 10.3945/an.116.012211] [Medline: 26980827]
7. Leiter U, Garbe C. Epidemiology of melanoma and nonmelanoma skin cancer—the role of sunlight. Adv Exp Med Biol 2008;624:89-103. [doi: 10.1007/978-0-387-77574-6_8] [Medline: 18348450]
8. Cakir B, Adamson P, Cingi C. Epidemiology and economic burden of nonmelanoma skin cancer. Facial Plast Surg Clin North Am 2012 Nov;20(4):419-422. [doi: 10.1016/j.fsc.2012.07.004] [Medline: 23084294]
9. Chiao EY, Krown SE. Update on non-acquired immunodeficiency syndrome-defining malignancies. Curr Opin Oncol 2003 Sep;15(5):389-397. [doi: 10.1097/00001622-200309000-00008] [Medline: 12960522]
10. Dubas LE, Ingraffea A. Nonmelanoma skin cancer. Facial Plast Surg Clin North Am 2013 Feb;21(1):43-53. [doi: 10.1016/j.fsc.2012.10.003] [Medline: 23369588]
11. Wu Y, Duan Z. Visualization analysis of author collaborations in schizophrenia research. BMC Psychiatry 2015 Feb 19;15:27 [FREE Full text] [doi: 10.1186/s12888-015-0407-z] [Medline: 25884451]
12. Chien T, Chang Y, Wang H. Understanding the productive author who published papers in medicine using National Health Insurance Database: a systematic review and meta-analysis. Medicine (Baltimore) 2018 Feb;97(8):e9967 [FREE Full text] [doi: 10.1097/MD.0000000000009967] [Medline: 29465594]
13. Dasgupta S, Vaughan AS, Kramer MR, Sanchez TH, Sullivan PS. Use of a Google Map tool embedded in an internet survey instrument: is it a valid and reliable alternative to geocoded address data? JMIR Res Protoc 2014;3(2):e24 [FREE Full text] [doi: 10.2196/resprot.2946] [Medline: 24726954]
14. Kobayashi S, Fujioka T, Tanaka Y, Inoue M, Niho Y, Miyoshi A. A geographical information system using the Google Map API for guidance to referral hospitals. J Med Syst 2010 Dec;34(6):1157-1160. [doi: 10.1007/s10916-009-9335-0] [Medline: 20703591]
15. Sekercioglu CH. Quantifying coauthor contributions. Science 2008 Oct 17;322(5900):371. [doi: 10.1126/science.322.5900.371a] [Medline: 18927373]

16. Vavryčuk V. Fair ranking of researchers and research teams. PLoS One 2018;13(4):e0195509 [FREE Full text] [doi: 10.1371/journal.pone.0195509] [Medline: 29621316]
17. Leydesdorff L, Wagner C, Park HW, Adams J. International collaboration in science: the global map and the network. 2013. URL: https://arxiv.org/pdf/1301.0801 [accessed 2019-10-10]
18. Glänzel W, Schlemmer B. National research profiles in a changing Europe (1983–2003): an exploratory study of sectoral characteristics in the Triple Helix. Scientometrics 2007 Feb;70(2):267-275. [doi: 10.1007/s11192-007-0203-8]
19. Fenner T, Harris M, Levene M, Bar-Ilan J. A novel bibliometric index with a simple geometric interpretation. PLoS One 2018;13(7):e0200098 [FREE Full text] [doi: 10.1371/journal.pone.0200098] [Medline: 29990357]
20. Zhang C. The h′-index, effectively improving the h-index based on the citation distribution. PLoS One 2013;8(4):e59912 [FREE Full text] [doi: 10.1371/journal.pone.0059912] [Medline: 23565174]
21. Kano N, Seraku N, Takahashi F, Tsuji S. Attractive quality and must-be quality. J Jap Soc Qual Cont 1984;14(2):39-48.
22. Kanomodel. URL: https://youtu.be/Ic9ixWxSfAc [accessed 2019-11-24]
23. Chien T, Chow JC, Chang Y, Chou W. Applying Gini coefficient to evaluate the author research domains associated with the ordering of author names: a bibliometric study. Medicine (Baltimore) 2018 Sep;97(39):e12418 [FREE Full text] [doi: 10.1097/MD.0000000000012418] [Medline: 30278518]
24. Chien T, Wang H, Chang Y, Kan W. Using Google Maps to display the pattern of coauthor collaborations on the topic of schizophrenia: a systematic review between 1937 and 2017. Schizophr Res 2019 Feb;204:206-213. [doi: 10.1016/j.schres.2018.09.015] [Medline: 30262255]
25. Chien T. Google Maps for author nationality on skin cancer. URL: http://www.healthup.org.tw/gps/dermatologycancer.htm [accessed 2019-10-10]
26. Chien T. Google Maps for author in the US on skin cancer. URL: http://www.healthup.org.tw/gps/dermatologycancerUS.htm [accessed 2019-10-10]
27. Sadoughi F, Valinejadi A, Shirazi MS, Khademi R. Social network analysis of Iranian researchers on medical parasitology: a 41 year co-authorship survey. Iran J Parasitol 2016;11(2):204-212 [FREE Full text] [Medline: 28096854]
28. Osareh F, Khademi R, Rostami MK, Shirazi MS. Co-authorship network structure analysis of Iranian researchers' scientific outputs from 1991 to 2013 based on the Social Science Citation Index (SSCI). Collnet J Scientometr Info Manag 2015 Feb 10;8(2):263-271. [doi: 10.1080/09737766.2014.1015301]
29. Liu X, Bollen J, Nelson ML, Van de Sompel H. Co-authorship networks in the digital library research community. Info Process Manag 2005 Dec;41(6):1462-1480. [doi: 10.1016/j.ipm.2005.03.012]
30. Hirsch JE. An index to quantify an individual's scientific research output. Proc Natl Acad Sci USA 2005 Nov 15;102(46):16569-16572 [FREE Full text] [doi: 10.1073/pnas.0507655102] [Medline: 16275915]
31. Egghe L, Rousseau R, Van Hooydonk G. Methods for accrediting publications to authors or countries: consequences for evaluation studies. J Am Soc Info Sci 2000;51(2):145-157. [doi: 10.1002/(sici)1097-4571(2000)51:2<145::aid-asi6>3.0.co;2-9]
32. Jin B, Liang L, Rousseau R, Egghe L. The R- and AR-indices: complementing the h-index. Chinese Sci Bull 2007 Mar;52(6):855-863. [doi: 10.1007/s11434-007-0145-9]
33. Zhang C. The e-index, complementing the h-index for excess citations. PLoS One 2009;4(5):e5429 [FREE Full text] [doi: 10.1371/journal.pone.0005429] [Medline: 19415119]
34. Gini C. [Concentration and dependency ratios]. English translation in Rivista di Politica Economica 1997;87:769-789.
35. Kendall MG, Smith BB. The problem of m rankings. Ann Math Statist 1939 Sep;10(3):275-287. [doi: 10.1214/aoms/1177732186]
36. Bornmann L, Haunschild R. Plots for visualizing paper impact and journal impact of single researchers in a single graph. Scientometrics 2018;115(1):385-394 [FREE Full text] [doi: 10.1007/s11192-018-2658-1] [Medline: 29527073]
37. Bornmann L, Daniel H. What do citation counts measure? A review of studies on citing behavior. J Documentat 2008 Jan 18;64(1):45-80. [doi: 10.1108/00220410810844150]
38. Onodera N, Yoshikane F. Factors affecting citation rates of research articles. J Assn Inf Sci Tec 2014 May 21;66(4):739-764. [doi: 10.1002/asi.23209]
39. Tahamtan I, Safipour Afshar A, Ahamdzadeh K. Factors affecting number of citations: a comprehensive review of the literature. Scientometrics 2016 Feb 15;107(3):1195-1225. [doi: 10.1007/s11192-016-1889-2]

Abbreviations

AWS: author-weighted scheme
JIF: journal impact factor

Comparing Risk Profiles in Critical Care Patients with Stage 2 and Deep Tissue Pressure Injuries: Exploratory Retrospective Cohort Study

Jenny Alderden[1], PhD; Linda Amoafo[1], MSTAT; Yue Zhang[1], MSTAT, PhD; Caroline Fife[2], MD; David Yap[1]; Tracey Yap[3], PhD

[1]University of Utah, Salt Lake City, UT, United States
[2]Intellicure, Inc, The Woodlands, TX, United States
[3]Duke University, Durham, NC, United States

Corresponding Author:
Jenny Alderden, PhD
University of Utah
10 S 2000 E
Salt Lake City, UT, 84112
United States

Email: jenny.alderden@utah.edu

Abstract

Background: Understanding hospital-acquired pressure injury (HAPrI) etiology is essential for developing effective preventive interventions. Pressure injuries are classified based on the degree of visible tissue damage; the two most commonly identified HAPrI stages in critical care patients are stage 2 and deep tissue injury (DTI). Some experts speculate that stage 2 and DTI have different etiologies, with stage 2 injuries formed from the "outside in" as a result of tissue deformation, decreased perfusion, and subsequent ischemia caused by external pressure and/or shear forces, whereas DTI emerges from the "inside out" due to inadequate perfusion to the deeper tissues causing tissue ischemia.

Objective: The purpose of this study was to compare risk profiles of intensive care unit (ICU) patients who developed stage 2 injuries versus DTIs.

Methods: This was a retrospective cohort study to compare the risk profiles of patients in the ICU with stage 2 injuries and DTIs using electronic health record data. Eligible patients were admitted to the surgical or cardiovascular ICU at an academic medical center in the United States between 2014 and 2018. Anatomic locations were examined, and differences in anatomic patterns were compared using the χ^2 test. Risk profile variables included demographic characteristics, Braden Scale scores, vasopressor infusions, hypotension, surgical factors, length of stay, BMI, laboratory values, diabetes, Charlson Comorbidity Index, and the levels of sedation or agitation. The distributions of potential risk variables between patients with stage 2 injuries and DTIs were summarized and compared. A logistic regression model with the least absolute shrinkage and selection operator method was developed to identify the critical risk factors for distinguishing stage 2 and DTI patients.

Results: A total of 244 patients developed a stage 2 injury or DTI during the study period. Of those, 38 patients with medical device–related pressure injury were excluded. The final study sample consisted of 206 patients (n=146 stage 2 and n=60 DTI). Compared with DTIs, stage 2 HAPrIs were more likely to be located on a bony prominence (n=206, χ^2_1=8.43, *P*=.03). The multivariate model showed that patients who developed stage 2 HAPrIs had a longer length of stay in the ICU than those with DTIs (odds ratio [OR] 1.001, 95% CI 1-1.002, *P*=.03) but were less likely than patients with DTIs to experience a diastolic blood pressure <50 mmHg (OR 0.179, 95% CI 0.072-0.416, *P*<.001) or receive an epinephrine infusion (OR 0.316, 95% CI 0.079-0.525, *P*=.008).

Conclusions: Stage 2 injuries and DTIs have different risk factors and different anatomic patterns. Patients who developed DTIs were more likely to experience low diastolic blood pressure and receive epinephrine, a potent vasopressor. Stage 2 injuries were more likely to occur on the bony prominences, whereas DTIs commonly occurred on the fleshy parts of the body such as the buttock.

KEYWORDS

pressure ulcer; pressure injury; critical care; intensive care; hospital-acquired pressure injury; tissue damage; electronic health records; EHRs

Introduction

The United States has an estimated cost burden exceeding US $26 billion for hospital-acquired pressure injury (HAPrI) treatment [1], although these injuries are considered to be mainly preventable. The prevailing belief about the development of HAPrIs is that a localized injury occurs to an area of the skin and underlying tissue—usually over a bony prominence—as a result of external pressure and sometimes shear forces, along with additional factors that have yet to be elucidated [2]. Patients admitted to the intensive care unit (ICU) are more likely than other hospitalized patients to experience hemodynamic instability and hypotension; in fact, their risk tends to double [3] given a constellation of other factors such as longer length of stay [4,5], surgical factors [6], vasopressor infusions [7,8] older age [9], increased severity of illness [10], and decreased mobility [8,9].

Understanding the etiology of HAPrI is foundational for developing effective preventive interventions. The National Pressure Injury Advisory Panel and the European Pressure Ulcer Advisory Panel provide a pressure injury (PrI) classification staging system (stages 1-4, deep tissue injury [DTI], and unstageable) along with common descriptions of the extent of the visible skin and tissue damage for the purpose of clinical practice, audits, and research [2]. Stage 2 and DTI, the two most commonly occurring injuries within the classification system, appear to be markedly different: stage 2 injuries are generally shallow ulcers, whereas DTIs present as discolored intact skin as a result of damage to the underlying tissue. Some experts speculate that stage 2 injuries and those considered to be DTIs have different etiologies, with stage 2 injuries forming from the "outside in" as a result of tissue deformation, decreased perfusion, and subsequent ischemia caused by external pressure and/or shear forces, whereas DTIs emerge from the "inside out" due to inadequate perfusion to the deeper tissues causing tissue ischemia [11]. If a stage 2 injury occurs from the "outside in" and a DTI forms from the "inside out," it is likely that ICU patients with a DTI would experience more perfusion-related risk factors. Therefore, the purpose of this study was to compare the risk profiles of ICU patients who developed stage 2 injuries and DTIs.

Methods

Design

This was a retrospective cohort study of electronic health record (EHR) data to establish risk factor profiles of ICU patients comparing stage 2 injuries and DTIs. The institutional review board of the University of Utah approved the study (IRB_00111380).

Sample and Setting

Eligible patients were those who were admitted to the surgical or cardiovascular ICU at an academic medical center in the United States between 2014 and 2018. Inclusion criteria were age >18 years and development of a nonmedical device–related stage 2 injury or DTI during the ICU stay. Exclusion criteria were pediatric patients (<18 years old) and the absence of an ICU-acquired stage 2 injury or DTI. Patients with a medical device–related PrI were included in the study only if they also developed a nonmedical device–related PrI of stage 2 or a DTI [12]. Patients with PrI present on admission to the ICU were only included in the study if they also subsequently developed an ICU-acquired PrI.

Critical care nurses at this institution conduct a head-to-toe skin assessment each shift and document results in the EHR, noting the location and stage of any HAPrI, which is then confirmed by a certified wound care nurse. Patients unable to reposition independently are repositioned every 2 hours, and skincare protocols are employed to encourage nurses to keep the skin as clean and dry as possible. All of the ICU beds are pressure redistribution/low air loss beds; bariatric pressure redistribution/low air loss beds are used for patients with obesity.

Data Collection

Data were obtained using a combination of a query of the institution's critical-care datamart cross-referenced with data maintained by the institution's quality department, along with a manual review of the EPIC EHR system when necessary. Data extracted were limited to the first ICU stay for patients with multiple ICU stays. To capture HAPrI risk factors, only data from the timeframe between ICU admission and HAPrI detection were included.

Measures

Stage 2 injury and DTI were defined according to the National Pressure Injury Advisory Panel definitions [13]; a PrI was considered to be hospital-acquired if it was detected ≥48 hours after admission. The anatomic location was recorded from structured fields in the EHR and also verified with photographic evidence when available. Risk profile variables included demographic characteristics [14], Braden Scale scores [15], vasopressor infusions [7], hypotension [16], surgical factors [6,16,17], length of stay [5,18], BMI [19], laboratory values [16], diabetes [4], Charlson Comorbidity Index (categorizing comorbidities of the patients' disease burden and their 1-year mortality risk) [20], and the Riker score (levels of sedation or agitation) [21].

Analysis

All statistical analyses were performed in R version 3.6.1. (R Foundation for Statistical Computing). First, the distributions of potential risk variables between patients with stage 2 injuries and DTIs were summarized and compared using t tests (or

Wilcoxon rank-sum tests) for continuous variables and with the χ^2 test (or Fisher exact test) for categorical variables. Variance inflation factors (VIFs) were calculated to detect if multicollinearity was present among the list of potential predictors. If none of the potential predictors had a VIF exceeding 5, we treated all predictors as independent predictors. We employed a logistic regression model with the least absolute shrinkage and selection operator (LASSO) method [22] to identify the critical risk factors for distinguishing stage 2 injury and DTI patients.

Unlike other variable selection approaches—such as the stepwise approach—the LASSO approach does not select important risk factors based on *P* values. Instead, by imposing a penalty in the regression model fitting, the LASSO approach shrinks the coefficients of unimportant predictors to zero while retaining the important coefficients [22]. The optimal penalty term was determined using 10-fold cross-validation criteria; the predictor was selected if, and only if, its coefficient was nonzero. The final model included all important predictors with parsimonious representation, enhanced interpretability, and improved precision. From the soft-thresholding property of LASSO in generalized linear regression models, the estimated regression coefficients from the penalized logistic regression were biased toward zero. To mitigate these bias problems, we report a more unbiased estimation of the regression coefficients from unpenalized logistic regression using the selected factors from the LASSO.

Results

A total of 244 patients developed a stage 2 injury or DTI during the study period. Of those, 38 patients with a medical device–related PrI were excluded. The final study sample consisted of 206 patients (n=146 stage 2 and n=60 DTI). Univariate relationships between study variables and HAPrI stage are presented in Table 1. The multivariate model for the effects of risk profiles on stage 2 versus DTI development is presented in Table 2.

Compared with DTIs, stage 2 HAPrIs were more likely to be located on a bony prominence (n=206, χ^2_1=8.43, *P*=.03). Among the 146 stage 2 HAPrIs, 93 (63.7%) were located on the sacrum or the coccyx and 11 (7.5%) were located on other bony prominences (ischium, heel, or spine). Among the 60 DTIs, 30 (50%) were found on a bony prominence (sacrum, coccyx, ischium, heel, or spine), whereas the other 30 (50%) occurred on fleshy parts of the body, particularly the buttock (n=23, 38%).

Table 1. Risk factor profiles in stage 2 and deep tissue hospital-acquired pressure injury.

Variable	Stage 2 injury (n=146)	Deep tissue injury (n=60)	*P* value
Demographic factors			
Age (years), mean (SD)	57.5 (16.4)	57.5 (14.0)	.99[a]
Sex (male), n (%)	86 (58.9)	43 (71.7)	.09[b]
Race (White), n (%)	117 (80.1)	48 (80.0)	.98[b]
Ethnicity (Non-Hispanic), n (%)	123 (84.2)	50 (83.3)	.87[b]
Hospital length of stay (days), mean (SD)	31 (23)	28 (19)	.52[c]
ICU[d] length of stay (days), mean (SD)	20 (18)	18 (18)	.35[c]
Surgical factors, mean (SD)			
Longest surgery (hours)	3 (3)	5 (4)	<.001[c]
Total surgical time (hours)	6 (4)	4 (5)	.001[c]
Laboratory values, mean (SD)			
Minimum albumin (g/dl)	2.7 (0.7)	2.6 (0.5)	.23[a]
Minimum hemoglobin (g/dl)	7.5 (2.1)	7.4 (2.2)	.76[a]
Maximum lactate (mmol/l)	7.3 (6.0)	5.1 (4.1)	.008[c]
Maximum creatinine mg/dL	2.9 (2.1)	2.9 (2.2)	.78[c]
Blood pressure, n (%)			
Systolic <90 mmHg	120 (82.2)	54 (90.0)	.16[b]
MAP[e] <60 mmHg	99 (67.8)	43 (71.7)	.59[b]
Diastolic <50 mmHg	60 (41.1)	44 (73.3)	<.001[b]
Epinephrine	49 (33.6)	40 (66.7)	<.001[b]
Norepinephrine	71 (48.6)	33 (55.0)	.41[b]
Dopamine	12 (8.2)	2 (3.3)	.36[f]
Vasopressin	63 (43.2)	41 (68.3)	.001[b]
Phenylephrine	8 (5.5)	3 (5.0)	.99[b]
Diagnosis and comorbidities			
Charlson Comorbidity Index, mean (SD)	4.3 (2.9)	4.5 (2.7)	.53[c]
Diabetes, n (%)	28 (19.2)	14 (23.3)	.50[b]
Minimum Braden scale score, mean (SD)	11.1 (3.0)	11.5 (2.8)	.32[c]
Minimum Riker score, mean (SD)	2.2 (1.2)	1.8 (1.0)	.08[c]

[a]Based on the *t* test.

[b]Based on the χ^2 test.

[c]Based on the Wilcoxon rank-sum test.

[d]ICU: intensive care unit.

[e]MAP: mean arterial pressure.

[f]Based on the Fisher exact test.

Table 2. Logistic regression model for stage 2 vs deep tissue injury after least absolute shrinkage and selection operator variable selection.

Variable	Odds ratio	95% CI	*P* value
Sex (reference: male)	0.335	0.14-0.755	.11
Hospital length of stay (days)	1.001	1-1.002	.03
Longest surgery (hours)	0.998	0.996-1	.06
Minimum albumin (g/dl)	0.696	0.353-1.351	.29
Diastolic blood pressure <50 mmHg	0.179	0.072-0.416	<.001
Epinephrine	0.316	0.079-0.525	.008
Dopamine	4.277	0.836-33.803	.11

Discussion

Principal Findings

This exploratory study investigated differences in risk factors and anatomic patterns between surgical and cardiovascular ICU patients who developed stage 2 injuries vs DTIs. Understanding HAPrI risk factors and the associated etiology is essential for developing effective prevention approaches. It is possible that etiological differences exist between different PrI stages, with stage 2 PrI resulting primarily from external pressure and/or shearing forces affecting perfusion to the superficial tissues and DTI resulting from inadequate blood flow (perfusion) to the deeper tissues [23]. ICU patients are an ideal population for studying perfusion in relation to HAPrIs because they are more likely to experience hypotension and hemodynamic instability.

In this exploratory study, low diastolic blood pressure had the strongest correlation with the development of a DTI. This finding is consistent with a prior study aimed at identifying risk factors for DTI in ICU patients [16], which found that for every 1 mmHg decrease in diastolic blood pressure, the odds of a DTI increased by about 8%. Considering that the heart is in diastole about 2/3 of the time (and in systole 1/3 of the time), it is logical that inadequate diastolic blood pressure is a significant factor contributing to tissue perfusion.

The finding that epinephrine, a potent vasopressor, was associated with DTI is further evidence for the importance of tissue perfusion in DTI etiology. Vasopressor drugs are administered to improve organ perfusion in patients with hypotension; however, the alpha-adrenergic properties of certain vasopressors, including epinephrine, cause arterial vasoconstriction and therefore decrease blood flow to the vessels in the muscles and peripheral tissues. Although it is well established that vasopressor drugs are risk factors for HAPrI, likely as a result of their indication (severe illness and hypotension) and the mechanism of action (arterial vasoconstriction) [8,9,24], this is the first study to examine vasopressors in relation to HAPrI stage.

This study showed that stage 2 HAPrIs were more likely than DTIs to be located on a bony prominence, whereas DTIs were mostly located on the fleshy parts of the body (primarily the buttock). This finding has important clinical implications for routine nursing care because routine skin assessment usually involves checking the bony prominences and not the fleshy areas [2]. Therefore, the fleshy areas, particularly the buttock, should be included in routine nursing skin assessments.

The differences in anatomic patterns, with stage 2 injuries mostly occurring on the bony prominences and DTIs mainly occurring on the fleshy areas, suggest a potential etiological difference between stage 2 injuries and DTIs. Stage 2 HAPrIs are likely primarily caused by pressure (tissue compression) between a surface (eg, a bed) and a bony prominence, or pressure combined with shear force [2]. However, fleshy areas are typically not exposed to significant external pressure, and therefore an "inside-out" etiology driven by perfusion should be considered [11,16,24].

Limitations

The study is limited by its small sample size, and therefore the results are considered exploratory. We were limited to the data contained in the EHR, and consequently unable to accurately obtain variables difficult to capture retrospectively, such as repositioning frequency. Moreover, these data are based on a single study site and therefore may not be generalizable to other institutions.

Conclusion

Results from this exploratory study performed in surgical and cardiovascular ICU patients showed that deep tissue and stage 2 HAPrIs have different risk factors and different anatomic patterns. Patients who developed DTIs were more likely than patients with stage 2 HAPrIs to experience low diastolic blood pressure and to have received epinephrine, a potent vasopressor. Stage 2 HAPrIs were more likely to occur on the bony prominences, whereas DTIs commonly occurred on the fleshy parts of the body such as the buttock. Future research is needed to elucidate the detailed etiologic differences between stages, which will lead to identifying effective preventive interventions.

Acknowledgments

The authors wish to thank Kendall Varin, BA, for her assistance in editing this manuscript.

References

1. Padula WV, Delarmente BA. The national cost of hospital-acquired pressure injuries in the United States. Int Wound J 2019 Jun 28;16(3):634-640 [FREE Full text] [doi: 10.1111/iwj.13071] [Medline: 30693644]
2. European Pressure Ulcer Advisory Panel, National Pressure Injury Advisory Panel, and Pan Pacific Pressure Injury Alliance. In: Haesler E, editor. Prevention and treatment of pressure ulcers/injuries: clinical practice guideline. The International Guideline: EPUAP/NPIAP/PPPIA; 2019.
3. Baumgarten M, Margolis DJ, Localio AR, Kagan SH, Lowe RA, Kinosian B, et al. Extrinsic risk factors for pressure ulcers early in the hospital stay: a nested case-control study. J Gerontol A Biol Sci Med Sci 2008 Apr 01;63(4):408-413 [FREE Full text] [doi: 10.1093/gerona/63.4.408] [Medline: 18426965]
4. Cox J. Pressure injury risk factors in adult critical care patients: a review of the literature. Ostomy Wound Manage 2017 Nov;63(11):30-43 [FREE Full text] [Medline: 29166261]
5. Alderden J, Cowan L, Dimas J, Chen D, Zhang Y, Cummins M, et al. Risk factors for hospital-acquired pressure injury in surgical critical care patients. Am J Crit Care 2020 Nov 01;29(6):e128-e134. [doi: 10.4037/ajcc2020810] [Medline: 33130863]
6. Chen H, Chen X, Wu J. The incidence of pressure ulcers in surgical patients of the last 5 years: a systematic review. Wounds 2012 Sep;24(9):234-241. [Medline: 25874704]
7. Cox J. Pressure ulcer development and vasopressor agents in adult critical care patients: a literature review. Ostomy Wound Manage 2013 Apr;59(4):50-56 [FREE Full text] [Medline: 23562874]
8. Alderden J, Rondinelli J, Pepper G, Cummins M, Whitney J. Risk factors for pressure injuries among critical care patients: A systematic review. Int J Nurs Stud 2017 Jun;71:97-114 [FREE Full text] [doi: 10.1016/j.ijnurstu.2017.03.012] [Medline: 28384533]
9. Lima Serrano M, González Méndez M, Carrasco Cebollero F, Lima Rodríguez J. Risk factors for pressure ulcer development in Intensive Care Units: A systematic review. Medicina Intensiva 2017 Aug;41(6):339-346. [doi: 10.1016/j.medine.2017.04.006]
10. Manzano F, Pérez-Pérez AM, Martínez-Ruiz S, Garrido-Colmenero C, Roldan D, Jiménez-Quintana MDM, et al. Hospital-acquired pressure ulcers and risk of hospital mortality in intensive care patients on mechanical ventilation. J Eval Clin Pract 2014 Aug 22;20(4):362-368. [doi: 10.1111/jep.12137] [Medline: 24854297]
11. Yap TL, Alderden J, Lewis M, Taylor K, Fife CE. Angiosomal vascular occlusions, deep-tissue pressure injuries, and competing theories: a case report. Adv Skin Wound Care 2021;34(3):157-164. [doi: 10.1097/01.asw.0000732804.13066.30]
12. Barakat-Johnson M, Lai M, Wand T, Li M, White K, Coyer F. The incidence and prevalence of medical device-related pressure ulcers in intensive care: a systematic review. J Wound Care 2019 Aug 02;28(8):512-521. [doi: 10.12968/jowc.2019.28.8.512] [Medline: 31393800]
13. Edsberg L, Black J, Goldberg M, McNichol L, Moore L, Sieggreen M. Revised National Pressure Ulcer Advisory Panel Pressure Injury Staging System: Revised Pressure Injury Staging System. J Wound Ostomy Continence Nurs 2016;43(6):585-597 [FREE Full text] [doi: 10.1097/WON.0000000000000281] [Medline: 27749790]
14. Strazzieri-Pulido KC, S González CV, Nogueira PC, Padilha KG, G Santos VLC. Pressure injuries in critical patients: Incidence, patient-associated factors, and nursing workload. J Nurs Manag 2019 Mar 20;27(2):301-310. [doi: 10.1111/jonm.12671] [Medline: 30238676]
15. Bergstrom N, Braden BJ, Laguzza A, Holman V. The Braden Scale for predicting pressure sore risk. Nurs Res 1987;36(4):205-210. [doi: 10.1097/00006199-198707000-00002]
16. Kirkland-Kyhn H, Teleten O, Wilson M. A retrospective, descriptive, comparative study to identify patient variables that contribute to the development of deep tissue injury among patients in intensive care units. Ostomy Wound Manage 2017 Feb;63(2):42-47 [FREE Full text] [Medline: 28267682]
17. Shen W, Chen H, Xu Y, Zhang Q, Wu J. The relationship between length of surgery and the incidence of pressure ulcers in cardiovascular surgical patients: a retrospective study. Adv Skin Wound Care 2015 Oct;28(10):444-450. [doi: 10.1097/01.ASW.0000466365.90534.b0] [Medline: 26375947]
18. Tayyib N, Coyer F, Lewis P. Saudi Arabian adult intensive care unit pressure ulcer incidence and risk factors: a prospective cohort study. Int Wound J 2016 Oct 09;13(5):912-919 [FREE Full text] [doi: 10.1111/iwj.12406] [Medline: 25662591]
19. Cowan L, Broderick V, Alderden JG. Pressure injury prevention considerations for older adults. Crit Care Nurs Clin North Am 2020 Dec;32(4):601-609. [doi: 10.1016/j.cnc.2020.08.009] [Medline: 33129417]
20. de Almeida Medeiros AB, da Conceição Dias Fernandes MI, de Sá Tinôco JD, Cossi MS, de Oliveira Lopes MV, de Carvalho Lira ALB. Predictors of pressure ulcer risk in adult intensive care patients: A retrospective case-control study. Intensive Crit Care Nurs 2018 Apr;45:6-10. [doi: 10.1016/j.iccn.2017.09.007] [Medline: 29223413]
21. Cox J, Roche S, Murphy V. Pressure injury risk factors in critical care patients: a descriptive analysis. Adv Skin Wound Care 2018 Jul;31(7):328-334. [doi: 10.1097/01.ASW.0000534699.50162.4e] [Medline: 29923903]
22. Tibshirani R. Regression shrinkage and selection via the lasso. J R Stat Soc B 2018 Dec 05;58(1):267-288. [doi: 10.1111/j.2517-6161.1996.tb02080.x]

23. Fife CE, Gkotsoulias E. On the origin of intraoperative pressure injury: an angiosomal theory of pressure injury formation. Adv Wound Care 2019 Nov 01;8(11):580-584 [FREE Full text] [doi: 10.1089/wound.2018.0905] [Medline: 31832271]
24. Cox J, Roche S. Vasopressors and development of pressure ulcers in adult critical care patients. Am J Crit Care 2015 Nov;24(6):501-510. [doi: 10.4037/ajcc2015123] [Medline: 26523008]

Abbreviations

DTI: deep tissue injury
EHR: electronic health record
HAPrI: hospital-acquired pressure injury
ICU: intensive care unit
LASSO: least absolute shrinkage and selection operator
PrI: pressure injury
VIF: variance inflation factor

22

Patient Factors Associated with Interest in Teledermatology

Maham Ghani[1*], BSc; Colin Adler[2*], MPH; Howa Yeung[2,3], MD, MSc

[1]City University of New York School of Medicine, City University of New York, New york, NY, United States
[2]Department of Dermatology, Emory University School of Medicine, Emory University, Atlanta, GA, United States
[3]Regional Telehealth Service, Veterans Affairs Veterans Integrated Service Network 7, Decatur, GA, United States
[*]these authors contributed equally

Corresponding Author:
Howa Yeung, MD, MSc
Department of Dermatology, Emory University School of Medicine
Emory University
1525 Clifton Rd NE Suite 100
Atlanta, GA, 30322
United States

Email: howa.yeung@emory.edu

Abstract

Background: Teledermatology is a conduit for patients communicating with dermatologists on the internet, which bypasses in-person visits. It holds promise to address access needs for dermatologic care; however, the interest in using teledermatology is unknown in underserved populations with potential barriers to the use of health care technology.

Objective: This study aimed to characterize the association between demographic characteristics with interest in exchanging digital images or videos of skin lesions with health care providers electronically.

Methods: We examined data from the Health Information National Trends Survey (HINTS) 4 cycle 4 (2014) of the National Cancer Institute. HINTS is a cross-sectional, nationally representative household survey conducted annually, which collects information on demographics, perceptions and use of health information, and provides information on how cancer risks are perceived. HINTS 4 cycle 4 had a sample of 3677 participants. We examined the outcome to the question, "how interested are you in exchanging digital images or videos (eg, photos of skin lesions) with a health care provider electronically?" We dichotomized the outcome by a high level of interest (responding with "very") and those who did not have a high level of interest (responding with "somewhat," "a little," or "not at all") in exchanging images or videos. We used a multivariable logistic regression model developed through backwards selection, with all final covariates associated with varying levels of teledermatology use at $P<.05$. Sensitivity analysis was performed by changing the outcome dichotomy to model those who were "not at all" interested. Two-sided tests were performed with $P<.05$ considered significant.

Results: Among 3447 respondents, 888 (weighted prevalence=26.2%) were "very" interested in participating in teledermatology. A higher interest in using teledermatology was associated with a younger age, higher educational attainment, higher household income, internet usage, type of mobile device ownership, history of electronic medical information exchange with a clinician within the past 12 months, and high level of trust in web-based information on cancer (for all, $P<.01$), but not with the female gender, race or ethnicity, health insurance status, or having a regular medical provider.

Conclusions: Modifiable access barriers to teledermatology adoption include trust, experience with teledermatology, and use of health apps. Teledermatology program implementation should address these specific factors within the digital divide to promote equitable access to care across diverse patient populations.

KEYWORDS

digital divide; e-health literacy; Internet; modifiable behaviors; teledermatology

Introduction

Teledermatology is a conduit for patients communicating with dermatologists on the internet, which bypasses in-person visits. It can occur through a live videoconferencing or by sending photographs for asynchronous review [1]. Patients may work with their general practitioners (GP) to contact a dermatologist via telehealth, or they can initiate the interaction themselves directly [2]. With evolving technology, camera phones can click photographs of sufficient quality to meet teledermatology standards, with potential for broad patient adoption without facilitation from an intermediary GP [2]. Implementation of teledermatology has recently been accelerated during the 2020 COVID-19 pandemic [3].

Teledermatology has the ability to increase medical care access to diverse populations at reduced costs and wait times [1,4]. High levels of concordance in diagnosis have been noted between teledermatology and in-person consultations [5]. However, there remains a knowledge gap in the characteristics of patients who use teledermatology. Previous studies suggest that demographics such as young age, high income, and high educational status are correlated with increased eHealth literacy, which refers to the ability to search, obtain, and understand web-based health information [6], as well as increased health app usage [7] and communication with physicians on the internet [8]. However, these studies did not explore the factors that influence patient interest in participating specifically in teledermatology.

Consideration of the identified characteristics of individuals who are less interested in using teledermatology in the context of the digital divide has implications for health equity as teledermatology expands. The digital divide encompasses a broad range of variables that contribute to the gap in the ability to access and use digital devices [9]. The exchange of images or videos distinguishes teledermatology from the more general telemedicine. Exchanging images requires more advanced technologic skills, with particular attention to be paid to aspects pertaining to image quality such as focus, lighting, and background [10]. Teledermatology requires a minimal bandwidth to adequately participate in videoconferencing [10]. Identifying the images of the patient may pose a potential vulnerability and require substantial patient trust in the technological platform.

In this study, we aimed to determine sociodemographic correlates with patient interest in exchanging images and videos electronically with health care providers in the nationally representative Health Information National Trends Survey (HINTS) of the National Cancer Institute. We hypothesized that teledermatology adoption by various subpopulations may be mediated by differential levels of access to and interest in exchanging images and videos with their health care providers.

Methods

Study Sample

We examined data from HINTS 4 cycle 4 (2014) of the National Cancer Institute. HINTS is a cross-sectional, nationally representative household survey conducted annually, which collects information on demographics and the perceptions and use of health information, and provides information on how cancer risks are perceived. HINTS 4 cycle 4 had a sample of 3677 participants. Data from 2014 were used because the outcome of interest, "How interested are you in exchanging digital images or video (eg, photos of skin lesions) with a health care provider electronically?" was only available in this cycle. Details about HINTS data collection, including weighting methodologies, is described elsewhere. The institutional review board of Emory University exempted this study from review.

Sociodemographic and Health Behavior Correlates

The covariates include sociodemographic variables as well as access and use of the internet such as the following: self-reported gender, age, education, race and ethnicity, annual household income level, seeing a health professional regularly, having health insurance, using the internet, using electronic devices to share medical information with a health professional, and using various devices (if any) with or without health apps on them. The survey question on devices was, "please indicate if you have one of the following electronic devices: tablet, smartphone, cellphone, etc." The responses were as follows: "(1) tablet computer like an iPad, Samsung, Galaxy Tab, Motorola Xoom, or Kindle Fire, only; (2) smartphone such as an iPhone, Android phone, Blackberry device, or a Windows phone; (3) basic cellphone only; and (4) multiple devices listed." The survey question regarding health apps contained on one's electronic device was, "on your tablet or smartphone, do you have any software apps related to health?" The answer choices were as follows: "yes," "no," and "don't know." These 2 questions were combined to generate 1 variable to specify the type of electronic device a participant owned and if there were health apps installed on that device.

We also assessed cancer information–seeking behavior, including, but not limited to, skin cancer. Cancer-related covariates included the following: seeking cancer information, trusting web-based information on cancer, and using the internet to obtain cancer-related information for oneself in the past 12 months.

Outcome: Interest in Using Teledermatology

The primary outcome was defined by the following question: "how interested are you in exchanging information like digital images or video (eg, photos of skin lesions) with a health care provider electronically?" We dichotomized the outcome by a high level of interest (responding with "very") and those who did not have a high level of interest (responding with "somewhat," "a little," or "not at all") in exchanging images and videos with health care providers.

Statistical Analysis

Statistical analyses were conducted using SAS (version 9.4, SAS Institute). Nationally representative prevalence estimates were obtained using jackknife replicate weights that accounted for the complex survey design. For bivariate analyses, the associations between specific sociodemographic groups and interest in sharing photographs or videos were assessed using unconditional logistic regression. We used complete cases analysis for logistic regression owing to the low proportion of missing data (6%). A multivariable logistic regression model was developed through backwards selection, with all final covariates associated with varying levels of teledermatology use at *P*<.05. Furthermore, sensitivity analysis was performed by changing the outcome dichotomy to model those who were "not at all" interested. Two-sided tests were performed with *P*<.05 indicating statistical significance.

Results

The response rate of HINTS 4 cycle 4 was 34%. In total, 3677 respondents fully completed 3529 surveys and partially completed 148 surveys. Demographic characteristics of survey respondents by the level of their interest in teledermatology are summarized in Table 1. A total of 888 of 3447 (weighted prevalence=26.2%) participants were very interested, 784 (22.8%) were somewhat interested, 515 (16.2%) were a little interested, and 1260 (34.8%) were not at all interested.

As shown in Table 1, the socioeconomic demographic characteristics associated with high levels of interest in sharing photographs or videos were the female gender (*P*=.02), young age (*P*<.001), high levels of education (*P*=.001), high annual household income range (*P*<.001), having a regular medical provider (*P*=.02), trusting web-based information on cancer (*P*<.001), using the internet (*P*<.001), sharing medical information with medical providers (*P*<.001), and having multiple electronic devices, including smartphones and tablets, with health apps (for both *P*<.001).

Multivariable modeling in Table 2 shows that trust in web-based information on cancer (odds ratio [OR] 1.9, 95% CI 1.3-2.8) is associated with high levels of interest in exchanging images.

Sharing medical information electronically with a health care professional (OR 2.1, 95% CI 1.5-2.9) is associated with high levels of interest in exchanging images (Table 2). Sensitivity analysis revealed that individuals who reported no interest in exchanging images were less likely to have shared medical information electronically with a health care professional (OR 0.3, 95% CI 0.2-0.4).

Having multiple devices with health apps (OR 2.6, 95% CI 1.5-4.6) is associated with high levels of interest in exchanging images (Table 2). Sensitivity analysis revealed that individuals reporting no interest in exchanging images were less likely to own multiple devices with health apps (OR 0.3, 95% CI 0.2-0.5), own multiple devices without health apps (OR 0.5, 95% CI 0.3-0.7), own a tablet device without health apps (OR 0.6, 95% CI 0.4-0.9), own a smartphone with health apps (OR 0.4, 95% CI 0.2-0.8), and own a smartphone without health apps (OR 0.5, 95% CI 0.3-0.7).

Age, gender, annual household income, education, having a regular medical provider, internet usage, having health insurance, and trusting web-based information on cancer were not significant predictors of a high level of interest in teledermatology after adjusting for the aforementioned variables.

Table 1. Patient factors associated with high levels of interest in exchanging digital images (eg, photographs of skin lesions) with a health care provider electronically.

Factors	Very interested (n=888), n (weighted %)	Not at all interested (n=2559), n (weighted %)	Total participants	*P* value
Gender				.02
Male	322 (25.1[a])	1018 (74.9)	1340	
Female	557 (27.7)	1495 (72.3)	2052	
Unknown	9 (9.2)	46 (90.8)	55	
Age (years)				<.001
18-34	153 (30.0)	310 (70.0)	463	
35-49	243 (32.2)	474 (67.8)	717	
50-64	295 (22.3)	876 (77.7)	1171	
≥65	166 (16.1)	780 (83.9)	946	
Unknown	31 (19.0)	119 (81.0)	150	
Education				.001
High school or below	56 (19.0)	200 (81.0)	256	
High School	126 (21.7)	479 (78.3)	605	
Some college degree	256 (24.4)	788 (75.6)	1044	
College or higher	424 (31.7)	994 (68.3)	1418	
Unknown	26 (18.8)	98 (81.2)	124	
Race and ethnicity				.61
Hispanic	143 (29.3)	343 (70.7)	486	
Non-Hispanic White	445 (24.6)	1447 (75.4)	1892	
Non-Hispanic Black	152 (30.4)	361 (69.9)	513	
Other	63 (28.8)	166 (71.2)	229	
Unknown	85 (25.9)	242 (74.1)	327	
Income range				<.001
<US $20,000	157 (24.8)	537 (75.2)	694	
US $20,000-$34,999	109 (22.2)	348 (77.8)	457	
US $35,000-$49,999	118 (24.2)	347 (75.8)	465	
US $50,000-$74,999	132 (26.5)	396 (73.5)	528	
≥US $75,000	321 (33.0)	643 (67.0)	964	
Unknown	51 (11.1)	288 (88.9)	339	
Having a regular medical provider				.02
Yes	627 (27.7)	1783 (72.3)	2410	
No	260 (23.7)	760 (76.3)	1020	
Unknown	1 (2.1)	16 (97.9)	17	
Having health insurance				.15
Yes	773 (25.7)	2263 (74.3)	3036	
No	113 (29.7)	284 (70.3)	397	
Unknown	2 (9.7)	12 (90.3)	14	
Trust in web-based information on cancer				<.001
A lot	231 (38.4)	407 (61.6)	638	
Not a lot	620 (23.8)	1997 (76.2)	2617	

Factors	Very interested (n=888), n (weighted %)	Not at all interested (n=2559), n (weighted %)	Total participants	*P* value
Unknown	37 (20.8)	155 (79.2)	192	
Using the internet				<.001
Yes	767 (27.5)	1977 (72.5)	2744	
No	117 (17.8)	580 (82.2)	697	
Unknown	4 (85.7)	2 (14.3)	6	
Owning electronic devices and using health apps				<.001
Multiple devices with health apps	220 (40.9)	292 (59.1)	512	
Multiple devices without health apps	187 (25.0)	508 (75.0)	693	
Tablet device with health apps	14 (30.6)	51 (69.4)	65	
Tablet device without health apps	68 (25.4)	213 (74.6)	281	
Smartphone with health apps	73 (34.4)	150 (65.6)	223	
Smartphone without health apps	142 (23.4)	421 (76.6)	563	
Basic cellphone	117 (15.2)	631 (84.8)	748	
None	42 (11.0)	249 (89.0)	291	
Unknown	25 (43.7)	44 (56.3)	69	
Sharing medical information with health care providers				<.001
Yes	371 (39.6)	572 (60.4)	943	
No	507 (20.9)	1954 (79.1)	2461	
Unknown	10 (13.9)	33 (86.1)	43	

[a]Weighted percentage to adjust for the nonresponse bias.

Table 2. Multivariable analysis of interest levels in exchanging digital images (eg, photographs of skin lesions) with a health care provider electronically.

Characteristics	Very interested		Not at all interested	
	Odds Ratio (95% CI)	*P* value	Odds ratio (95% CI)	*P* value
Gender	N/A[a]	.51		.20
Male	Ref[b]		Ref	
Female	1.1 (0.8-1.7)		1.2 (0.9-1.6)	
Age (years)		.06		.10
18-34	Ref		Ref	
35-49	1.2 (0.8-1.9)		0.9 (0.7-1.4)	
50-64	0.8 (0.5-1.2)		1.3 (0.9-1.8)	
≥65	0.7 (0.4-1.2)		1.5 (1.0-2.1)	
Trusting web-based information on cancer		.002		.80
Yes	1.9 (1.3-2.8)		0.9 (0.7-1.3)	
No	Ref		Ref	
Sharing medical information with health care providers		<.001		<.001
Yes	2.1 (1.5-2.9)		0.3 (0.2-0.4)	
No	Ref		Ref	
Owning devices with or without health apps		<.001		<.001
Multiple devices with health apps	2.6 (1.5-4.6)		0.3 (0.2-0.5)	
Multiple devices without health apps	1.5 (0.8-2.7)		0.5 (0.3-0.7)	
Tablet device with health apps	1.7 (0.6-4.5)		0.9 (0.3-2.6)	
Tablet device without health apps	1.6 (0.8-3.3)		0.6 (0.4-0.9)	
Smartphone with health apps	2.0 (0.9-4.0)		0.4 (0.2-0.8)	
Smartphone without health apps	1.3 (0.7-2.4)		0.5 (0.3-0.7)	
Basic cellphone	Ref		Ref	
None	0.7 (0.3-1.4)		1.5 (1.0-2.1)	

[a]N/A: not applicable.

[b]Ref: Reference group for comparison.

Discussion

Principal Findings

High levels of interest in using teledermatology were associated with modifiable behaviors such as the use of devices with health apps, trust in web-based information on cancer, and prior experiences in exchanging health information with physicians on the internet. Sociodemographic factors such as young age, female gender, high education, and high household income were not associated with an increased interest in exchanging images of skin lesions with health care providers after adjusting for these modifiable variables. Future implementation of teledermatology should address these identified factors within the digital divide to provide equitable access to care across diverse patient populations.

Access to devices and how they are used are aspects of the digital divide, which can be adjusted. Physical access to the internet was found to be the most significant predictor of web-based patient-provider communication [9]. Once access is established, usage becomes the rate-limiting factor, which depends on the ability to retrieve and search for information on the internet and to use mobile health apps [11,12]. Users of mobile health apps are more likely to exhibit health-promoting behaviors than those who own similar devices but do not use health apps [11]. A potential barrier to the use of health apps is privacy concerns with inputting personal data into digital devices. Digital health information requires high levels of eHealth literacy to effect action [13]. Mobile device and health app usage is associated with characteristics previously linked to increased eHealth literacy, such as young age, higher education, and high income [7,14]. However, unlike age, education, and income, access and usage of devices can be modified to enhance teledermatology implementation.

Trust in web-based information on cancer can be directed to mediate interest in teledermatology usage. Trust is a necessary antecedent to the development of eHealth literacy and engagement with health information [15,16]. Trust in web-based health information is associated with higher education and the disclosure of health information on the internet, which are factors linked to eHealth literacy [17]. Even among groups with increased eHealth literacy, young individuals have higher trust in web-based health care services than their older counterparts [18]. Patient trust in a telemedicine service can be broken down into their trust in the organization, treatment, care professional, and technology [19]. Increased trust in the telehealth service can be gained when patients are referred by other health care professionals [20]. Moreover, face-to-face interactions with the provider prior to a web-based consultation also increases patient trust [21]. The provider should ensure that patient concerns are being addressed as this will increase trust in the telehealth provider and the treatment plan [21].

Prior experience in exchanging health information on the internet is an adjustable factor that can be targeted to increase interest in exchanging digital images. Lack of knowledge and experience with web-based patient-provider communication is found to impede its use [9], while prior experience with sharing medical information electronically is associated with higher interest in exchanging digital images with providers [15]. As patients expand their experiences with digital technology within and outside of the health care context, patients will have the opportunity to develop trust in teledermatology services [19].

Teledermatology interventions are implemented and expanded across populations to bridge the digital divide [22]. For example, the US Department of Veteran Affairs has expanded the reach of teledermatology by loaning electronic devices to veterans and provided training in using the devices so that veterans can more easily connect with the existing telehealth networks [23]. They have also attempted to evaluate the effectiveness of these measures through a survey on patient satisfaction with teledermatology use and its contributory factors [24]. Our study found that factors malleable to influence—use of health apps, trust, and experience—are barriers that can be mediated to increase the reach, adoption, and effectiveness of teledermatology.

Limitations

There were some limitations to this study. The cross-sectional nature of the HINTS data precluded the establishment of causal relationships between the usage, trust, and prior experience in using health apps and the interest in teledermatology. The measured outcome was available only in HINTS 4 cycle 4 (2014); more recent data were not available to address the study question. All survey responses were self-reported and subject to information bias. We could not exclude residual confounding variables from additional unmeasured or unexamined variables. We were unable to distinguish the history of skin cancer from that of other cancers when controlling for covariates related to information-seeking behaviors associated with cancer. Interest in exchanging images on the internet might differ if the patient worked with GPs to send images to a teledermatology service or if the service is directly patient-initiated, and this aspect should be examined in future studies. Future studies should explore how well patients and GPs follow teledermatology guidelines on taking adequate images. We were unable to assess if interests in teledermatology translated directly to teledermatology usage or adherence to recommendations from teledermatology services.

Conclusions

In conclusion, modifiable access barriers to teledermatology adoption included experience with exchanging health information on the internet, trust in web-based information on cancer, and the use of mobile health apps. Future implementation of teledermatology should address these identified factors within the digital divide to provide equitable access to care across diverse patient populations.

Acknowledgments

This study was supported in part by the Dermatology Foundation and the National Institute of Arthritis and Musculoskeletal and Skin Diseases (L30 AR076081) (HY). The content of this manuscript is solely the responsibility of the authors and does not necessarily represent the official views of the National Institutes of Health or the Department of Veterans Affairs.

References

1. Coates SJ, Kvedar J, Granstein RD. Teledermatology: from historical perspective to emerging techniques of the modern era: part I: History, rationale, and current practice. J Am Acad Dermatol 2015 Apr;72(4):563-574. [doi: 10.1016/j.jaad.2014.07.061] [Medline: 25773407]
2. Walocko FM, Tejasvi T. Teledermatology Applications in Skin Cancer Diagnosis. Dermatol Clin 2017 Oct;35(4):559-563. [doi: 10.1016/j.det.2017.06.002] [Medline: 28886813]
3. Hollander JE, Carr BG. Virtually Perfect? Telemedicine for Covid-19. N Engl J Med 2020 Mar 11;382(18):1679-1681. [doi: 10.1056/NEJMp2003539] [Medline: 32160451]
4. Uscher-Pines L, Malsberger R, Burgette L, Mulcahy A, Mehrotra A. Effect of Teledermatology on Access to Dermatology Care Among Medicaid Enrollees. JAMA Dermatol 2016 Aug 01;152(8):905-912. [doi: 10.1001/jamadermatol.2016.0938] [Medline: 27144986]
5. Bashshur RL, Shannon GW, Tejasvi T, Kvedar JC, Gates M. The Empirical Foundations of Teledermatology: A Review of the Research Evidence. Telemed J E Health 2015 Dec;21(12):953-979 [FREE Full text] [doi: 10.1089/tmj.2015.0146] [Medline: 26394022]

6. Kontos E, Blake KD, Chou WS, Prestin A. Predictors of eHealth usage: insights on the digital divide from the Health Information National Trends Survey 2012. J Med Internet Res 2014 Jul 16;16(7):e172 [FREE Full text] [doi: 10.2196/jmir.3117] [Medline: 25048379]
7. Carroll JK, Moorhead A, Bond R, LeBlanc WG, Petrella RJ, Fiscella K. Who Uses Mobile Phone Health Apps and Does Use Matter? A Secondary Data Analytics Approach. J Med Internet Res 2017 Apr 19;19(4):e125 [FREE Full text] [doi: 10.2196/jmir.5604] [Medline: 28428170]
8. Graham AL, Amato MS. Twelve Million Smokers Look Online for Smoking Cessation Help Annually: Health Information National Trends Survey Data, 2005-2017. Nicotine Tob Res 2019 Jan 04;21(2):249-252 [FREE Full text] [doi: 10.1093/ntr/nty043] [Medline: 29660037]
9. Jiang S, Street RL. Factors Influencing Communication with Doctors via the Internet: A Cross-Sectional Analysis of 2014 HINTS Survey. Health Commun 2017 Feb;32(2):180-188. [doi: 10.1080/10410236.2015.1110867] [Medline: 27196037]
10. McKoy K, Antoniotti NM, Armstrong A, Bashshur R, Bernard J, Bernstein D, et al. Practice Guidelines for Teledermatology. Telemed J E Health 2016 Dec;22(12):981-990. [doi: 10.1089/tmj.2016.0137] [Medline: 27690203]
11. Mahmood A, Kedia S, Wyant DK, Ahn S, Bhuyan SS. Use of mobile health applications for health-promoting behavior among individuals with chronic medical conditions. Digit Health 2019;5:2055207619882181 [FREE Full text] [doi: 10.1177/2055207619882181] [Medline: 31656632]
12. Connolly KK, Crosby ME. Examining e-Health literacy and the digital divide in an underserved population in Hawai'i. Hawaii J Med Public Health 2014 Feb;73(2):44-48 [FREE Full text] [Medline: 24567867]
13. Cosco TD, Firth J, Vahia I, Sixsmith A, Torous J. Mobilizing mHealth Data Collection in Older Adults: Challenges and Opportunities. JMIR Aging 2019 Mar 19;2(1):e10019 [FREE Full text] [doi: 10.2196/10019] [Medline: 31518253]
14. Tennant B, Stellefson M, Dodd V, Chaney B, Chaney D, Paige S, et al. eHealth literacy and Web 2.0 health information seeking behaviors among baby boomers and older adults. J Med Internet Res 2015 Mar 17;17(3):e70. [doi: 10.2196/jmir.3992] [Medline: 25783036]
15. Serrano KJ, Yu M, Riley WT, Patel V, Hughes P, Marchesini K, et al. Willingness to Exchange Health Information via Mobile Devices: Findings From a Population-Based Survey. Ann Fam Med 2016;14(1):34-40 [FREE Full text] [doi: 10.1370/afm.1888] [Medline: 26755781]
16. Strekalova YA. When Trust Is Not Enough: A Serial Mediation Model Explaining the Effect of Race Identity, eHealth Information Efficacy, and Information Behavior on Intention to Participate in Clinical Research. Health Educ Behav 2018 Dec;45(6):1036-1042 [FREE Full text] [doi: 10.1177/1090198118757822] [Medline: 29478354]
17. AlGhamdi KM, Moussa NA. Internet use by the public to search for health-related information. Int J Med Inform 2012 Jun;81(6):363-373. [doi: 10.1016/j.ijmedinf.2011.12.004] [Medline: 22217800]
18. Paige SR, Krieger JL, Stellefson ML. The Influence of eHealth Literacy on Perceived Trust in Online Health Communication Channels and Sources. J Health Commun 2017 Jan;22(1):53-65 [FREE Full text] [doi: 10.1080/10810730.2016.1250846] [Medline: 28001489]
19. Velsen LV, Tabak M, Hermens H. Measuring patient trust in telemedicine services: Development of a survey instrument and its validation for an anticoagulation web-service. Int J Med Inform 2017 Jan 01;97:52-58. [doi: 10.1016/j.ijmedinf.2016.09.009] [Medline: 27919395]
20. Van Velsen L, Wildevuur S, Flierman I, Van Schooten B, Tabak M, Hermens H. Trust in telemedicine portals for rehabilitation care: an exploratory focus group study with patients and healthcare professionals. BMC Med Inform Decis Mak 2016 Jan 27;16:11 [FREE Full text] [doi: 10.1186/s12911-016-0250-2] [Medline: 26818611]
21. Almathami HKY, Win KT, Vlahu-Gjorgievska E. Barriers and Facilitators That Influence Telemedicine-Based, Real-Time, Online Consultation at Patients' Homes: Systematic Literature Review. J Med Internet Res 2020 Feb 20;22(2):e16407 [FREE Full text] [doi: 10.2196/16407] [Medline: 32130131]
22. Peracca S, Jackson G, Weinstock M, Oh D. Implementation of Teledermatology: Theory and Practice. Curr Derm Rep 2019 May 2;8(2):35-45. [doi: 10.1007/s13671-019-0252-2]
23. At Home. US Department of Veterans Affairs. 2016. URL: https://telehealth.va.gov/type/home [accessed 2019-12-23]
24. Baranowski MLH, Balakrishnan V, Chen SC. Patient Satisfaction with the Veteran's Administration Teledermatology Service. J Am Acad Dermatol 2019 Jan 28. [doi: 10.1016/j.jaad.2019.01.036] [Medline: 30703451]

Abbreviations

GP: general practitioner
HINTS: Health Information National Trends Survey

23

Exploring Access to Surgical Interventions for Hidradenitis Suppurativa: Retrospective Population-Based Analysis

Alexandra Finstad[1], BSc, BA; Alex Lee[1], BSc; Ralph George[2,3], MD; Raed Alhusayen[4,5], MD, MSc

[1]Faculty of Medicine, University of Ottawa, Ottawa, ON, Canada

[2]Division of General Surgery, Department of Surgery, University of Toronto, Toronto, ON, Canada

[3]Department of Surgery, Canadian Imperial Bank of Commerce Breast Centre, St. Michael's Hospital, Toronto, ON, Canada

[4]Division of Dermatology, Department of Medicine, University of Toronto, Toronto, ON, Canada

[5]Division of Dermatology, Department of Medicine, Sunnybrook Health Sciences Centre, Toronto, ON, Canada

Corresponding Author:
Raed Alhusayen, MD, MSc
Division of Dermatology
Department of Medicine
Sunnybrook Health Sciences Centre
2075 Bayview Avenue
Toronto, ON, M4N 3M5
Canada

Email: Raed.Alhusayen@sunnybrook.ca

Abstract

Background: Hidradenitis suppurativa (HS) is a painful inflammatory disorder that confers significant distress to patients, with surgery as an integral treatment modality.

Objective: To inform improvements in care, patterns in HS surgery were assessed.

Methods: A retrospective population-based analysis was performed on Ontario billing claims for HS surgery across a period of 10 years from January 1, 2008 to December 31, 2017. HS surgery was defined as the excision of inguinal, perineal, or axillary skin and sweat glands for hidradenitis. The top 5 billing specialties, including general and plastic surgery, were analyzed. The total number of procedures performed as well as the number performed per physician were investigated. Patient and physician locations were compared.

Results: A total of 7195 claims for the excision of inguinal, perineal, or axillary skin and sweat glands for HS were submitted across the study period. Annual HS surgery claims showed an increasing trend across 10 years, ranging between 4.9 and 5.8 per 100,000 population. However, overall, for every additional year, the number of claims per 100,000 population only increased slightly, by 0.03 claims. The number of providers steadily decreased, ranging between 1.7 and 1.9 per 100,000, with approximately twice as many general than plastic surgeons. However, again overall, for every additional year, the number of providers per 100,000 population decreased slightly, by 0.002 physicians. The mean annual number of procedures per physician rose from 2.8 to 3.1. In rural areas, analyzed per claim, general surgeons performed the majority of surgeries (1318/2003, 65.8%), while in urban areas, surgeries were more equally performed by general (2616/5192, 50.4%) and plastic (2495/5192, 48.1%) surgeons. Of HS surgery claims, 25.7%-35.9% were provided by a physician residing in a different area than the patient receiving care.

Conclusions: No significant improvements in access to HS surgery were seen across the study period, with access potentially worsening with annual HS claims rising overall and number of providers decreasing, with patients travelling further to access surgery. System barriers across the continuum of HS diagnosis and management must be evaluated to improve access to surgical care.

KEYWORDS

hidradenitis suppurativa; surgery; dermatology; access; epidemiology; universal health care

Introduction

Hidradenitis suppurativa (HS) is a painful, inflammatory disorder involving a dysfunction of the pilosebaceous unit, which confers significant distress to patients due to its relapsing and remitting nature [1-3]. HS management is complex, with both medical and surgical treatment options and the first North American clinical management guidelines only recently published in 2019 [4,5]. A variety of options for medical treatment is available depending on the severity of disease, including topical and intralesional therapies, systemic antibiotics, hormonal therapies, retinoids, immunosuppressants, and biologics [4,5]. However, surgery remains an integral treatment modality regardless of disease severity [4-6]. Approximately 80% of patients were shown to be satisfied with surgical treatment of HS and considered it as the best treatment option [6].

Unfortunately, the diagnosis of HS is relatively rare, and it is often mistaken for a simple infection, limiting access to proper treatment [7]. HS is commonly diagnosed after a significant delay, with one multinational study reporting a mean delay of 10.2 years [8] and Canadian data reporting a median delay of 7 years with an average of 3 misdiagnoses [9]. Treatment has also been found to be fragmented over multiple specialties, including dermatology, primary care, general surgery, and plastic surgery [10,11], with patients trying an average of 15 different methods to manage their HS symptoms [9]. The absence of a designated specialty for HS management has been suggested to further delay diagnosis and treatment [12,13].

The prevalence of HS has been reported to range from 0.03% to 4.10% [14]. Although guidelines have been published for the surgical management of HS, they commonly rely on low-quality, uncontrolled, retrospective reports, and whether there is adequate access to HS surgery is unknown [5]. Moreover, although early surgical interventions are believed to potentially prevent progression of disease, data are sparse, and the extent of adoption of surgical management for HS is unclear [15].

To inform improvements in HS care, patterns in current and past HS surgery must be assessed. The objectives of this study were to evaluate patient access to surgical procedures for HS and investigate trends in HS surgery across different specialties and geographical regions.

Methods

Data Source

Ontario was chosen as the study setting as it is the most populous province in Canada with approximately 14.7 million inhabitants [16] and provides its citizens with universal health care through the Ontario Health Insurance Plan (OHIP). Data on OHIP medical claims were obtained from the Medical Services and Population data source within IntelliHealth, a province-wide data repository operated by the Ontario Ministry of Health and Long-Term Care containing information on physician billing. IntelliHealth has been utilized in prior population-based studies on physician billing and practices [17-22]. Research ethics board approval was not required for this study as information obtained through IntelliHealth is anonymized and publicly available.

Study Population

A retrospective, population-based analysis was performed on Ontario physicians who surgically treated HS. Data were collected across 10 years from January 1, 2008 to December 31, 2017. Physicians who surgically treated HS or hyperhidrosis were identified by procedure codes R059 (unilateral excision of inguinal, perineal, or axillary skin and sweat glands for hyperhidrosis and/or hidradenitis) and R060 (excision of inguinal, perineal, or axillary skin and sweat glands for hyperhidrosis and/or hidradenitis with skin graft(s) or rotation flap(s)) [23]. From these, claims billed under diagnostic code 799 for "excessive sweating" (hyperhidrosis) were excluded to further isolate those for HS, as no OHIP diagnostic code currently exists for HS [24]. The top 5 billing specialties were analyzed, excluding family physicians and anaesthesiologists, to further ensure that the procedure was being performed for the purposes of HS.

Data Analysis

Data were exported from IntelliHealth's online system and analyzed using Microsoft Excel version 16.36. Physician specialty was defined as the specialty billed for the procedure. The number, location, and specialty of physicians who performed the excision of inguinal, perineal, or axillary skin and sweat glands for HS were analyzed. The total number of procedures performed as well as the number performed per physician were investigated. Patient and physician locations were compared. Location was determined based on the assigned Local Health Integration Network (LHIN). Each LHIN was further classified as rural or urban following previously applied methodology in which a LHIN is deemed rural if its population is less than 1,000,000 and urban if greater [17,20,21].

Results

Demographics

Across the study period, a total of 12,539 claims were submitted for the excision of inguinal, perineal, or axillary skin and sweat glands for hyperhidrosis and/or HS. Of these cases, 1758 were excluded because they were submitted for hyperhidrosis (excessive sweating). A further 3586 claims were excluded based on specialty billed. A final total of 7195 claims was included in the study (Figure 1). Patient demographics are shown in Table 1 for patients with a valid health card number. Approximately 10% of patients had multiple surgeries over the study period.

Figure 1. Cohort formation flowchart. OHIP: Ontario Health Insurance Plan.

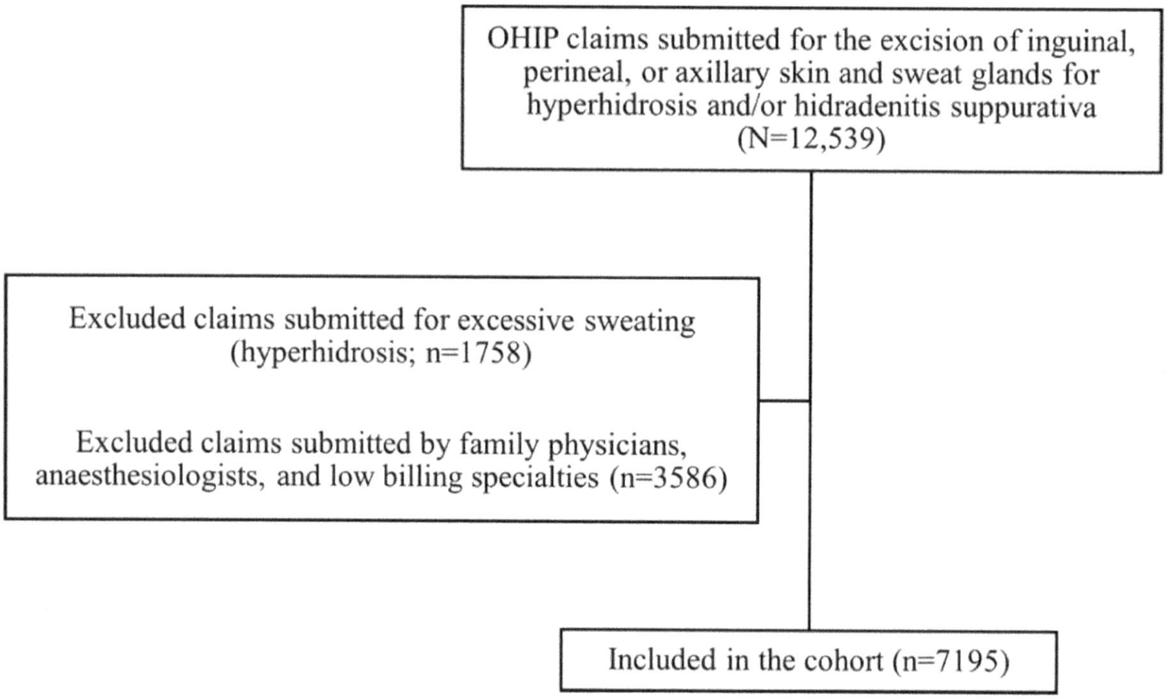

Table 1. Ontario hidradenitis suppurativa surgery patient demographics.

Characteristics	2008 (n=569)	2009 (n=628)	2010 (n=624)	2011 (n=631)	2012 (n=704)	2013 (n=667)	2014 (n=669)	2015 (n=640)	2016 (n=668)	2017 (n=670)
Sex, n (%)										
Female	366 (64.3)	427 (68.0)	441 (70.7)	433 (68.6)	458 (65.1)	453 (67.9)	454 (67.9)	415 (64.8)	426 (63.8)	419 (62.5)
Male	203 (35.7)	201 (32.0)	183 (29.3)	198 (31.4)	246 (34.9)	214 (32.1)	215 (32.1)	225 (35.2)	242 (36.2)	251 (37.5)
Age (years), mean	40.4	40.8	41.0	40.7	40.2	40.3	39.9	41.8	41.6	42.8
Age (years), n (%)										
0-19	41 (7.2)	26 (4.1)	31 (5.0)	36 (5.7)	55 (7.8)	36 (5.4)	32 (4.8)	30 (4.7)	30 (4.5)	31 (4.6)
20-44	306 (53.8)	350 (55.7)	349 (55.9)	351 (55.6)	386 (54.8)	372 (55.8)	396 (59.2)	347 (54.2)	381 (57.0)	340 (50.7)
45-64	181 (31.8)	215 (34.2)	203 (32.5)	194 (30.7)	216 (30.7)	217 (32.5)	192 (28.7)	219 (34.2)	197 (29.5)	234 (34.9)
65-74	23 (4.0)	24 (3.8)	25 (4.0)	36 (5.7)	29 (4.1)	29 (4.3)	36 (5.4)	28 (4.4)	35 (5.2)	46 (6.9)
≥75	18 (3.2)	13 (2.1)	16 (2.6)	14 (2.2)	18 (2.6)	13 (1.9)	13 (1.9)	16 (2.5)	25 (3.7)	19 (2.8)

Providers of HS Surgery

The top 5 billing specialties for HS surgery were general surgery, plastic surgery, obstetrics and gynecology, urology, and dermatology (Multimedia Appendix 1, Supplemental Table 1). Over the course of the entire study period, general and plastic surgeons submitted the vast majority of claims for surgical treatment of HS, at 3934 and 3107 claims, respectively. General surgeons performed the majority of unilateral excision procedures (R059), while plastic surgeons performed the majority of procedures that involved a skin graft or rotation flap (R060). The annual number of claims submitted for HS surgery experienced an overall slight increase across the study period when standardized by population, ranging between 4.9 (2008) and 5.8 (2012) claims per 100,000 population (Figure 2). However, overall, for every additional year, the number of claims per 100,000 population only slightly increased, by 0.03 claims.

Figure 2. Submission of claims for hidradenitis suppurativa surgery over time per 100,000 population.

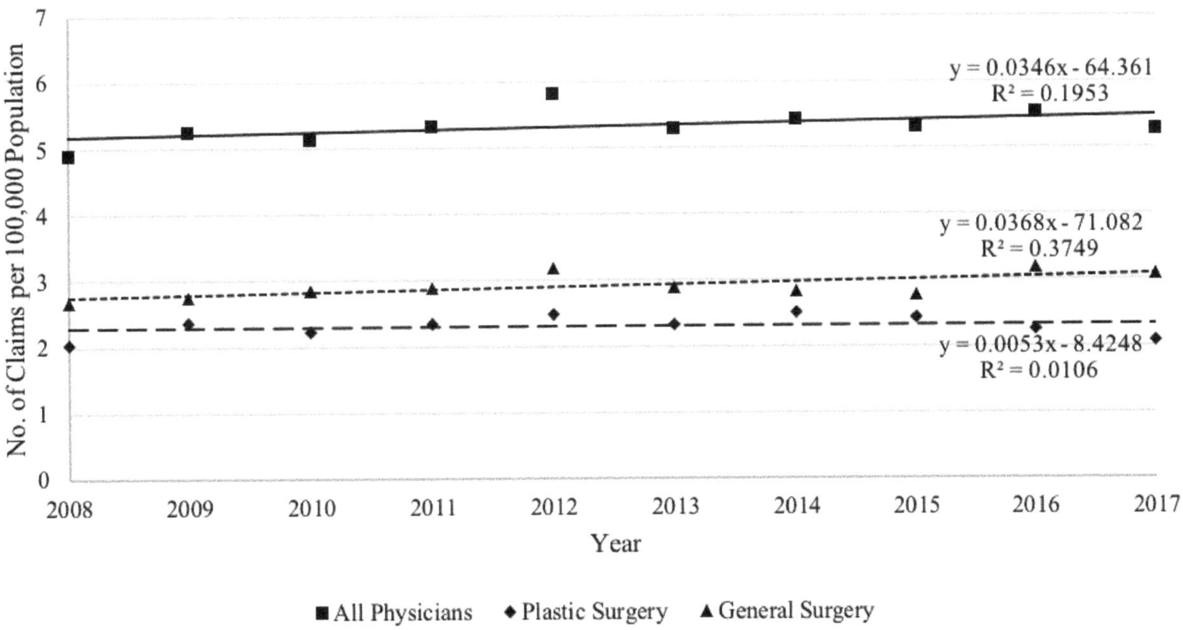

By specialty, annual claims submitted by general surgeons increased slightly more than those by plastic surgeons. The number of HS surgery providers per 100,000 population ranged from 1.7 to 1.9, with general surgeons ranging from 1.1 to 1.3 and plastic surgeons ranging from 0.5 to 0.6 (Figure 3). However, overall, for every additional year, the number of providers per 100,000 population decreased slightly, by 0.002 physicians.

Figure 3. Providers of hidradenitis suppurativa surgery over time per 100,000 population.

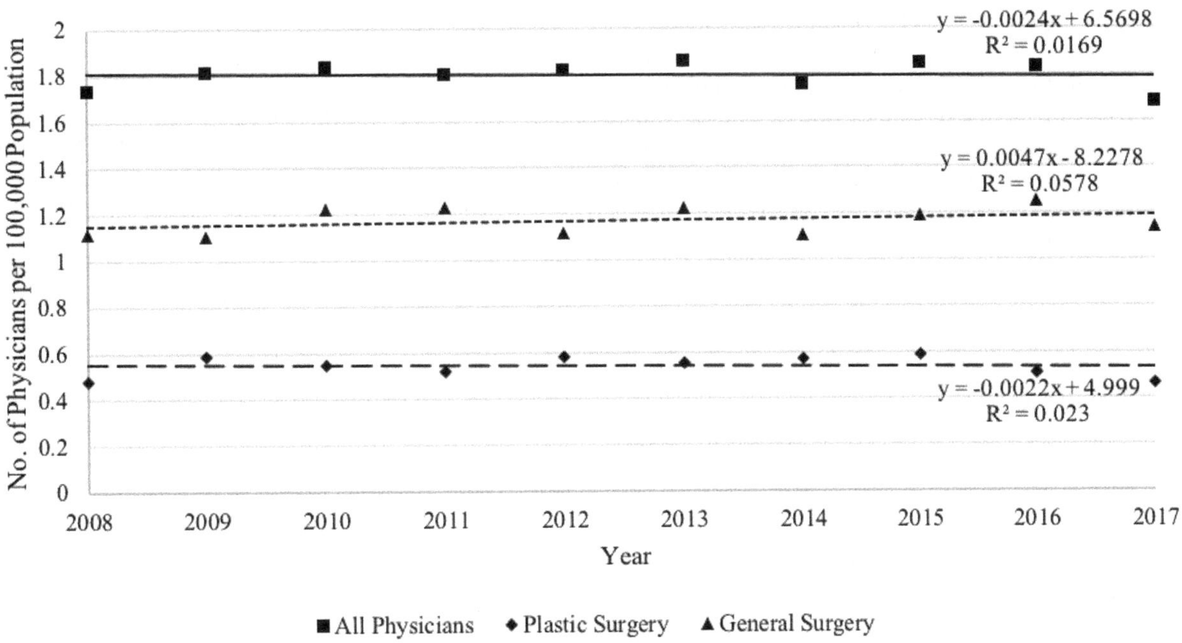

The mean number of procedures performed annually per physician rose from 2.8 to 3.1 across 10 years (Figure 4). Plastic surgeons performed more procedures per physician than did general surgeons, ranging from 4.0 to 4.5 compared with 2.3 to 2.8. However, the change in procedures per physician over time for all providers, as well as plastic surgeons and general surgeons, was not statistically significant. It is also important to note that, averaged across the 10 years, 85.2% (2069/2427) of physicians submitted <5 claims per year, while only 14.8% (358/2427) submitted ≥5 claims per year. Furthermore, many only performed 1 HS surgery per year, therefore not necessarily qualifying as a specialized provider of HS care.

Figure 4. Annual hidradenitis suppurativa surgeries performed per physician.

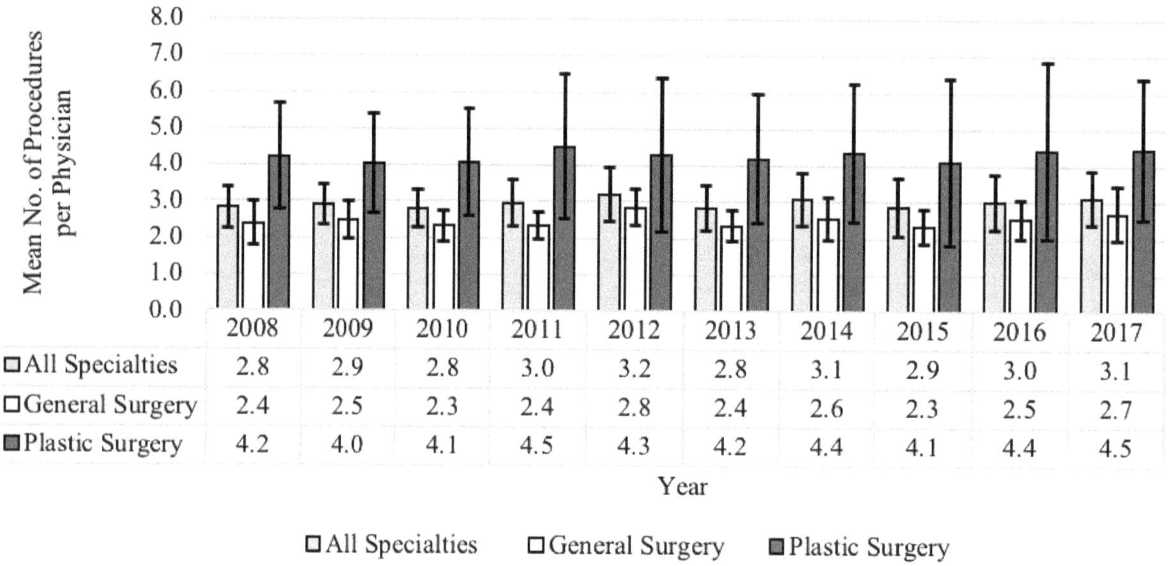

	2008	2009	2010	2011	2012	2013	2014	2015	2016	2017
All Specialties	2.8	2.9	2.8	3.0	3.2	2.8	3.1	2.9	3.0	3.1
General Surgery	2.4	2.5	2.3	2.4	2.8	2.4	2.6	2.3	2.5	2.7
Plastic Surgery	4.2	4.0	4.1	4.5	4.3	4.2	4.4	4.1	4.4	4.5

Geographic Distribution of Claims

In total, analyzed per claim, more patients (2281/7195, 31.7%) than physicians (2003/7195, 27.8%) resided in a rural area, while more physicians (5192/7195, 72.2%) than patients (4914/7195, 68.3%) resided in an urban area (see Multimedia Appendix 2, Supplemental Figure 1a). Furthermore, over time, HS surgeries were increasingly being performed by physicians residing in a different geographic region than the patient receiving care (low of 176/684, 25.7% in 2009 to a high of 269/749, 35.9% in 2017; Multimedia Appendix 3, Supplemental Figure 2). When comparing surgeries performed in rural areas to those in urban areas, in rural areas, surgery was most often performed by a general surgeon (1318/2003, 65.8%), while in urban areas, surgeries were more equally performed by general surgeons (2616/5192, 50.4%) and plastic surgeons (2495/5192, 48.1%; Multimedia Appendix 2, Supplemental Figure 1b).

Discussion

Principal Findings

In this population-based analysis of HS surgical care in Canada, there was a slight trend towards increasing number of claims for HS surgery per 100,000 population over the 10-year study period, while the number of providers per 100,000 population decreased, particularly in general surgery. However, procedures performed per physician increased overall, although the increase was not statistically significant. Geographically, patients were also travelling further to access surgery. These findings suggest that overall access to HS surgery has not significantly improved over the study period and in fact may be decreasing as more and more patients seek care away from home as the number of clinicians providing surgery decreases.

The female:male ratio of patients included in this study was similar to that of a previous report on surgical interventions for HS patients in Ontario [25]. In comparison, the general female:male ratio among all HS patients is 3:1 [26-28], suggesting that men diagnosed with HS are more likely to undergo surgery than women. This is possibly due to men generally experiencing more severe disease [28,29], underestimation and dismissal of pain in female patients [30], or a lack of surgical expertise for female care due to common lesion localization to the inguinofemoral area [28], as well as low numbers of gynecologists providing HS surgery. This emphasizes the need for improved access to care for female patients through improved surgical expertise and increased awareness surrounding perception of pain in women.

The mean age of disease onset has been reported as 20.5 (SD 9.3) years, with a mean age at diagnosis of 30.7 (SD 10.9) years, representing a mean delay from onset of symptoms to diagnosis of 10.2 (SD 8.9) years [8]. In our study, the mean age at the time of surgery was in the early 40s and increased by 2 years during the study period, representing a duration of potentially 10 more years from diagnosis to surgical treatment. One reason for the general rise in the mean age of patients undergoing HS surgery and the decrease in claims among patients 20-44 years old may be that medical therapy for control of early disease is increasingly being utilized over surgery, which remains a necessary adjunct intervention for refractory HS cases [6,10,31,32]. The mean age of surgery may also be increasing as patients may be receiving multiple surgeries, found to be approximately 10% in this study, with surgical intervention potentially starting at a later age due to surgical options only being explored once the disease has progressed to a more severe state. Furthermore, in Canada, 3.8% of the population, or approximately 3800 per 100,000 persons, are estimated to be living with HS [33]. Exact estimates of HS severity still vary widely, with reports of 3.9% to 23.7% of HS patients diagnosed with Hurley Stage III [28,29,34]. However, in this study, only 4.9 to 5.8 claims per 100,000 persons were submitted annually for the surgical excision of HS. Despite the considerable number of severe cases reported in the literature, surgical management of HS may therefore be underutilized.

Other recent advances in HS care have focused on new systemic drugs that target different immune mediators in the pathogenesis of HS [35]. Research on various monoclonal antibodies and small molecules are currently underway, while the use of anti-tumor necrosis factor biologic therapy has already demonstrated reductions in HS severity in clinical trials [35]. However, patients have reported high satisfaction with surgical management and experience relatively low recurrence of HS [5,6,36,37]. This suggests the need to consider surgery earlier as part of HS management to limit the long-term morbidity and prolonged progression of the disease. Combined management with biologic therapy has also been advocated in the setting of moderate-to-severe disease [38].

HS surgery was found to be primarily performed by general and plastic surgeons, consistent with previous literature [13]. Although general surgeons were the primary providers of HS surgical care, plastic surgeons submitted more claims per physician. Plastic surgeons also performed the majority of procedures that involved a skin graft or rotation flap, with a previous study showing that flap reconstructions by plastic surgeons had significantly shorter operation times and lower transfusion rates than those by general surgeons, reflecting the specialized training plastic surgeons receive in reconstructive procedures [13]. Investigation into the education of relevant surgical programs on specialized HS surgical care may highlight areas of training requiring further improvement.

Furthermore, it is likely that more surgeons are choosing narrower scopes of practice, especially in general surgery where broader scopes of surgical services are diminishing with highly specialized postresidency fellowships [39]. This is reflected in the study, with more HS surgery claims being accompanied by more claims per provider but fewer providers overall. Increased specialization and narrowing scopes of practice may also lead to patients having to travel further to receive care from an available provider. Accordingly, approximately one-third of patients received care away from their home, with this number also increasing over time. This has important implications for postsurgical follow-up care, with HS being a chronic relapsing disease requiring months to even years of follow-up post-surgical excision [6,31]. This highlights the need for recruitment of more surgeons to perform HS surgery as well as the training of rural surgeons on the surgical treatment of HS.

Strengths and Limitations

This study benefited from the use of a comprehensive, large, longitudinal database, allowing for future comparison studies. However, a limitation to this study was the lack of a specific diagnostic code for HS. Therefore, we were unable to evaluate and compare changes in HS surgery over time to changes in HS claims. Future studies should explore this association, to further help characterize patient access to HS surgical care. Second, the two billing codes used in this study, R059 and R060, do not reflect the entirety of procedures that can be offered for HS, such as abscess drainage, laser treatments, or electrosurgical peeling procedures [5,40]. However, these treatment modalities are relatively novel and are rarely performed as standard of care. Procedures such as abscess drainage also have high recurrence rates of up to 100% and are not performed as a curative option [5,41]. Furthermore, we were unable to assess demographic factors of patients and physicians such as gender, race, and ethnicity, limiting our analysis. However, evidence suggests unequal access leading to racial disparities in surgical care [42]. Further investigation into HS patient and physician demographic factors would be impactful to analyze in future studies.

Comparison With Prior Work

Barriers to seeking HS care have previously been reported to include a lack of knowledge about HS among providers, difficulty accessing specialists, poor patient-physician communication, distrust in the medical community, and patients' experiences with HS [43]. This can be amplified by the significant delay to diagnosis that adds to patient frustration and disease severity and affects the likelihood of receiving well-planned, individual management [35]. Despite ongoing research on new treatment modalities, there is also a need to evaluate the circumstances of these barriers including access to operating room time, extent of provider education on HS, role of subspecialization among surgical providers, and public awareness around HS. This also translates to potential areas for public health authorities and hospital administrations to improve HS care, specifically in regard to increasing operating room time for HS surgeries.

Conclusions

Unfortunately, no significant improvements in patient access to surgery were seen across the study period, with annual HS claims rising overall, number of providers decreasing, and patients travelling further to access surgery. A lack of access to operating room time and narrowing scopes of practice may be contributing factors potentially worsening access over time. Further research on HS surgery, including evaluation into system barriers across the continuum of HS diagnosis and management, are required in order to improve access to surgical care for HS patients.

Acknowledgments

This study made use of data from the Ontario Ministry of Health and Long-Term Care: IntelliHealth Ontario. No financial support was provided.

Authors' Contributions

RA conceived the study. All authors contributed to the study design. AF acquired the data through IntelliHealth. AF and AL contributed to analysis and interpretation of data and drafting of the article. RA and RG critically revised the article. All authors approved the final version to be published.

References

1. Parks R, Parks T. Pathogenesis, clinical features and management of hidradenitis suppurativa. Ann R Coll Surg Engl 1997 Mar;79(2):83-89 [FREE Full text] [Medline: 9135232]
2. Napolitano M, Megna M, Timoshchuk E, Patruno C, Balato N, Fabbrocini G, et al. Hidradenitis suppurativa: From pathogenesis to diagnosis and treatment. CCID 2017 Apr;Volume 10:105-115. [doi: 10.2147/ccid.s111019]
3. Alavi A, Anooshirvani N, Kim WB, Coutts P, Sibbald RG. Quality-of-life impairment in patients with hidradenitis suppurativa: A Canadian study. Am J Clin Dermatol 2015 Feb 29;16(1):61-65. [doi: 10.1007/s40257-014-0105-5] [Medline: 25432664]
4. Alikhan A, Sayed C, Alavi A, Alhusayen R, Brassard A, Burkhart C, et al. North American clinical management guidelines for hidradenitis suppurativa: A publication from the United States and Canadian Hidradenitis Suppurativa Foundations: Part II: Topical, intralesional, and systemic medical management. J Am Acad Dermatol 2019 Jul;81(1):91-101. [doi: 10.1016/j.jaad.2019.02.068] [Medline: 30872149]
5. Alikhan A, Sayed C, Alavi A, Alhusayen R, Brassard A, Burkhart C, et al. North American clinical management guidelines for hidradenitis suppurativa: A publication from the United States and Canadian Hidradenitis Suppurativa Foundations: Part I: Diagnosis, evaluation, and the use of complementary and procedural management. J Am Acad Dermatol 2019 Jul;81(1):76-90. [doi: 10.1016/j.jaad.2019.02.067] [Medline: 30872156]
6. Fertitta L, Hotz C, Wolkenstein P, Méningaud JP, Sawan D, Hersant B, et al. Efficacy and satisfaction of surgical treatment for hidradenitis suppurativa. J Eur Acad Dermatol Venereol 2020 Apr;34(4):839-845. [doi: 10.1111/jdv.16135] [Medline: 31799758]
7. Jemec GB. Hidradenitis Suppurativa. N Engl J Med 2012 Jan 12;366(2):158-164. [doi: 10.1056/nejmcp1014163]
8. Garg A, Neuren E, Cha D, Kirby JS, Ingram JR, Jemec GB, et al. Evaluating patients' unmet needs in hidradenitis suppurativa: Results from the Global Survey Of Impact and Healthcare Needs (VOICE) Project. J Am Acad Dermatol 2020 Feb;82(2):366-376. [doi: 10.1016/j.jaad.2019.06.1301] [Medline: 31279015]
9. Scarred for Life: 2020 Update: A National Report of Patients' Experiences Living with Hidradenitis Suppurativa. Canadian Skin Patient Alliance. 2020 May. URL: https://canadianskin.ca/images/HS_Report/CSPA_HS_Report_May_22_2020_Final.pdf [accessed 2021-11-01]
10. Wang S, Wang S, Alavi A, Alhusayen R, Bashash M, Sibbald R. Hidradenitis suppurativa: A frequently missed diagnosis, Part 2: Treatment options. Adv Skin Wound Care 2015 Aug;28(8):372-80; quiz 381. [doi: 10.1097/01.ASW.0000466712.21948.8a] [Medline: 26181861]
11. Zouboulis C, Desai N, Emtestam L, Hunger R, Ioannides D, Juhász I, et al. European S1 guideline for the treatment of hidradenitis suppurativa/acne inversa. J Eur Acad Dermatol Venereol 2015 Apr 30;29(4):619-644. [doi: 10.1111/jdv.12966] [Medline: 25640693]
12. McMillan K. Hidradenitis suppurativa: Number of diagnosed patients, demographic characteristics, and treatment patterns in the United States. Am J Epidemiol 2014 Jun 15;179(12):1477-1483. [doi: 10.1093/aje/kwu078] [Medline: 24812161]
13. Ruan QZ, Chen AD, Singhal D, Lee BT, Fukudome EY. Surgical management of hidradenitis suppurativa: Procedural trends and risk factors. J Surg Res 2018 Sep;229:200-207. [doi: 10.1016/j.jss.2018.04.007] [Medline: 29936991]
14. Jemec GB, Kimball AB. Hidradenitis suppurativa: Epidemiology and scope of the problem. J Am Acad Dermatol 2015 Nov;73(5 Suppl 1):S4-S7. [doi: 10.1016/j.jaad.2015.07.052] [Medline: 26470614]
15. Alavi A, Lynde C, Alhusayen R, Bourcier M, Delorme I, George R, et al. Approach to the management of patients with hidradenitis suppurativa: A consensus document. J Cutan Med Surg 2017 Jun 22;21(6):513-524. [doi: 10.1177/1203475417716117] [Medline: 28639459]
16. Table 17-10-0009-01: Population estimates, quarterly. Statistics Canada. URL: https://www150.statcan.gc.ca/t1/tbl1/en/tv.action?pid=1710000901 [accessed 2021-11-01]
17. Micieli JA, Micieli R, Margolin EA. A review of specialties performing temporal artery biopsies in Ontario: A retrospective cohort study. CMAJ Open 2015 Jul 30;3(3):E281-E285 [FREE Full text] [doi: 10.9778/cmajo.20140108] [Medline: 26442226]
18. Micieli JA, Micieli A, Schlenker MB, Kertes PJ. Growth of medical and surgical vitreoretinal subspecialization in Ontario over 12 years. Can J Ophthalmol 2014 Aug;49(4):312-319. [doi: 10.1016/j.jcjo.2014.02.010] [Medline: 25103646]
19. Micieli JA, Trope GE, Buys YM. Gender gap and declining surgical activity among new graduates: Cataract surgery in Ontario. Can J Ophthalmol 2016 Jun;51(3):154-160. [doi: 10.1016/j.jcjo.2016.04.013] [Medline: 27316260]
20. Micieli JA. Geographic distribution of ophthalmologists in Ontario: A 10-year review. Can J Ophthalmol 2014 Jun;49(3):283-286. [doi: 10.1016/j.jcjo.2014.01.006] [Medline: 24862776]
21. Micieli R, Alhusayen R. Changes in the practice patterns and demographics of Ontario dermatologists. J Cutan Med Surg 2018 Mar 08;22(4):390-399. [doi: 10.1177/1203475418762719] [Medline: 29519145]
22. Micieli JA, Buys YM. Proportion of medical-only versus surgical ophthalmology practices: Associations and trends. Can J Ophthalmol 2016 Jun;51(3):161-167. [doi: 10.1016/j.jcjo.2016.04.005] [Medline: 27316261]
23. Ontario Ministry of Health and LTC. Schedule of Benefits. Physician Services Under the Health Insurance Act 2011:1-874.

24. Resource Manual for Physicians: Section 4 Claims Submission. Ontario Ministry of Health and Long-Term Care. 2015. URL: https://www.health.gov.on.ca/English/providers/pub/ohip/physmanual/download/section_4.pdf [accessed 2021-11-01]
25. Mehdizadeh A, Rosella L, Alavi A, Sibbald G, Farzanfar D, Hazrati A, et al. A Canadian population-based cohort to the study cost and burden of surgically resected hidradenitis suppurativa. J Cutan Med Surg 2018 Mar 11;22(3):312-317. [doi: 10.1177/1203475418763536] [Medline: 29528753]
26. Garg A, Kirby JS, Lavian J, Lin G, Strunk A. Sex- and age-adjusted population analysis of prevalence estimates for hidradenitis suppurativa in the United States. JAMA Dermatol 2017 Aug 01;153(8):760-764 [FREE Full text] [doi: 10.1001/jamadermatol.2017.0201] [Medline: 28492923]
27. Cosmatos I, Matcho A, Weinstein R, Montgomery MO, Stang P. Analysis of patient claims data to determine the prevalence of hidradenitis suppurativa in the United States. J Am Acad Dermatol 2013 Mar;68(3):412-419. [doi: 10.1016/j.jaad.2012.07.027] [Medline: 22921795]
28. Canoui-Poitrine F, Revuz JE, Wolkenstein P, Viallette C, Gabison G, Pouget F, et al. Clinical characteristics of a series of 302 French patients with hidradenitis suppurativa, with an analysis of factors associated with disease severity. J Am Acad Dermatol 2009 Jul;61(1):51-57. [doi: 10.1016/j.jaad.2009.02.013] [Medline: 19406505]
29. Schrader AM, Deckers IE, van der Zee HH, Boer J, Prens EP. Hidradenitis suppurativa: A retrospective study of 846 Dutch patients to identify factors associated with disease severity. J Am Acad Dermatol 2014 Sep;71(3):460-467. [doi: 10.1016/j.jaad.2014.04.001] [Medline: 24880664]
30. Zhang L, Losin EAR, Ashar YK, Koban L, Wager TD. Gender biases in estimation of others' pain. J Pain 2021 Sep;22(9):1048-1059 [FREE Full text] [doi: 10.1016/j.jpain.2021.03.001] [Medline: 33684539]
31. Kagan RJ, Yakuboff KP, Warner P, Warden GD. Surgical treatment of hidradenitis suppurativa: A 10-year experience. Surgery 2005 Oct;138(4):734-40; discussion 740. [doi: 10.1016/j.surg.2005.06.053] [Medline: 16269303]
32. Scuderi N, Monfrecola A, Dessy LA, Fabbrocini G, Megna M, Monfrecola G. Medical and surgical treatment of hidradenitis suppurativa: A review. Skin Appendage Disord 2017 May 21;3(2):95-110 [FREE Full text] [doi: 10.1159/000462979] [Medline: 28560220]
33. Lachaine J, Miron A, Shear N, Alhusayen R. The prevalence and incidence of hidradenitis suppurativa in Canada: Results from a population-based survey. Value in Health 2016 May;19(3):A123. [doi: 10.1016/j.jval.2016.03.495]
34. Bianchi L, Caposiena Caro RD, Ganzetti G, Molinelli E, Dini V, Oranges T, et al. Sex-related differences of clinical features in hidradenitis suppurativa: Analysis of an Italian-based cohort. Clin Exp Dermatol 2019 Jul 28;44(5):e177-e180. [doi: 10.1111/ced.13861] [Medline: 30593710]
35. Sabat R, Jemec GBE, Matusiak L, Kimball AB, Prens E, Wolk K. Hidradenitis suppurativa. Nat Rev Dis Primers 2020 Mar 12;6(1):18. [doi: 10.1038/s41572-020-0149-1] [Medline: 32165620]
36. Mehdizadeh A, Hazen PG, Bechara FG, Zwingerman N, Moazenzadeh M, Bashash M, et al. Recurrence of hidradenitis suppurativa after surgical management: A systematic review and meta-analysis. J Am Acad Dermatol 2015 Nov;73(5 Suppl 1):S70-S77. [doi: 10.1016/j.jaad.2015.07.044] [Medline: 26470621]
37. Kohorst JJ, Baum CL, Otley CC, Roenigk RK, Pemberton JH, Dozois EJ, et al. Patient satisfaction and quality of life following surgery for hidradenitis suppurativa. Dermatol Surg 2017;43(1):125-133. [doi: 10.1097/dss.0000000000000942]
38. Falola RA, DeFazio MV, Anghel EL, Mitnick CDB, Attinger CE, Evans KK. What heals hidradenitis suppurativa: Surgery, immunosuppression, or both? Plastic and Reconstructive Surgery 2016;138:219S-229S. [doi: 10.1097/prs.0000000000002671]
39. Doherty GM. Call to action for general surgery-trained specialists: Maintain both breadth and depth. JAMA Surg 2016 Mar 01;151(3):209-210. [doi: 10.1001/jamasurg.2015.4653] [Medline: 26650975]
40. Saunte DML, Jemec GBE. Hidradenitis suppurativa: Advances in diagnosis and treatment. JAMA 2017 Nov 28;318(20):2019-2032. [doi: 10.1001/jama.2017.16691] [Medline: 29183082]
41. Ritz J, Runkel N, Haier J, Buhr HJ. Extent of surgery and recurrence rate of hidradenitis suppurativa. Int J Colorectal Dis 1998;13(4):164-168. [doi: 10.1007/s003840050159] [Medline: 9810520]
42. Haider AH, Scott VK, Rehman KA, Velopulos C, Bentley JM, Cornwell EE, et al. Racial disparities in surgical care and outcomes in the United States: A comprehensive review of patient, provider, and systemic factors. J Am Coll Surg 2013 Mar;216(3):482-92.e12 [FREE Full text] [doi: 10.1016/j.jamcollsurg.2012.11.014] [Medline: 23318117]
43. Shukla N, Paul M, Halley M, Lowes M, Hester V, Aguilar C, et al. Identifying barriers to care and research in hidradenitis suppurativa: Findings from a patient engagement event. Br J Dermatol 2020 Jun 29;182(6):1490-1492 [FREE Full text] [doi: 10.1111/bjd.18818] [Medline: 31883104]

Abbreviations

HS: hidradenitis suppurativa
LHIN: Local Health Integration Network
OHIP: Ontario Health Insurance Plan

24

Nonprescription Products of Internet Retailers for the Prevention and Management of Herpes Zoster and Postherpetic Neuralgia: Analysis of Consumer Reviews on Amazon

Pengyi Zhu[1,2*], BS; Benjamin K P Woo[1*], MD

[1]Olive View-University of California Los Angeles Medical Center, Sylmar, CA, United States

[2]College of Osteopathic Medicine of the Pacific, Western University of Health Sciences, Pomona, CA, United States

[*]all authors contributed equally

Corresponding Author:
Pengyi Zhu, BS
College of Osteopathic Medicine of the Pacific
Western University of Health Sciences
309 E 2nd St
Pomona, CA, 91766
United States

Email: sharonpzhu2@gmail.com

Abstract

Background: Herpes zoster affects approximately 1 million people annually in the United States, with postherpetic neuralgia as the most common complication. The frequent prescription of opioids as the first-line medication for herpes zoster or postherpetic neuralgia contributes to the increasing health care costs of their treatment. Despite the advent of internet retailers providing alternative products for the prevention and management these conditions, there are limited studies on the availability, ingredients, and consumer preference for the products.

Objective: This study used the internet retailer Amazon to determine the availability of products for the management of herpes zoster and postherpetic neuralgia, and assessed consumer preference based on listed ingredients.

Methods: The internet retailer Amazon was used to perform a search for products related to "shingles" in September 2020. Top products sorted by reviews and ratings were determined to be either shingles-specific (including "shingles" in either the product title or description) or shingles-nonspecific. Analysis of price, rating, type of vehicle, and ingredients was performed. The types of vehicles, ingredients, and percentages of positive and negative reviews related to "shingles" of the product groups were analyzed with a two-tailed two-sample proportions *Z*-test to assess the difference between shingles-specific and shingles-nonspecific products. Statistical significance was judged at $P<.05$.

Results: The top 131 products among over 3000 products retrieved were determined based on a rating of 4 or more stars after searching for the term "shingles" on Amazon. Forty-six of the 131 products (35.1%) were shingles-specific. Shingles-nonspecific products were more likely to have positive reviews mentioning "shingles" ($P=.005$). Vehicles, balms ($P=.02$), and salves ($P=.04$) were more likely to be shingles-specific, whereas tablets or capsules ($P=.002$) were more likely to be shingles-nonspecific. Among the ingredients analyzed, aloe vera was the top-ranked ingredient, included in 29 of the 131 total products (22.1%). Aloe vera ($P=.01$), lemon balm ($P<.001$), vitamin E ($P=.03$), and peppermint oil ($P=.008$) were more likely to be included in the shingles-specific products, whereas magnesium ($P=.01$) was more likely to be included in shingles-nonspecific products.

Conclusions: There is an abundance of products and ingredients being used for the management and treatment of shingles with certain ingredients preferred by consumers. There is a discrepancy between approved ingredients and the ingredients preferred by consumers. Furthermore, there are insufficient studies on ingredients used by consumers on internet retailers such as Amazon, and future studies can focus on the effectiveness of popular ingredients to decrease misinformation on the internet.

KEYWORDS

Amazon; consumer preference; herpes zoster; postherpetic neuralgia; shingles; internet; customer; herpes; ingredients; treatment

Introduction

Shingles, or herpes zoster (HZ), is caused by reactivation of latent varicella zoster virus (VZV) in the sensory neurons, typically after the primary infection of chicken pox in childhood [1,2]. Previous studies have shown that more than 95% of adults across North America and Europe are at risk for HZ, and approximately 1 million people are affected by HZ in the United States annually [2,3]. Stress, aging, illness, medication, or other causes of decreased immunity can cause the activation of dormant VZV that commonly affects the cervical, thoracic, and trigeminal nerves [3,4]. Acute herpes zoster (AHZ) manifests as a painful blistering rash along a dermatome, initially presenting as a maculopapular rash that develops into vesicles and pustules [4,5]. Postherpetic neuralgia (PHN) is the most common complication of HZ, which is defined as the persistence of acute HZ pain in a dermatomal distribution that lasts over 3 months [1,3,6,7]. PHN is due to damage to the nerves from an inflammatory response caused by viral replication within the nerve [8]. PHN can cause allodynia, hyperalgesia, anesthesia, and other sensory deficits of the affected dermatome [3,9]. Owing to the debilitating nature of PHN, patients seek medications to manage the pain.

The therapies for AHZ include antivirals, corticosteroids as adjunctive therapy, acetaminophen or nonsteroidal anti-inflammatory drugs (NSAIDs) for analgesia, and capsaicin or lidocaine as topical treatment [8]. For PHN, first-line medications include calcium channel blockers (gabapentin and pregabalin), tricyclic antidepressants, and a lidocaine patch [10]. Second-line treatments include opioid analgesics and a capsaicin patch or cream [10]. A previous study showed that opioids were commonly prescribed as the initial treatment for PHN, followed by gabapentin, prescription NSAIDs, lidocaine patch, pregabalin, tricyclic antidepressant, topical lidocaine, and capsaicin, respectively [3].

However, with the advent of internet information and shopping through internet retailers such as Amazon, patients can now easily access nonprescription remedies for the rashes and neuropathic pain caused by shingles or PHN. Amazon has recently been utilized as a data source in studies to analyze consumer perception and preference for health-related products [11-13]. Some natural treatment choices offered on internet retailers have been studied for either PHN or neuropathic pain, including vitamins and nutrients such as zinc, licorice, honey, aloe vera, and St John's wort [14-16]. However, most herbal remedies such as St John's wort have not been assessed in proper clinical trials or have not been proven to be useful [17].

Given the readily available nonprescription options that claim effectiveness for shingles and PHN pain, it is important to understand what products are available for patients and the efficacy of the ingredients in these products. In this study, we evaluated the products that are available and preferred by customers through analyzing the vehicle types, ingredients, and customer reviews of shingles-related products sold on Amazon. Finally, we sought to understand the different factors and ingredients of products used for shingles or PHN prevention and treatment.

Methods

Amazon, the internet retailer, was accessed in September 2020 to search for products related to shingles. "Shingles" was used as the keyword to search in the "Health & Household" department of the website. The searches were screened for customer ratings of 4 stars and above. Products such as bandages or household items were excluded. Finally, only products that included the term "shingles" in the product title, description, Customer Reviews, or Customer Question and Answer were included in the final analysis. Product listings without mention of "shingles" in the product title, description, Customer Reviews, or Customer Question and Answer were excluded. For product listings with different quantities and sizes, only the listing with the most reviews was included. From the overall products, the average price, median price per unit, average ratings, average number of reviews, type of vehicle, and ingredients were determined. Several ingredients studied previously for shingles were analyzed in this study [14,17,18].

Two groups were derived from the original sample set. First, products that included the term "shingles" in either the product title or description were classified as shingles-specific products. Second, products that did not include the term "shingles" in either the product title or description, but included the term in either the Customer Reviews or the Customer Question and Answer sections were classified as shingles-nonspecific products. A two-tailed two-sample proportions *Z*-test was used to determine if a product specific to "shingles" was more likely to be a specific vehicle or to include certain ingredients. The numbers of positive and negative reviews in Customer Reviews including the term "shingles" were counted. The two-tailed two-sample proportions *Z*-test was also used to compare the means of percentages of positive and negative reviews among all reviews of products including "shingles" for shingles-specific and shingles-nonspecific products. A P value <.05 was considered to indicate a statistically significant difference.

Results

Over 3000 results were populated on the Amazon internet retailer when searching for the key term "shingles." There were 742 results in the "Health & Household" department that received a rating of 4 stars and above. Among the 131 top-rated products, there was a total of 215,225 reviews with a median of 698 reviews (range 24-16,523 reviews) and an average rating of 4.4 (out of 5) stars with a median of 4.4 (range 4-4.9 stars). Different types of vehicles for shingles were counted and categorized. Among the 131 total products, 44 (33.6%) were creams or lotions, 30 (22.9%) were tablets or capsules, 11 (8.4%) were gels, 10 (7.7%) were balms, 8 (6.1%) were bath products, 7 (5.3%) were ointments, 6 (4.6%) were oils, 5 (3.8%) were salves, and the remaining 10 products (7.6%) included powders, wipes, pump dispensers, liquids, and sprays. Among all reviews for the products that mentioned "shingles," there was an average of 82.6% positive reviews and 10% negative reviews.

Among the 131 products, 46 (35.1%) products that included "shingles" in either the title or product description comprised shingles-specific products and 85 (64.9%) that did not include "shingles" in either the title or product description comprised the shingles-nonspecific products. Table 1 shows the top 10 most reviewed overall shingles products and Table 2 shows the top 10 most reviewed shingles-specific products. Comparison of the two tables reveals only three products among both the top 10 most reviewed overall products and the top 10 most reviewed shingles-specific products: Leven Rose Store's Jojoba Oil, Emuaid's EmuaidMAX Ointment, and Quantum Health's Super Lysine.

Table 1. Top 10 most reviewed overall products.

Rank	Manufacturer	Product name	Number of reviews	Mean rating (out of 5)
1	Leven Rose Store	Jojoba Oil	16,523	4.7
2	Puriya	Mother of All Creams	11,139	4.3
3	Sun Essential Oils	Geranium	9046	4.2
4	Emuaid	EmuaidMAX Ointment	8974	4.0
5	Truremedy	Remedy Soap	8800	4.5
6	Mederma	Mederma Advanced Scar Gel	8063	4.2
7	Ramina	Natural Hemp Cream	6377	4.3
8	Puriya	Wonder Balm	6050	4.3
9	Quantum Health	Super Lysine	5875	4.6
10	NOW Foods	Double Strength L-Lysine	5607	4.7

Table 2. Top 10 most reviewed shingles-specific products.

Rank	Manufacturer	Product name	Number of reviews	Mean rating (out of 5)
1	Leven Rose Store	Jojoba Oil	16,523	4.7
2	Emuaid	EmuaidMAX Ointment	8974	4.0
3	Quantum Health	Super Lysine	5875	4.6
4	Blue Emu	Original Blue-Emu Super Strength	4723	4.5
5	Dermachange	Shingles	3254	4.2
6	Wild Naturals	Eczema & Psoriasis Cream	2896	4.1
7	Clearbody Organics	Hemp Relief Cream	2828	4.4
8	Era Organics	Relief	1885	4.0
9	Emuaid	Emuaid	1794	4.2
10	Frankincense & Myrrh	Neuropathy Rubbing Oil	1574	4.3

When analyzing customer reviews including "shingles" among the shingles-specific products, there was an average of 69.5% positive reviews and 10.1% negative reviews among the total shingles-related reviews per product. Among the shingles-nonspecific products, there was an average of 89.9% positive reviews and 10% negative reviews out of the total shingles-related reviews per product. Shingles-nonspecific products were more likely to have positive customer reviews mentioning "shingles" based on the Z-test analysis (P=.005), whereas there was no significant difference in negative customer reviews between shingles-specific and shingles-nonspecific groups (P=.99).

Out of the 46 shingles-specific products, 18 (39%) were creams or lotions, 7 (15%) were balms, 4 (9%) were oils, 4 (9%) were salves, 3 (7%) were tablets or capsules, 3 (7%) were gels, 3 (7%) were ointments, 1 (2%) was a bath product, and 3 (7%) were other products, including pump dispenser, spray, and liquid. Among the 85 shingles-nonspecific products, 27 (32%) were tablets or capsules, 26 (31%) were creams or lotions, 8 (9%) were gels, 7 (8%) were bath products, 4 (5%) were ointments, 3 (4%) were balms, 2 (2%) were oils, 1 (1%) was a salve, and 7 (8%) were other products, including powders, liquid, sprays, wipes, and solutions. Balms (P=.02) and salves (P=.04) were more likely to be shingles-specific, whereas tablets or capsules (P=.002) were more likely to be shingles-nonspecific.

Based on previous studies related to treatment for shingles, several ingredients were assessed from the products [14,17,18]. Among all 131 products, 29 (22.1%) contained aloe vera, 18 (13.7%) contained honey, 17 (13.0%) contained magnesium, 16 (12.2%) contained lemon balm, 14 (10.7%) contained L-lysine, 13 (9.9%) contained menthol, 11 (8.4%) contained lidocaine, 10 (7.6%) contained zinc, 9 (6.9%) contained oatmeal or oat straw extract, 7 (7.6%) contained St John's wort, 6 (4.6%) contained licorice, 2 (1.5%) contained capsaicin, 2 (1.5%) contained Reishi mushroom, and 1 (0.8%) contained aspirin.

Out the 46 shingles-specific products, 16 (34.8%) contained aloe vera, 10 (21.7%) contained honey, 1 (2.2%) contained magnesium, 12 (26.1%) contained lemon balm, 5 (10.9%) contained L-lysine, 3 (6.5%) contained menthol, 2 (4.3%) contained lidocaine, 4 (8.7%) contained zinc, 2 (4.3%) contained oatmeal or oat straw extract, 4 (8.7%) contained St John's wort, 3 (6.5%) contained licorice, and none of the products contained capsaicin, Reishi mushroom, or aspirin. Among the 85 shingles-nonspecific products, 13 (15.3%) contained aloe vera, 8 (9.4%) contained honey, 16 (18.8%) contained magnesium, 4 (4.7%) contained lemon balm, 9 (10.6%) contained L-lysine, 10 (11.8%) contained menthol, 9 (10.6%) contained lidocaine, 6 (7.1%) contained zinc, 7 (8.2%) contained oatmeal or oat straw extract, 3 (3.5%) contained St John's wort, 3 (3.5%) contained licorice, 2 (2.4%) contained capsaicin, 2 (2.4%) contained Reishi mushroom, and 1 (1.2%) contained aspirin. Among all ingredients, aloe vera (P=.01) and lemon balm (P<.001) were more likely to be included in shingles-specific products, whereas magnesium (P=.01) was more likely to be included in shingles-nonspecific products.

Vitamins were assessed individually [15,16,18]. Among all 131 products, 4 (3.1%) included vitamin A, 3 (2.3%) included vitamin B2, 4 (3.1%) included vitamin B6, 2 (1.5%) included vitamin B9, 2 (1.5%) included vitamin B12, 15 (11.5%) included vitamin C, 3 (2.3%) included vitamin D, and 28 (21.4%) included vitamin E. Among the 46 shingles-specific products, 8 (17%) included vitamin C and 15 (33%) included vitamin E, whereas no products included vitamins A, B2, B6, B9, B12, or D. Of the 85 shingles-nonspecific products, 4 (5%) included vitamin A, 3 (4%) included vitamin B2, 4 (4%) included vitamin B6, 2 (2%) included vitamin B9, 2 (2%) included vitamin B12, 7 (8%) included vitamin C, 3 (4%) included vitamin D, and 13 (15%) included vitamin E. Vitamin E was more likely to be used in shingles-specific products (P=.03).

Specific oils were assessed based off prior studies, including peppermint oil, geranium oil, and hemp oil [19-21]. Among all 131 products, 19 (14.5%) included peppermint oil, 5 (3.8%) included geranium oil, and 15 (11.5%) included hemp oil. Of the 46 shingles-specific products, 12 (26%) included peppermint oil, none included geranium oil, and 8 (17%) included hemp oil. Out the 85 shingles-nonspecific products, 7 (8%) included peppermint oil, 5 (6%) included geranium oil, and 7 (8%) included hemp oil. Peppermint oil was more likely to be included in shingles-specific products (P=.008).

Discussion

Principal Findings

With nearly 1 million cases of HZ diagnosed annually in the United States, HZ can affect up to 20% of individuals within their lifetimes [22,23]. HZ is a large health care burden, with opioids prescribed as the most common first-line treatment, further contributing to the already high health insurance cost of opioids [3]. Patients inflicted by PHN can spend 2-4 times more on health costs than patients with only HZ [24]. As such, internet retailers such as Amazon provide other options for the management and treatment of HZ or PHN that can provide relief for patients. However, with the wide variety of products and ingredients available, it can be difficult for patients to determine which products would be effective. This study showed that among the variety of vehicles available, Amazon customers preferred creams or lotions, which comprised 33.6% of the 131 products, with tablets or capsules coming in second comprising 22.9% of the 131 products. Tablets or capsules were more likely to be shingles-nonspecific products, whereas balms and salves were more likely to be shingles-specific products. This suggests a lack of consensus regarding products recommended for shingles and products that patients prefer.

Over 3000 products were retrieved when searching "shingles" on Amazon. "Shingles" was used as the keyword as it is a term more widely known in the general population. Among the products indicated for shingles treatment, there were also household cleaning products, which raises concern that such products are being suggested for shingles use on the internet retailer. Out of the 131 products, only 35.1% included products that specifically mentioned shingles in either the title or product description, and the majority (64.9%) of products did not. Furthermore, only 3 products from the top 10 most reviewed overall shingles products were within the top 10 most reviewed shingles-specific products. This highlights the discrepancy between products that are suggested for shingles use and products that are labeled for shingles use. When comparing customer reviews that mention shingles between shingles-nonspecific and shingles-specific products, shingles-nonspecific products were more likely to have more positive customer reviews (89.9%) compared with shingles-specific products (69.5%). This suggests that customer reviews play a larger role in product selection compared to a specified product indication for shingles. Interestingly, there was no significant difference in customer reviews of shingles-specific and shingles-nonspecific products, further compounding the importance of reviews in the consumer selection of products.

Various ingredients were analyzed that were previously studied in relation to shingles or PHN treatment. A 5% lidocaine patch and 0.075% capsaicin cream are among first- or second-line topical treatment options for PHN [8]. In our analysis of the 131 products, 8.4% contained lidocaine and 1.5% contained capsaicin. Of the shingles-specific products, only 4.3% contained lidocaine and none contained capsaicin, whereas of the shingles-nonspecific products, 10.6% contained lidocaine and 2.4% contained capsaicin. Lidocaine acts as a local anesthetic with a mechanism of action involving partial inhibition of voltage-gated calcium channels and reducing the discharge of activity in afferent pain receptors [25]. Lidocaine is considered a first-line therapy for PHN despite limited studies on its effectiveness [26,27]. The lidocaine products found in the Amazon products were between 4% and 5% in concentration; however, none of the top products recommended including lidocaine was a patch, which is recommended in the literature [8]. The products including lidocaine were creams, gels, or sprays, which suggests that lidocaine administered using these vehicles was preferred among customers instead of patches. Topical capsaicin is an activator of the TRPV1 channel of nociceptor nerve fibers, leading to an influx of calcium that decreases the function of nociceptor nerve fibers [25]. Studies have shown that a higher concentration of capsaicin was effective for PHN [28]. The concentration of capsaicin in the products found on Amazon was either 0.025% or 0.1%, whereas high-dose capsaicin products have a concentration of 8%. This may explain why capsaicin was not a highly preferred or recommended product as the smaller concentration only provides moderate relief for patients [25].

Other natural ingredients have been studied for their effects against HZ, such as licorice and Reishi mushroom [14]. Ingredients that have shown efficacy against herpes simplex virus (HSV) may also have a benefit for HZ, such as honey, aloe vera, and St John's wort [14,29]. Licorice may be able to inactivate viral particles and was reported to show in vitro antiviral activity against VZV, although further studies are needed to evaluate its use as a topical agent [14]. Reishi mushroom was tested in a small clinical trial and a case study, demonstrating relief of pain [14]. Honey has shown faster healing times for patients with HSV infection, suggesting a possible benefit against HZ [14]. Aloe vera is a known ingredient for wound healing, and St John's wort has shown antiviral activity against HSV-1 [14]. In this study, aloe vera was one of the top ingredients used among the 131 products, accounting for 22.1%, and is more likely to be used as an ingredient in shingles-specific products. This indicates that customers also prefer aloe vera for the treatment of shingles. Honey comprised 13.7% of all products, making it the second most likely included ingredient, suggesting that more studies should be performed to assess the efficacy of honey against HZ. St John's wort, licorice, and Reishi mushroom were less commonly used as ingredients; however, more studies can reveal if these ingredients will be of benefit to patients with HZ or PHN. Lemon balm was also more likely to be included in shingles-specific products; despite few studies regarding the use of lemon specifically for this condition, it is likely preferred for shingles owing to its high vitamin C level.

Decreased immunity is a known risk factor for HZ and PHN, with nutritional deficiency being a major cause [18]. Vitamin and nutrient deficiencies, such as zinc and magnesium, and their effect on HZ have been studied to assess their efficacy as potential treatments [18,30,31]. Low vitamin C levels have been found to play a role in the development of herpes infection and PHN, with trials of intravenous vitamin C demonstrating efficacy in relieving pain [16]. Hypovitaminosis D has been associated with the development of neuropathic pain due to various mechanisms, including inflammatory processes and an increase of reactive oxygen species [15,32]. Vitamin B such as cobalamin (vitamin B12) was shown to be effective for painful neuropathies, and deficiency of folic acid (vitamin B9) causes peripheral neuropathy [33,34]. Vitamin E has also been shown to act as an analgesic in rat models with neuropathic pain [35]. Zinc deficiency has been shown to be a risk factor for PNH [30]. Magnesium has been found to block the N-methyl-D-aspartate receptor, which is associated with hypersensitivity [30,36]. Among the ingredients assessed, magnesium was more likely to be included in shingles-nonspecific products, whereas vitamin E was more likely to be included in shingles-specific products. Given the sparsity of studies on the efficacy of either magnesium or vitamin E, these results suggest that more studies are warranted for assessing these nutrients in the treatment of HZ and PHN. Vitamin C was the second-ranked nutrient among the 131 products, although it was not necessarily preferred in shingles-specific products despite studies showing its role in HZ and PHN. This discrepancy could be due to the lower concentration of vitamin C as either an oral supplement or within topical agents compared to a higher available systemic dose as an intravenous treatment.

Finally, certain oils were assessed, including peppermint oil, geranium oil, and hemp oil [19-21]. Peppermint oil was more likely to be used as an ingredient in shingles-specific products. The main ingredient of peppermint oil is menthol, which is commonly used for musculoskeletal pain [19]. The possible mechanism of action of peppermint oil is the inhibition of sensitized nociceptors [19]. However, few studies have assessed peppermint oil; thus, its common use in shingles-specific products warrants more studies on its effect on HZ and PHN. Geranium oil was found to relieve pain quickly in a small study [16]; however, it was not widely used in shingles products available on Amazon. Hemp oil was used a primary ingredient in several products (11.5% of 131 total products); however, few studies have focused on its effect for shingles. A small trial showed the effectiveness of a cannabinoid receptor agonist topical for PHN [21]. Given that it is commonly used, hemp oil should be further studied to better understand if it is effective for the treatment of shingles.

Limitations

The main limitation of the study is that not all of the products related to "shingles" from Amazon were included in the analysis since there was over 3000 products found. Only the top 131 products were included with products receiving a rating of less than 4 stars excluded. Furthermore, products that did not include "shingles" in either the product name, description, or mentioned in the customer reviews were excluded. This excluded products that were suggested by the internet retailer algorithm but may not have been suggested by the manufacturer or customers to be used for shingles. Another limitation was that only "shingles" was used as the keyword to narrow down the search based on what the general populace would search. Searching for "postherpetic neuralgia" and "herpes zoster" could potentially produce more results. Furthermore, we did not analyze all of the active ingredients used by all of the products analyzed. Finally, we did not compare ingredients of the products with the amount of positive and negative reviews related to "shingles" that the product received. This comparison would allow for further analysis of whether specific ingredients were perceived to be effective to the general population.

Conclusion

Our analysis of "shingles" products on the internet retailer Amazon demonstrated an abundance of products and available ingredients used for shingles treatment. Although there are already available treatments that are approved for the management of AHZ and PHN, because these are conditions that are typically managed by several treatments, understanding over-the-counter management would benefit patients. Using Amazon to understand what is available to and preferred by customers can allow us to assess which ingredients require further studies to better educate our patients on what would be effective for AHZ and PHN and to target potential misinformation online.

References

1. Rahmatpour Rokni G, Rathod D, Tabarestani M, Mirabi A, Jha A, de Vita V, et al. Postherpetic neuralgia and recalcitrant cystic lesions following herpes zoster: A case report and review of treatment options. Dermatol Ther 2020 Jul 12;33(4):e13793. [doi: 10.1111/dth.13793] [Medline: 32510833]
2. Johnson RW, Rice AS. Postherpetic neuralgia. N Engl J Med 2014 Oct 16;371(16):1526-1533. [doi: 10.1056/nejmcp1403062]
3. Gudin J, Fudin J, Wang E, Haylon T, Patel K, Goss TF. Treatment patterns and medication use in patients with postherpetic neuralgia. J Manag Care Spec Pharm 2019 Dec;25(12):1387-1396. [doi: 10.18553/jmcp.2019.19093] [Medline: 31589557]
4. Argoff CE. Review of current guidelines on the care of postherpetic neuralgia. Postgrad Med 2011 Sep 13;123(5):134-142. [doi: 10.3810/pgm.2011.09.2469] [Medline: 21904096]
5. Ngo AL, Urits I, Yilmaz M, Fortier L, Anya A, Oh JH, et al. Postherpetic neuralgia: current evidence on the topical film-forming spray with bupivacaine hydrochloride and a review of available treatment strategies. Adv Ther 2020 May 15;37(5):2003-2016 [FREE Full text] [doi: 10.1007/s12325-020-01335-9] [Medline: 32297285]
6. Cunningham AL, Lal H, Kovac M, Chlibek R, Hwang S, Díez-Domingo J, ZOE-70 Study Group. Efficacy of the herpes zoster subunit vaccine in adults 70 years of age or older. N Engl J Med 2016 Sep 15;375(11):1019-1032. [doi: 10.1056/NEJMoa1603800] [Medline: 27626517]
7. Xing X, Sun K, Yan Y. Postherpetic Neuralgia. Topics in Pain Management 2001;17(4):13-17. [doi: 10.1097/00587875-200111000-00001]
8. Saguil A, Kane S, Mercado M, Lauters R. Herpes zoster and postherpetic neuralgia: prevention and management. Am Fam Physician 2017 Nov 15;96(10):656-663. [doi: 10.1093/med/9780190298357.003.0011]
9. Lin C, Lin Y, Lao H, Chen C. Interventional Treatments for Postherpetic Neuralgia: A Systematic Review. Pain Physician 2019 May;22(3):209-228 [FREE Full text] [Medline: 31151330]
10. Mallick-Searle T, Snodgrass B, Brant J. Postherpetic neuralgia: epidemiology, pathophysiology, and pain management pharmacology. J Multidiscip Healthc 2016;9:447-454. [doi: 10.2147/JMDH.S106340] [Medline: 27703368]
11. Xu S, Kwa M, Agarwal A, Rademaker A, Kundu RV. Sunscreen Product Performance and Other Determinants of Consumer Preferences. JAMA Dermatol 2016 Aug 01;152(8):920-927. [doi: 10.1001/jamadermatol.2016.2344] [Medline: 27385189]
12. Zhu P, Fung A, Woo BKP. Consumer preference of products for the prevention and treatment of stretch marks: systematic product search. JMIR Dermatol 2020 Jun 4;3(1):e18295 [FREE Full text] [doi: 10.2196/18295]
13. Chong KPL, Guo JZ, Deng X, Woo BKP. Consumer perceptions of wearable technology devices: retrospective review and analysis. JMIR Mhealth Uhealth 2020 Apr 20;8(4):e17544 [FREE Full text] [doi: 10.2196/17544] [Medline: 32310148]
14. Roxas M. Herpes zoster and postherpetic neuralgia: diagnosis and therapeutic considerations. Altern Med Rev 2006 Jun;11(2):102-113 [FREE Full text] [Medline: 16813460]
15. Chao C, Chiang C, Huang J, Hung K. Vitamin D is closely linked to the clinical courses of herpes zoster: From pathogenesis to complications. Med Hypotheses 2015 Oct;85(4):452-457. [doi: 10.1016/j.mehy.2015.06.027] [Medline: 26163058]
16. Kim MS, Kim DJ, Na CH, Shin BS. A Study of Intravenous Administration of Vitamin C in the Treatment of Acute Herpetic Pain and Postherpetic Neuralgia. Ann Dermatol 2016 Dec;28(6):677-683 [FREE Full text] [doi: 10.5021/ad.2016.28.6.677] [Medline: 27904265]
17. Boyd A, Bleakley C, Hurley D, Gill C, Hannon-Fletcher M, Bell P, et al. Herbal medicinal products or preparations for neuropathic pain. Cochrane Database Syst Rev 2019 Apr 02;4:CD010528 [FREE Full text] [doi: 10.1002/14651858.CD010528.pub4] [Medline: 30938843]
18. Chen J, Chu C, Lin Y, So EC, Shieh J, Hu M. Nutrient deficiencies as a risk factor in Taiwanese patients with postherpetic neuralgia. Br J Nutr 2011 Sep;106(5):700-707. [doi: 10.1017/S0007114511000481] [Medline: 21473799]
19. Davies SJ, Harding LM, Baranowski AP. A novel treatment of postherpetic neuralgia using peppermint oil. Clin J Pain 2002;18(3):200-202. [doi: 10.1097/00002508-200205000-00011] [Medline: 12048423]
20. Greenway FL, Frome BM, Engels TM, McLellan A. Temporary relief of postherpetic neuralgia pain with topical geranium oil. Am J Med 2003 Nov;115(7):586-587. [doi: 10.1016/s0002-9343(03)00434-0] [Medline: 14599644]
21. Phan N, Siepmann D, Gralow I, Ständer S. Adjuvant topical therapy with a cannabinoid receptor agonist in facial postherpetic neuralgia. J Dtsch Dermatol Ges 2010 Mar;8(2):88-91. [doi: 10.1111/j.1610-0387.2009.07213.x] [Medline: 19744255]
22. Insinga RP, Itzler RF, Pellissier JM, Saddier P, Nikas AA. The incidence of herpes zoster in a United States administrative database. J Gen Intern Med 2005 Aug;20(8):748-753 [FREE Full text] [doi: 10.1111/j.1525-1497.2005.0150.x] [Medline: 16050886]
23. Thompson R, Kong C, Porco T, Kim E, Ebert C, Acharya N. Herpes zoster and post-herpetic neuralgia: changing incidence rates from 1994 to 2018 in the United States. Clin Infect Dis 2020 Aug 23:ciaa1185. [doi: 10.1093/cid/ciaa1185] [Medline: 32829399]

24. Dworkin R, White R, O'Connor AB, Baser O, Hawkins K. Healthcare costs of acute and chronic pain associated with a diagnosis of herpes zoster. J Am Geriatr Soc 2007 Aug;55(8):1168-1175. [doi: 10.1111/j.1532-5415.2007.01231.x] [Medline: 17661954]
25. Shrestha M, Chen A. Modalities in managing postherpetic neuralgia. Korean J Pain 2018 Oct;31(4):235-243 [FREE Full text] [doi: 10.3344/kjp.2018.31.4.235] [Medline: 30310548]
26. Davies PS, Galer BS. Review of lidocaine patch 5% studies in the treatment of postherpetic neuralgia. Drugs 2004;64(9):937-947. [doi: 10.2165/00003495-200464090-00002] [Medline: 15101784]
27. Derry S, Wiffen P, Moore R, Quinlan J. Topical lidocaine for neuropathic pain in adults. Cochrane Database Syst Rev 2014 Jul 24(7):CD010958 [FREE Full text] [doi: 10.1002/14651858.CD010958.pub2] [Medline: 25058164]
28. Derry S, Sven-Rice A, Cole P, Tan T, Moore R. Topical capsaicin (high concentration) for chronic neuropathic pain in adults. Cochrane Database Syst Rev 2013 Mar 28(2):CD007393. [doi: 10.1002/14651858.CD007393.pub3] [Medline: 23450576]
29. Morelli V, Calmet E, Jhingade V. Alternative therapies for common dermatologic disorders, part 1. Prim Care 2010 Jun;37(2):269-283. [doi: 10.1016/j.pop.2010.02.004] [Medline: 20493336]
30. Lin Y, Lan K, Wang L, Chen J. Treatment of postherpetic neuralgia with intravenous administration of zinc sulfate: a case report. A A Pract 2018 Jul 01;11(1):8-10. [doi: 10.1213/XAA.0000000000000712] [Medline: 29634548]
31. Kim YH, Lee PB, Oh TK. Is magnesium sulfate effective for pain in chronic postherpetic neuralgia patients comparing with ketamine infusion therapy? J Clin Anesth 2015 Jun;27(4):296-300. [doi: 10.1016/j.jclinane.2015.02.006] [Medline: 25792176]
32. Chen J, Lin Y, Wang L, Hung K, Lan K, Ho C, et al. Hypovitaminosis din postherpetic neuralgia-high prevalence and inverse association with pain: a retrospective study. Nutrients 2019 Nov 15;11(11):2787 [FREE Full text] [doi: 10.3390/nu11112787] [Medline: 31731694]
33. Xu G, Lv Z, Xu G, Tang W. Thiamine, cobalamin, locally injected alone or combination for herpetic itching: a single-center randomized controlled trial. Clin J Pain 2014 Mar;30(3):269-278. [doi: 10.1097/AJP.0b013e3182a0e085] [Medline: 23887347]
34. Xu G, Lv Z, Feng Y, Tang W, Xu GX. A single-center randomized controlled trial of local methylcobalamin injection for subacute herpetic neuralgia. Pain Med 2013 Jun 08;14(6):884-894. [doi: 10.1111/pme.12081] [Medline: 23566267]
35. Kim HK, Kim JH, Gao X, Zhou J, Lee I, Chung K, et al. Analgesic effect of vitamin E is mediated by reducing central sensitization in neuropathic pain. Pain 2006 May;122(1-2):53-62. [doi: 10.1016/j.pain.2006.01.013] [Medline: 16524661]
36. Brill S, Sedgwick PM, Hamann W, Di Vadi PP. Efficacy of intravenous magnesium in neuropathic pain. Br J Anaesth 2002 Nov;89(5):711-714 [FREE Full text] [Medline: 12393768]

Abbreviations

AHZ: acute herpes zoster
HSV: herpes simplex virus
HZ: herpes zoster
NSAIDs: nonsteroidal anti-inflammatory drugs
PHN: postherpetic neuralgia
VZV: varicella zoster virus

Permissions

All chapters in this book were first published by JMIR Publications; hereby published with permission under the Creative Commons Attribution License or equivalent. Every chapter published in this book has been scrutinized by our experts. Their significance has been extensively debated. The topics covered herein carry significant findings which will fuel the growth of the discipline. They may even be implemented as practical applications or may be referred to as a beginning point for another development.

The contributors of this book come from diverse backgrounds, making this book a truly international effort. This book will bring forth new frontiers with its revolutionizing research information and detailed analysis of the nascent developments around the world.

We would like to thank all the contributing authors for lending their expertise to make the book truly unique. They have played a crucial role in the development of this book. Without their invaluable contributions this book wouldn't have been possible. They have made vital efforts to compile up to date information on the varied aspects of this subject to make this book a valuable addition to the collection of many professionals and students.

This book was conceptualized with the vision of imparting up-to-date information and advanced data in this field. To ensure the same, a matchless editorial board was set up. Every individual on the board went through rigorous rounds of assessment to prove their worth. After which they invested a large part of their time researching and compiling the most relevant data for our readers.

The editorial board has been involved in producing this book since its inception. They have spent rigorous hours researching and exploring the diverse topics which have resulted in the successful publishing of this book. They have passed on their knowledge of decades through this book. To expedite this challenging task, the publisher supported the team at every step. A small team of assistant editors was also appointed to further simplify the editing procedure and attain best results for the readers.

Apart from the editorial board, the designing team has also invested a significant amount of their time in understanding the subject and creating the most relevant covers. They scrutinized every image to scout for the most suitable representation of the subject and create an appropriate cover for the book.

The publishing team has been an ardent support to the editorial, designing and production team. Their endless efforts to recruit the best for this project, has resulted in the accomplishment of this book. They are a veteran in the field of academics and their pool of knowledge is as vast as their experience in printing. Their expertise and guidance has proved useful at every step. Their uncompromising quality standards have made this book an exceptional effort. Their encouragement from time to time has been an inspiration for everyone.

The publisher and the editorial board hope that this book will prove to be a valuable piece of knowledge for researchers, students, practitioners and scholars across the globe.

List of Contributors

Irene S Gabashvili
Aurametrix, MEBO Research, Miami, FL, United States

Ingrid Muller, Adam W A Geraghty, Kate Rumsby, Beth Stuart, Paul Little and Miriam Santer
Primary Care, Population Sciences and Medical Education, University of Southampton, Southampton, United Kingdom

Athena Ip
Primary Care, Population Sciences and Medical Education, University of Southampton, Southampton, United Kingdom
School of Health Sciences, University of Surrey, Guildford, United Kingdom

Mary K Hill
Department of Dermatology, University of Colorado Anschutz Medical Campus, Aurora, CO, United States

Melissa R Laughter
School of Medicine, University of Colorado, Aurora, CO, United States
Department of Dermatology, University of Colorado Anschutz Medical Campus, Aurora, CO, United States

Cecile I Harmange
School of Medicine, University of Colorado, Aurora, CO, United States

Robert P Dellavalle
Department of Dermatology, University of Colorado Anschutz Medical Campus, Aurora, CO, United States
Dermatology Service, United States Department of Veterans Affairs, Eastern Colorado Health Care System, Aurora, CO, United States
Department of Epidemiology, Colorado School of Public Health, University of Colorado Anschutz Medical Campus, Aurora, CO, United States

Cory A Dunnick
Department of Dermatology, University of Colorado Anschutz Medical Campus, Aurora, CO, United States
Dermatology Service, United States Department of Veterans Affairs, Eastern Colorado Health Care System, Aurora, CO, United States

Chandler W Rundle
School of Medicine, Loma Linda University, Loma Linda, CA, United States
Department of Medicine, St. Joseph's Hospital, Denver, CO, United States

Michelle S Lee
Harvard Medical School, Boston, MA, United States

Robert Stavert
Department of Dermatology, Cambridge Health Alliance, Somerville, MA, United States

Mercedes Sendín-Martín, Julian Conejo-Mir and Jose Juan Pereyra-Rodriguez
University Hospital Virgen del Rocio, Sevilla, Spain

Ana Jiménez-Zarco
Faculty of Economic and Business Sciences, Universitat Oberta de Cataluña, Barcelona, Spain

Francesc Saigí-Rubió
Faculty of Health Sciences, Universitat Oberta de Cataluña, Barcelona, Spain

Judy Hamad, Amy Fox, Maria Suzanne Kammire and Alison Nancy Hollis
Department of Dermatology, School of Medicine, University of North Carolina at Chapel Hill, Chapel Hill, NC, United States

Saif Khairat
Carolina Health Informatics Program, University of North Carolina at Chapel Hill, Chapel Hill, NC, United States
Healthcare Systems, School of Nursing, University of North Carolina at Chapel Hill, Chapel Hill, NC, United States

Trevor Champagne
Division of Dermatology, Women's College Hospital, University of Toronto, Toronto, ON, Canada

Peter G Rossos
Institute of Health Policy, Management and Evaluation, Dalla Lana School of Public Health, University of Toronto, Toronto, ON, Canada
Centre for Global eHealth Innovation, University Health Network and Techna Institute, Toronto, ON, Canada
Department of Medicine, Dalla Lana School of Public Health, University of Toronto, Toronto, ON, Canada

Veronica Kirk
Institute of Health Policy, Management and Evaluation, Dalla Lana School of Public Health, University of Toronto, Toronto, ON, Canada

Emily Seto
Institute of Health Policy, Management and Evaluation, Dalla Lana School of Public Health, University of Toronto, Toronto, ON, Canada
Centre for Global eHealth Innovation, University Health Network and Techna Institute, Toronto, ON, Canada

Arnab Ray, Aman Gupta and Amutha Al
SRM Institute of Science and Technology, Chennai, India

Emily Habgood
Department of General Practice and Centre for Cancer Research, University of Melbourne, Melbourne, Australia

Christopher McCormack
Department of Surgical Oncology, Peter MacCallum Cancer Centre, Melbourne, Australia

Fiona M Walter
Department of General Practice and Centre for Cancer Research, University of Melbourne, Melbourne, Australia
Primary Care Unit, Department of Public Health and Primary Care, University of Cambridge, Cambridge, United Kingdom
Wolfson Institute of Population Health, Queen Mary University of London, London, United Kingdom

Jon D Emery
Department of General Practice and Centre for Cancer Research, University of Melbourne, Melbourne, Australia
Primary Care Unit, Department of Public Health and Primary Care, University of Cambridge, Cambridge, United Kingdom

Robyn-Jenia Wilcha
Faculty of Biology, Medicine and Health, University of Manchester, Manchester, United Kingdom

Kayd J Pulsipher
College of Osteopathic Medicine, Rocky Vista University, Parker, CO, United States

Mindy D Szeto
Department of Dermatology, University of Colorado Anschutz Medical Campus, Aurora, CO, United States

Colby L Presley
Division of Dermatology, Lehigh Valley Health Network, Allentown, PA, United States

Ashley M Snyder and Aaron M Secrest
Department of Dermatology, University of Utah, Salt Lake City, UT, United States
Department of Population Health Sciences, University of Utah, Salt Lake City, UT, United States

Vanina L Taliercio, Lisa B Webber, Abram P Beshay and Jamie L W Rhoads
Department of Dermatology, University of Utah, Salt Lake City, UT, United States

Joshua E Biber
Department of Population Health Sciences, University of Utah, Salt Lake City, UT, United States

Adelheid U Brandenberger and Bianca E Rich
School of Medicine, University of Utah, Salt Lake City, UT, United States

Rachel Hess
Department of Population Health Sciences, University of Utah, Salt Lake City, UT, United States
Department of Internal Medicine, University of Utah, Salt Lake City, UT, United States

Taylor C Rogers
Oklahoma State University Center for Health Sciences, Tulsa, OK, United States

Andrew Fung and Benjamin K P Woo
Olive View–University of California Los Angeles Medical Center, Sylmar, CA, United States

Ryan Ottwell, Benjamin Heigle, Arjun K Reddy, Nicholas Sajjadi, Alexis Wirtz, Courtney Cook and Hannah Howard
Oklahoma State University Center for Health Sciences, Tulsa, OK, United States

Caitlin Horsham, Helen Ford and Elke Hacker
School of Public Health and Social Work, Queensland University of Technology, Brisbane, Australia

Jeremy Herbert and Alexander Wall
Designworks Group Pty Ltd, Brisbane, Australia

Sebastian Walpole
Genetics & Population Health Division, QIMR Berghofer, Brisbane, Australia

Jennifer Costigan and Sue S Feldman
Department of Health Services Research, School of Health Professions, University of Alabama at Birmingham, Birmingham, AL, United States

Mark Lemak
University of Alabama at Birmingham Health System, Birmingham, AL, United States

Jalal Maghfour
Department of Dermatology, Henry Ford Hospital, Detroit, MI, United States

Torunn Elise Sivesind and Cory Dunnick
Department of Dermatology, University of Colorado School of Medicine, Aurora, CO, United States

Robert Paul Dellavalle
Department of Dermatology, University of Colorado School of Medicine, Aurora, CO, United States
Dermatology Service, Rocky Mountain Regional Veterans Affairs Medical Center, Aurora, CO, United States

Zane Rulon, J Michael Anderson, Austin Johnson, Micah Hartwell and Matt Vassar
Center for Health Sciences, Oklahoma State University, Tulsa, OK, United States

Kalyn Powers
College of Pharmacy, Southwestern Oklahoma State University, Weatherford, OK, United States

Michael Weaver
College of Osteopathic Medicine, Kansas City University of Medicine and Biosciences, Joplin, OK, United States

Tsair-Wei Chien
Department of Dermatology, Chi-Mei Medical Center, Tainan, Taiwan

Hsien-Yi Wang
Department of Nephrology, Chi-Mei Medical Center, Tainan, Taiwan
Department of Sports Management, Chia-Nan University of Pharmacy and Science, Tainan, Taiwan

Feng-Jie Lai
Department of Dermatology, Chi-Mei Medical Center, Tainan, Taiwan
Center for General Education, Southern Taiwan University of Science and Technology, Tainan, Taiwan

Jenny Alderden, Linda Amoafo, Yue Zhang and David Yap
University of Utah, Salt Lake City, UT, United States

Caroline Fife
Intellicure, Inc, The Woodlands, TX, United States

Tracey Yap
Duke University, Durham, NC, United States

Maham Ghani
City University of New York School of Medicine, City University of New York, New york, NY, United States

Colin Adler
Department of Dermatology, Emory University School of Medicine, Emory University, Atlanta, GA, United States

Howa Yeung
Department of Dermatology, Emory University School of Medicine, Emory University, Atlanta, GA, United States
Regional Telehealth Service, Veterans Affairs Veterans Integrated Service Network 7, Decatur, GA, United States

Alexandra Finstad and Alex Lee
Faculty of Medicine, University of Ottawa, Ottawa, ON, Canada

Ralph George
Division of General Surgery, Department of Surgery, University of Toronto, Toronto, ON, Canada
Department of Surgery, Canadian Imperial Bank of Commerce Breast Centre, St. Michael's Hospital, Toronto, ON, Canada

Raed Alhusayen
Division of Dermatology, Department of Medicine, University of Toronto, Toronto, ON, Canada
Division of Dermatology, Department of Medicine, Sunnybrook Health Sciences Centre, Toronto, ON, Canada

Pengyi Zhu
Olive View-University of California Los Angeles Medical Center, Sylmar, CA, United States
College of Osteopathic Medicine of the Pacific, Western University of Health Sciences, Pomona, CA, United States

Index

www.ingramcontent.com/pod-product-compliance
Lightning Source LLC
LaVergne TN
LVHW082139200926
848484LV00008B/2079